The World Health Report 1998

Life in the 21st century
A vision for all

Report of the Director-General

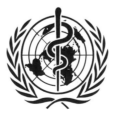

World Health Organization
Geneva
1998

9811111
WX 90

WHO Library Cataloguing in Publication Data

The world health report 1998 – Life in the 21st century: a vision for all
    1. World health   2. Public health – history   3. Public health - trends
    4. Health status   5. Forecasting   6. World Health Organization
    I. Title: Life in the 21st century: a vision for all

ISBN 92 4 156189 0   (NLM Classification: WA 540.1)
ISSN 1020-3311

Information concerning this publication can be obtained from:
Office of World Health Reporting
World Health Organization
1211 Geneva 27, Switzerland
Fax: (41-22) 791 4870

Design and layout by WHO
Printed in France
98/11891 – Sadag – 20000

Contents

Synopsis of the report

Chapter 1 *(Leading and responding)*
examines the origins of WHO and its history from 1948 to 1998, and describes how the Organization works and what it does.

Chapter 2 *(Measuring health)*
summarizes the main trends in mortality since 1955, and gives an overview of disease trends during the same period.

Chapter 3 *(Health across the life span)*
looks at the health problems encountered and progress made in the past 50 years for all age groups – infants and small children under 5, older children of school age and adolescents (5-19), adults (20-64 years) and older people (over 65).

Chapter 4 *(The changing world)*
discusses the three main global trends that affect health: economic trends, population trends and social trends.

Chapter 5 *(Achieving health for all)*
reports on the evolution of health systems and health care, including primary health care, since the launching of the global strategy for Health for All at the Alma-Ata Conference in 1978.

Chapter 6 *(WHO worldwide)*
summarizes health trends since 1948 for each of the six WHO regions, as well as current activities or problems.

Chapter 7 *(Global partnerships for health)*
gives examples of cooperation since 1948 with the United Nations and other entities within the system, as well as with NGOs, international and national research institutions and collaborating centres.

Chapter 8 *(Health agenda for the 21st century)*
considers the unfinished agenda and shows the way to enhance health potential worldwide in the future.

Message from the Director-General

The desire for a healthier and better world in which to live our lives and raise our children is common to all people and all generations. Now, as we near the end of one century and enter the next, our past achievements and technological advances make us more optimistic about our future than perhaps at any stage in recent history.

Despite being threatened by two devastating world wars in the first half of this century, and by many other conflicts and catastrophes in the second, humanity has, in general, not merely survived; it has thrived. Today, at least 120 countries (total population above 5 billion) have a life expectancy at birth of more than 60 years; the global average is 66 years compared to only 48 years in 1955; it is projected to reach 73 years in 2025.

However, one of the main messages of *The World Health Report 1997* was the need to recognize that increased longevity without quality of life is an empty prize – that *health* expectancy is more important than *life* expectancy. It is therefore particularly encouraging to show evidence in this year's report of remarkable declines in disability over periods of time among older people in some populations.

In an era of global population ageing, this is not just good news for the individuals concerned and the societies in which they live. It may be a vital signal for us all. It suggests that we are slowly learning one of life's most important lessons: not just how to live longer, but also how to stay longer in good health with less disability, and therefore, less dependence on others.

Issued as the World Health Organization marks its 50th anniversary, *The World Health Report 1998* offers a cautiously optimistic vision of the future up to the year 2025. It gives us hope that longer life can be a prize worth winning.

Based on a review of health trends in the past 50 years, it finds that overall, remarkable improvements in health have been due to socioeconomic development, the wider provision of safe water, sanitation facilities and personal hygiene, and the establishment and expansion of national health services.

Major infectious diseases, such as poliomyelitis, leprosy, guinea-worm disease, Chagas disease and river blindness, are steadily being defeated. There have been spectacular advances in the development of vaccines and medicines, and countless other innovations in the investigation, diagnosis and treatment of illness, in the reduction of disability and in rehabilitation.

Tragically, however, while average life expectancy has been increasing throughout the 20th century, 3 out of 4 people in the least developed countries today are dying before the age of 50 – the global life expectancy figure of half a century ago. This year, 21 million deaths – 2 out of every 5 worldwide – will be among the under-50s, including 10 million small children who will never see their fifth birthday though most children worldwide are now immunized against major childhood killers. Over 7 million will be men and women in what should be some of the best and most productive years of their lives. Reducing these premature deaths is one of the greatest challenges facing humanity at the dawn of the 21st century.

There are others challenges. For while health globally has steadily improved over the years, great numbers of people have seen little if any improvement at all. The gaps between the health status of rich and poor are at least as wide as they were half a century ago, and are becoming wider still.

The prime concern of the international community must be the plight of those most likely to be left furthest behind as the rest of the world steps confidently into the future. These are the many hundreds of millions of men, women and children still trapped in the past by the grimmest poverty. They live mainly in the least developed countries, where the burdens of ill-health, disease and inequality are heaviest, the outlook is bleakest, and life is shortest.

Worldwide, the majority of premature deaths are preventable. At least 2 million children a year die from diseases for which there are vaccines. The report gives encouraging evidence that premature deaths among adults, too, can be significantly reduced. Deaths from heart disease have been dramatically reduced in many countries which are experiencing a transition from high incidence of circulatory diseases to low incidence, mainly due to the adoption of healthier lifestyles. It is imperative that such a favourable shift, conducive to further reductions in the incidence of these diseases, should be sustained and if possible accelerated.

Infectious diseases, meanwhile, remain leading causes of premature death among adults in much of the developing world. Reducing these tolls depends largely on the political will and commitment of individual governments, and the active support of the international community.

This means putting health high on the agenda of all countries, rich and poor, and keeping it there. It is time to realize that health is a global issue; it should be considered as an essential component of the continuing globalization process that is reshaping our world; it should be included in the growing interaction between countries that currently exists in terms of world trade, services, foreign investment and capital markets.

With the help of instant international communications and information technologies, and global surveillance systems to detect problems, prepare for them and respond to them, a wonderful opportunity now exists to build the new international partnerships for health, based on social justice, equity and solidarity, that the world of the 21st century will so urgently need.

They are partnerships involving all countries, their governments, their civil societies, and their individuals. All can be partners who are willing to share and exchange the life-enhancing information and technology that is already at the fingertips of the rich but as yet beyond the reach of the poor. Such a political vision is fundamental to ensure a participatory approach to peace and development at local, national and international levels and thus enhance the welfare of the individual and society.

The progress and achievements of the past 50 years are solid foundations for a healthier and better world. It is already time to build on them. Life in the 21st century could and should be better for all. We can pass no greater gift to the next generation than a healthier future. That is our vision. Together, the people of the world can make it a reality.

Hiroshi Nakajima, M.D., Ph.D.
Director-General
World Health Organization

Introduction

The most important

pattern of progress

now emerging is an

unmistakable trend

towards healthier,

longer life.

Looking forward to health

The 21st century offers a bright vision of better health for all. It holds the prospect not merely of longer life, but superior quality of life, with less disability and disease. As the new millennium approaches, the global population has never had a healthier outlook.

Weighing the evidence of the past and the present, *The World Health Report 1998* shows that humanity has many good reasons for hope in the future. Such an optimistic view must be tempered by recognition of some harsh realities. Nevertheless, unprecedented advances in health during the 20th century have laid the foundations for further dramatic progress in the years ahead.

This report provides the latest expert assessment of the global health situation, and uses that as a basis for projecting health trends to the year 2025. Examining the entire human life span, and sifting data gathered in the past 50 years, it studies the well-being of infants and children, adolescents and adults, older people and the "oldest old", and identifies priority areas for action in each age group. Women's health is given special emphasis. The future of human health in the 21st century depends a great deal on a commitment to investing in the health of women in the world today. Their health largely determines the health of their children, who are the adults of tomorrow.

The report's most disturbing finding is that, despite increasing life expectancy, two-fifths of all deaths in the world this year can be considered premature, in that more than 20 million people a year are dying before the age of 50, while average life expectancy has risen to 66 years. Ten million of these deaths are among children under 5 years; 7.4 million others are among adults aged 20-49.

Even so, the most important pattern of progress now emerging is an unmistakable trend towards healthier, longer life. Supported by solid scientific evidence of declines in disability among older people in some populations, this has considerable implications for individuals and for societies.

The explanation for this trend lies in the social and economic advances that the world has witnessed during the late 20th century – advances that have brought better living standards to many, but not all, people. The world saw a golden age of unparalleled prosperity between 1950 and 1973, followed by an economic slump that lasted 20 years. A global economic recovery has been under way since 1994. The long-term benefits are now becoming apparent. While they are most evident in the industrialized world, they are slowly but surely materializing in many poorer countries, too.

For example, food supply has more than doubled in the past 40 years, much faster than population growth. Per capita GDP in real terms has risen by at least 2.5 times in the past 50 years. Adult literacy rates have increased by more than 50% since 1970. The proportion of children at school has risen while the proportion

In many ways,

the face of humanity

is being rapidly

reshaped.

of people chronically undernourished has fallen.

These trends are changing the world. Without question, the world of 2025 will be significantly different from today's, and almost unrecognizable from that of 1950. The stunning technological advances of recent years, particularly in global telecommunications, have made the planet seem smaller than ever before. By the year 2025, it is likely to seem smaller still – and, with continuing population growth, it will certainly be much more crowded. In many ways, the face of humanity is being rapidly reshaped.

Two main trends – increasing life expectancy and falling fertility rates – mean that by 2025:

- Worldwide life expectancy, currently 66 years, will reach 73 years – a 50% improvement on the 1955 average of only 48 years.
- The global population, about 5.8 billion in 1997, will increase to about 8 billion. Every day in 1997, about 365 000 babies were born, and about 140 000 people died, giving a natural increase of about 220 000 people a day.
- There will never have been so many older people and so relatively few young ones.
- The number of people aged over 65 will have risen from 390 million in 1997 to 800 million – from 6.6% of the total population to 10%.
- The proportion of young people under 20 years will have fallen from 40% in 1997 to 32% of the total population, despite reaching 2.6 billion – an actual increase of 252 million.

These demographic trends, which have profound implications for human health in all age groups, follow on the many positive changes that have occurred in the past 50 years. More people than ever before now have access to at least minimum health care, safe water supplies and

sanitation facilities. Most of the world's children are now immunized against the six major diseases of childhood – measles, poliomyelitis, tuberculosis, diphtheria, pertussis and neonatal tetanus.

During the same period there have been steady and sometimes spectacular advances in the control and prevention of other diseases, the development of vaccines and medicines, and countless other medical and scientific innovations. The past decades have seen the final defeat of smallpox, one of the oldest diseases of humanity, and the gradual reduction in several others, including leprosy and poliomyelitis.

Crossing the threshold

Together, these and related achievements should help humankind to step confidently across the threshold into the new century. However, the future will pose many new as well as continuing challenges.

The war against ill-health in the 21st century will have to be fought simultaneously on two main fronts: infectious diseases and chronic, noncommunicable diseases. Many developing countries will come under greater attack from both, as heart disease, cancer and diabetes and other "lifestyle" conditions become more prevalent, while infectious illnesses remain undefeated. Of this latter group, HIV/AIDS will continue to be the deadliest menace.

This double threat imposes the need for difficult decisions about the allocation of scarce resources. Experience shows that reduced spending on controlling infectious diseases can cause them to return with a vengeance, while globalization – particularly expanding international travel and trade, including the transportation of foodstuffs – increases the risks of their global spread. At the same time, the stealthy onset of chronic conditions also saps a nation's strength. This trend will increasingly be the main focus of attention in industrialized countries which, however, must not lower their guard against infectious diseases.

The past few decades have seen the growing impact on health of poverty and malnutrition; widening health inequalities between rich and poor; the emergence of "new" diseases such as HIV/AIDS; the growing problem of antibiotic-resistant infections; and the epidemic of tobacco-related diseases.

These are only some of the problems representing the unfinished agenda of public health actions at the end of one century and requiring urgent action at the beginning of the next.

This report looks at the health implications for all age groups – infants and small children under 5; older children of school age and adolescents (5-19 years); adults (20-64 years); and older people (65 and over). Some of the main findings of the report, as they apply to each age group, are summarized below.

Infants and small children

- Spectacular progress in reducing under-5 mortality achieved in the past few decades is projected to continue, and could even accelerate. There were about 11 million deaths among children under 5 in 1995 compared to 21 million in 1955; there will only be 5 million deaths in 2025.
- The infant mortality rate per 1000 live births was 148 in 1955; 59 in 1995; and is projected to be 29 in 2025.
- The under-5 mortality rates per 1000 live births for the same years are 210, 78 and 37 respectively.
- In 1997, there were 10 million

deaths among children under 5 – 97% of them in the developing world, and most of them due to infectious diseases such as pneumonia and diarrhoea, combined with malnutrition.

- Most of these under-5 deaths are preventable. At least 2 million a year could be prevented by existing vaccines.
- Some 25 million low-birth-weight babies are born every year. They are more likely to die early, and those who survive may suffer illness, stunted growth or other health problems, even as adults.
- While most premature and low-birth-weight babies are born in the developing world, many born in industrialized countries owe their survival to high-technology neonatal care. Such care may have increasingly complex ethical implications.
- Tomorrow's small children face a "new morbidity" of illnesses and conditions that are linked to social and economic changes, including rapid urbanization. These include neglect, abuse and violence, especially among the growing numbers of street children.
- One of the biggest hazards to children in the 21st century will be the continuing spread of HIV/AIDS. In 1997, 590 000 children aged under 15 became infected with HIV. The disease could reverse some of the major gains achieved in child health over the last 50 years.
- Better prevention and treatment of some hereditary diseases in small children is likely.

Older children and adolescents

Traditionally regarded as enjoying the healthiest phase of life, these youngsters have tended to receive insufficient public health attention. But today theirs is a "prime time" for health

HIV/AIDS could reverse some of the major gains achieved in child health over the last 50 years.

promotion to encourage them to establish healthy patterns of behaviour that will influence their development and health in later years.

- There will be an even greater need than at present for education and advice on unhealthy diet, inadequate exercise, unsafe sexual activity and smoking, all of which provoke disease in adulthood but have their roots in these early formative years.
- Research suggests that stress, poor physical surroundings and an inadequate care-giving environment during early childhood are related to violent and criminal behaviour at later ages. More children than ever are growing up in such circumstances.
- The transition from childhood to adulthood will be marked for many in the coming years by such potentially deadly "rites of passage" as violence, delinquency, drugs, alcohol, motor-vehicle accidents and sexual hazards. For many, especially those growing up in poor urban areas, adolescence will represent the most dangerous years of life.
- Sexuality and sexual activity, key aspects of affirming maturity and adulthood, are becoming more dangerous due to HIV and other sexually transmitted diseases, while globally there is still enormous ignorance about sex among young people, particularly adolescent males.
- In 1995, girls aged 15-19 gave birth to 17 million babies. That number is expected to drop only to 16 million in 2025. Pregnancy and childbirth in adolescence pose higher risks for both mother and child. Earlier sexual activity increases health hazards for women.

> The continuing gains
>
> in the survival of
>
> infants and young
>
> children means that
>
> the adult population
>
> is increasing.

Adults

Globally, adults are now surviving longer, largely because during the past half century, when they were children, epidemics of infectious diseases such as tuberculosis and respiratory disease were being better controlled. The continuing gains in the survival of infants and young children means that the adult population is increasing.

- Currently, just over half the population is of working age, 20-64; by 2025 the proportion will have reached 58%.
- The proportion of older people requiring support from adults of working age will have increased from 10.5% in 1955 and 12.3% in 1995 to 17.2% in 2025.
- The health of the adult population of working age will be vitally important if this age group is to support growing numbers of dependants, both young and old.
- However, more than 15 million adults aged 20-64 are dying every year. Most of these deaths are preventable.
- Among the most tragic of these deaths are those of 585 000 young women who die each year in pregnancy or childbirth.
- 2-3 million adults a year are dying of tuberculosis, despite the existence of a strategy that could effectively cure all cases.
- About 1.8 million adults died of AIDS in 1997 and the annual death toll is likely to rise.

The successes achieved in the past 50 years against microbial and parasitic diseases stem from the creation of a healthier environment, with improvements in hygiene and sanitation; treatment with effective and affordable antibiotic and antiparasitic drugs; and the availability of vaccines. Unfortunately, these types of drugs cannot be relied on to the same extent in the future – because of the spread of strains of pneumonia, tuberculosis and malaria that are resistant to the most powerful medicines. Steady increases in cases of and deaths from tuberculosis are evidence of this trend.

- The future of infectious disease control is likely to lie with vaccines rather than drugs.
- In general, noncommunicable diseases such as coronary heart disease, cancer, diabetes and mental disorders are more common than infectious diseases in the industrialized world. Coronary heart disease and stroke have declined as causes of death in these countries in recent decades, while death rates from some cancers have risen.
- In developing countries, as their economies grow, noncommunicable diseases will become more prevalent, largely because of the adoption of "western" lifestyles and their accompanying risk factors – smoking, high-fat diet, lack of exercise. But infectious diseases will still be a major burden, none more so than HIV/AIDS.
- Cancer will remain one of the leading causes of death worldwide. Despite much progress in research, prevention and treatment, only one-third of all cancers can be cured by earlier detection combined with effective treatment. However, many of the remaining cancers could be prevented by a range of measures, including avoiding tobacco use and adopting a healthier diet.

Some likely trends to 2025 are given below:

- Overall, the risk of cancer will continue to increase in developing countries, with stable if not declining rates in industrialized countries. In individual countries, some cancers will become more common, others less common.
- Cases of and deaths from lung cancer and colorectal cancer will increase, largely due to smoking and unhealthy diet. Lung cancer deaths among women will rise in virtually all industrialized countries.
- Stomach cancer will become less common, mainly because of improved food conservation, dietary changes and declining related infection.
- Cervical cancer is expected to decrease further in industrialized countries due to screening; the possible advent of a vaccine would greatly benefit both developed and developing countries.
- Liver cancer will decrease as a consequence of current and future immunization against the hepatitis B virus in many countries and of screening for hepatitis C.
- Diabetes cases in adults will more than double globally, from 143 million in 1997 to 300 million in 2025, largely because of dietary and other lifestyle factors.

Older people

- By 2025 there will be more than 800 million people over 65 in the world, two-thirds of them in developing countries.
- There will be 274 million people over the age of 60 in China alone – more than the total present population of the United States.
- Increases of up to 300% of the older population are expected in many developing countries, especially in Latin America and Asia, within the next 30 years.
- Population ageing has immense implications for all countries. In the 21st century, one of the biggest challenges will be how best to prevent and postpone disease and disability and to maintain the health, independence and mobility of an ageing population.

Population ageing has immense implications for all countries.

- Even in wealthy countries, most old and frail people cannot meet more than a small fraction of the costs of the health care they need. In the coming decades, few countries will be able to provide specialized care for their large population of aged individuals.
- Some European countries already acknowledge that there is insufficient provision to meet with dignity the needs of all those over the age of 75, who currently consume many times more medical and social services than those under 75.
- Developing countries will face even more serious challenges, given their economic difficulties, the rapidity with which populations age, the lack of social service infrastructures, and the decline of traditional caring provided by family members.
- Many of the chronic conditions of old age can be successfully detected, prevented and treated, given sufficient resources and access to care.
- Worldwide, circulatory disease is the leading cause of death and disability in people over 65 years, but there is great potential for preventing and treating it.

Women

Women's health is inextricably linked to their status in society. It benefits from equality, and suffers from discrimination. Today, the status and well-being of countless millions of women worldwide remain tragically low. As a result, human well-being in general suffers, and the prospects for future generations are dimmer.

In many parts of the world, discrimination against women begins before they are born and stays with them until they die. Throughout history, female babies have been unwanted in some societies and are at a disadvantage from the moment of birth. Today, girls and women are still denied the same rights and privileges as their brothers, at home, at work, in the classroom or the clinic. They suffer more from poverty, low social status and the many hazards associated with their reproductive role. As a result, they bear an unfair burden of disadvantage and suffering, often throughout their lives.

Global population ageing is resulting in the evolution towards societies which are, for the most part, female. Yet while women generally live longer than men, for many of them greater life expectancy carries no real advantage in terms of additional years lived free of disability.

The status of women's health in old age is shaped throughout their lives by factors over which they have little if any control. If longer lives for women are to be years of quality, policies must be aimed at ensuring the best possible health for women as they age. These policies should be geared towards the problems that begin in infancy or childhood, and should cover the whole life span, through adolescence and adulthood into old age.

Infancy and childhood. The health of parents, particularly the mother before and during pregnancy, and the services available to her throughout her pregnancy, especially at delivery, are important determinants of the health status of their children. Infants whose health status is compromised at birth are more vulnerable to various health problems later in life. Girls who are inadequately fed in childhood may have impaired intellectual capacity, delayed puberty, possibly impaired fertility and stunted growth, leading to higher risks of complications during childbirth. Female genital mutilation, of which 2 million girls are at risk every year, or sexual abuse during

Today, the status and well-being of countless millions of women worldwide remain tragically low.

childhood, increase the risk of poor physical and mental health in later years.

Adolescence. Most reproductive health and family planning programmes have not paid enough attention to the special needs of adolescents. Premature entry into sexual relationships, high-risk sexual behaviour and lack of education, basic health information and services all compromise the current and future well-being of girls in this age group.

These girls are at increased risk of sexually transmitted diseases, including HIV/AIDS, early pregnancy and motherhood, and unsafe abortion. Adolescent girls are not physically prepared for childbirth, and are much more at risk of maternal death than women in their twenties. Inadequate diet during adolescence can jeopardize girls' health and physical development, with permanent consequences. Iron-deficiency anaemia is particularly common among adolescent girls.

Adulthood. The consequences of poor health in childhood and adolescence, including malnutrition, become apparent in adulthood, particularly during the childbearing years. This time is a particularly dangerous phase in the lives of many women in developing countries, where health care services, especially reproductive health facilities, are often inadequate and where society puts pressure on couples to have many children. More than 50% of pregnant women in the developing world are anaemic.

About 585 000 women die each year of pregnancy-related causes. Where women have many pregnancies the risk of related death over the course of their lifetime is compounded. While the risk in Europe is one in 1400, in Asia it is one in 65, and in Africa, one in 16.

An estimated 50 million adult women in developing countries are classified as being severely underweight, and about 450 million suffer from goitre.

Older women. Many millions of women are made old before their time by the daily harshness and inequalities of their earlier lives, beginning in childhood. They experience poor nutrition, reproductive ill-health, dangerous working conditions, violence and lifestyle-related diseases, all of which exacerbate the likelihood of breast and cervical cancers, osteoporosis and other chronic conditions after menopause. In old age poverty, loneliness and alienation are common.

Health agenda for the 21sr century

The World Health Report 1998 and its three predecessors have helped create a comprehensive map of the major issues that have dominated world health in the second half of the 20th century. The priorities for international action recommended in these four reports chart the future for health action in the 21st century.

The World Health Report 1995 – Bridging the gaps, identified poverty as the greatest cause of suffering and showed the widening health gaps between rich and poor. It recommended using available resources as effectively as possible and redirecting them to those who need them most.

The World Health Report 1996 – Fighting disease, fostering development identified three main priorities: completing the unfinished business of eradication and elimination of specific diseases; tackling "old" diseases such as tuberculosis and malaria, and the problems of antimicrobial resistance; and combating newly-emerging diseases.

The World Health Report 1997 – Conquering suffering, enriching hu-

Where women have

many pregnancies

the risk of related

death over the

course of their lifetime

is compounded.

On the unfinished

agenda for health,

poverty remains

the main item.

manity stressed the importance of health expectancy over life expectancy in the context of chronic noncommunicable diseases. Its main recommendation was the integration of disease-specific interventions into a comprehensive chronic disease control package incorporating prevention, diagnosis, treatment, rehabilitation and improved training of health professionals.

This year's report has shown the major developments and achievements in health in the past 50 years and described the economic trends, population trends and social trends which will influence health in the early 21st century. The third evaluation of progress in implementation of the health for all strategy, carried out in 1997, has shown substantial gains in life expectancy and in infectious disease control and reductions in infant and under-5 mortality. There have also been great improvements in immunization coverage, as well as in access to maternal care (including family planning services) and to essential drugs. These need to be safeguarded.

On the ***unfinished agenda*** for health, poverty remains the main item. The priority must be to reduce it in the poorest countries of the world, and to eliminate the pockets of poverty that exist within countries. Policies directed at improving health and ensuring equity are the keys to economic growth and poverty reduction.

Safeguarding the gains already achieved in health depends largely on sharing health and medical knowledge, expertise and experience on a global scale. Industrialized countries can play a vital part in helping solve global health problems. It is in their own interests as well as those of developing countries to do so.

Increased international cooperation in health can be facilitated by a managed global network making use of the latest communication technologies. Global surveillance for the detection of and response to emerging infectious diseases is essential. As a result of increased global trade and travel, the prevention of foodborne infections in particular is of increasing importance. Wars, conflicts, refugee movements and environmental degradation also facilitate the spread of infections as well as being health hazards in themselves.

Enhancing health potential in the future depends on preventing and reducing premature mortality, morbidity and disability. It involves enabling people of all ages to achieve over time their maximum potential, intellectually and physically through education, the development of life skills and healthy lifestyles.

The implications of ***healthy ageing*** – the physical and mental characteristics of old age and their associated problems – need to be better understood. Much more research is required in order to reduce disability among older age groups.

Concern for the older members of today's society is part of the intergenerational relationships that need to be developed in the 21st century. These relationships, vital for social cohesion, should be based on equity, solidarity and social justice.

The young and old must learn to understand each other's differing aspirations and requirements. The young have the skills and energies to enhance the life quality of their elders. The old have the wisdom of their experience of life to pass on to the children of today and of coming generations.

Chapter 1
Leading and responding

The origins of WHO

> The health of all
>
> peoples was
>
> considered to
>
> be fundamental to the
>
> attainment of peace
>
> and security
>
> in the world.

Public health beyond national borders was considered in 1851 at an international sanitary conference held in Paris. Five of the 12 participating countries signed an international sanitary convention to which was annexed the text of international sanitary regulations. After a succession of international sanitary conferences, 12 States signed the Rome Agreement in 1907, which provided for the setting up in Paris of an international office of public hygiene (*Office international d'hygiène publique – OIHP*). Its function was to provide general information to participating countries on public health, especially infectious diseases, while retaining a diplomatic orientation (as illustrated by the majority decision against restricting its directorship to a physician). Progress was made on control of the main infectious diseases, including yellow fever, cholera, malaria and tuberculosis. Activities also covered food safety, hospital building and administration, school health, industrial hygiene, and from 1909, biological standardization. Landmarks in international health are given in *Box 1*.

When the League of Nations was formed, there was a proposal to transform the OIHP into the health organ of the League, but this never happened. The Health Organization of the League of Nations thus existed independently in Geneva. The OIHP's publications included a weekly epidemiological bulletin which was eventually incorporated in the *Weekly epidemiological record* of the League of Nations (now published by WHO). It was not until after the Second World War that the functions of both bodies were combined to form a new organization able to deal with large epidemics through a coordinated international effort. Meanwhile several regional sanitary bodies were set up, including a sanitary council in Egypt, and an international sanitary office in the Americas, which became the Pan American Sanitary Bureau in 1923 (concerned mainly with combating yellow fever).

In 1945, a United Nations conference was held in San Francisco to consider the possibility of setting up an international health organization. The health of all peoples was considered to be fundamental to the attainment of peace and security in the world. In 1946, a preparatory technical commission was instituted, comprising not representatives of States but experts selected on the basis of their technical competence. This commission proposed the name "World Health Organization" and suggested that the organization should be run by three bodies: a World Health Assembly, an Executive Board and a Secretariat *(Box 2)*.

The International Health Conference, the first international conference to be held under the aegis of the United Nations, took place in 1946 in New York. The 51 Member States of the United Nations were represented, as well as 13 non-members and various specialized agencies and

Box 1. Landmarks in international health

1830 Cholera overruns Europe,

1851 The first International Sanitary Conference is held in Paris to produce an international sanitary convention, but fails.

1892 The International Sanitary Convention, restricted to cholera, is adopted.

1897 Another international convention dealing with preventive measures against plague is adopted.

1902 The International Sanitary Bureau, later renamed Pan American Sanitary Bureau, and subsequently Pan American Sanitary Organization, is set up in Washington, DC.

1907 *L'Office international d'hygiène publique* (OIHP) is established in Paris, with a permanent secretariat and a permanent committee of senior public health officials of Member governments.

1919 The League of Nations is created and is charged, among other tasks, with taking steps in matters of international concern for the prevention and control of disease. The Health Organization of the League of Nations is set up in Geneva, in parallel with the OIHP.

1926 The International Sanitary Convention is revised to include provisions against smallpox and typhus.

1935 The International Sanitary Convention for aerial navigation comes into force.

1945 A United Nations conference in San Francisco unanimously approves the establishment of a new, autonomous, international health organization.

1946 The International Health Conference in New York approves the Constitution of the World Health Organization (WHO).

1948 The WHO Constitution comes into force on 7 April (now marked as World Health Day each year).

1951 The text of new *International sanitary regulations* is adopted by the World Health Assembly, replacing the previous International Sanitary Conventions.

1969 These Regulations are renamed the *International health regulations*, covering only cholera, plague, smallpox and yellow fever.

1978 A Joint WHO/UNICEF International Conference in Alma-Ata, adopts a Declaration on Primary Health Care as the key to attaining the goal of Health for All by the Year 2000.

1979 A Global Commission certifies the worldwide eradication of smallpox, the last known natural case having occurred in 1977.

1981 The Global Strategy for Health for All by the Year 2000 is adopted by the World Health Assembly and endorsed by the United Nations General Assembly, which urges other international organizations concerned to collaborate with WHO.

1988 The World Health Assembly resolves that poliomyelitis will be eradicated by the year 2000.

1994 WHO's Executive Board launches reform of the Organization in response to global change.

nongovernmental organizations. Within four and a half weeks, the conference drafted the Constitution, as well as a protocol that brought the Rome Agreement to an end and transferred OIHP's duties and responsibilities to the new organization. The Constitution expressed clearly the principles that were to govern the new organization and went a long way towards fulfilling the wishes of those who favoured the creation of a single body for world health matters.

One recurrent theme in all international discussions, that of nonintervention in internal affairs of States, played an important part at the conference. WHO was requested to act as the directing and coordinating authority on international health work, but its assistance to governments was to be subject to those governments' request or acceptance. The World Health Assembly was given authority to adopt regulations concerning certain technical matters. This was tantamount to investing it with legislative powers, a measure allowing governments to accept international sanitary arrangements simultaneously and with minimum delay.

It was agreed that the organization should be open to all States without exception. No provision was made for expelling a Member State, only to suspend the voting rights of those who fail to meet their financial obligations.

WHO's first 30 years

On 7 April 1948, the Constitution was accepted by the required number of Member States of the United Nations (26). There were 48 Members by the opening of the First World Health Assembly and 55 when it closed a month later. Many more Members subsequently joined the Organization, bringing the total to 191 as of 1 January 1998 (*Table 1* and *Annex 1*).

Box 2. The World Health Assembly, Executive Board and Secretariat

According to Article 9 of WHO's Constitution, the work of the Organization shall be carried out by the World Health Assembly, the Executive Board and the Secretariat.

The World Health Assembly

The Assembly is composed of delegates representing Members, and meets once a year in regular session at the Palais des Nations, Geneva. The length of its sessions has been considerably reduced since the early days of WHO, and now ranges between six and nine days. The functions of the Assembly include: determining the policies of the Organization; the naming of Members entitled to designate a person to serve on the Executive Board; and appointing the Director-General.

Each Assembly elects a President and five vice-presidents, who hold office until their successors are elected. The work of the Assembly is conducted by two main Committees: Committee A to deal predominantly with programme and budget matters, and Committee B to deal predominantly with administrative, financial and legal matters.

Decisions are taken through the adoption of resolutions, which may be tabled by any Member. There must be a two-thirds majority of the Members present and voting for important questions such as the adoption of conventions or agreements and fixing the amount of the effective working budget. Decisions on other questions require a simple majority.

The Executive Board

The first Executive Board comprised 18 Members – the number has now increased to 32, to reflect the growing number of Members since 1948. The World Health Assembly, taking into account an equitable geographical distribution, elects the Members entitled to designate a person technically qualified in the field of health to serve on the Board: Members are elected for three years. The Board elects its Chairman, who serves for one year, and meets twice a year, traditionally at WHO headquarters in Geneva. Its functions include: giving effect to the decisions and policies of the World Health Assembly, acting as its executive organ; and taking emergency measures – for example, to combat epidemics.

The Secretariat

The Secretariat comprises the Director-General and such technical and administrative staff as the Organization may require. The paramount consideration in the employment of the staff is to ensure that the efficiency, integrity and internationally representative character of the Secretariat is maintained at the highest level, with due regard being paid to the importance of recruiting staff on as wide a geographical basis as possible.

The First World Health Assembly was held in Geneva, at the Palais des Nations, on 24 June 1948. One of its tasks was to elect the first Director-General, Dr Brock Chisholm, who remained in office until 1953. Current health problems were divided into six groups according to priority: malaria, maternal and child health, tuberculosis, venereal diseases, nutrition and sanitation; public health administration; parasitic diseases; viral diseases; mental health; and various other activities. It soon appeared that this classification did not correspond to the extreme diversity of national health needs. It was therefore replaced later by a more flexible method, better suited to the real needs of Member States and to their requests for assistance, which allowed the stage of development and the problems of each country to be taken into account.

The decentralization of activities was one of the most tricky problems facing the First World Health Assembly, which had to decide how many regions should be created, which countries they should include, how soon the regional organizations should be instituted, and what financial arrangements should be made. The Assembly suggested that the following factors should be taken into

One of the main

purposes of regional

offices was to provide

effective contact

between WHO and

national governments.

account: the health level of the countries to be included; the possible existence in those countries of a permanent epidemic focus; the extent to which those countries had managed to overcome the health consequences of war; the efficiency of their health administration; and their capacity to resolve their problems.

Finally the six WHO regions (Africa, the Americas, Eastern Mediterranean, Europe, South-East Asia, Western Pacific) were established. The Assembly's decision concerning Europe was limited to the setting-up of a temporary office to deal with the health rehabilitation of war-devastated countries. In the Eastern Mediterranean area, it was decided to integrate with WHO the existing Maritime and Quarantine Sanitary Council of Egypt located in Alexandria. An agreement was concluded with the Pan American Sanitary Organization: the Pan American Sanitary Bureau in Washington, DC, was to assume, in addition to its former functions, the new role of WHO Regional Office for the Americas. For further details, see *Chapter 6*.

Between 1949 and 1952, a certain number of transfers took place between the regions. In 1953, the World Health Assembly reaffirmed the principles that had prompted regionalization, found that they had been justified in practice, requested the Executive Board periodically to review and report on regionalization, and requested the Director-General to provide the regional offices with guidance and assistance, to ensure that they conformed with the principles and policies established by the governing bodies. The World Health Assembly recommended the interchange of staff among regions and between headquarters and regions. The Executive Board felt that there should be no rigid allocation of functions between the central and re-

gional offices, and it was also opposed to the decentralization of certain functions which in its opinion could only be efficiently discharged centrally. In 1953, the Executive Board carried out a full-scale organizational study of the regional structure. Its report gave a complete functional description for a composite or model regional office. One of the main purposes of regional offices was to provide effective contact between WHO and national governments. To meet their many requests for advice, regional advisers were attached to regional offices.

The working methods of WHO which were established in the early years are generally still in use today. To meet a request from a country, the regional director would consult with the national authorities to determine the form of international assistance to be supplied. On the basis of the requests received, the regional programme was planned, examining the various projects with regard to their conformity with policy guidelines and their suitability for inclusion in a coordinated plan of development for the region and country in question. For specific projects, the Organization would recruit and brief a suitable expert or team. The regional office ensured liaison and cooperation with the national counterparts and local services. International staff were assigned to assist the government, not to control the project, the course of which was determined by the local needs, environment and epidemiological conditions. Once the international staff were withdrawn, the local services applied, extended and continued the work, which became an integral part of the national health services.

Technical and scientific meetings were used to give authoritative technical direction to the policies and programmes of WHO, to pool and exchange information, to suggest

Table 1. Members and Associate Members of WHO [a]

1946	Canada, China, Iran (Islamic Republic of), New Zealand, Syrian Arab Republic, United Kingdom of Great Britain and Northern Ireland
1947	Albania, Austria, Egypt, Ethiopia, Finland, Haiti, Iraq, Ireland, Italy, Jordan, Liberia, Netherlands, Norway, Saudi Arabia, South Africa, Sweden, Switzerland, Thailand, Yugoslavia
1948	Afghanistan, Argentina, Australia, Belarus, Belgium, Brazil, Bulgaria, Chile, Denmark, Dominican Republic, El Salvador, France, Greece, Hungary, Iceland, India, Mexico, Monaco, Myanmar, Pakistan, Philippines, Poland, Portugal, Romania, Russian Federation, Sri Lanka, Turkey, Ukraine, United States of America, Venezuela
1949	Bolivia, Costa Rica, Ecuador, Guatemala, Honduras, Israel, Lebanon, Luxembourg, Paraguay, Peru, Republic of Korea, Uruguay
1950	Cambodia, Cuba, Indonesia, Lao People's Democratic Republic, Nicaragua, Viet Nam
1951	Germany, Japan, Panama, Spain
1952	Libyan Arab Jamahiriya
1953	Nepal, Yemen
1956	Morocco, Sudan, Tunisia
1957	Ghana
1958	Malaysia
1959	Colombia, Guinea
1960	Benin, Burkina Faso, Cameroon, Central African Republic, Congo, Côte d'Ivoire, Gabon, Kuwait, Mali, Niger, Nigeria, Senegal, Togo
1961	Chad, Cyprus, Democratic Republic of the Congo, Madagascar, Mauritania, Sierra Leone, Somalia
1962	Algeria, Burundi, Mongolia, Rwanda, Samoa, United Republic of Tanzania
1963	Jamaica, Trinidad and Tobago, Uganda
1964	Kenya
1965	Malawi, Maldives, Malta, Zambia
1966	Guyana, Singapore
1967	Barbados, Lesotho
1968	Mauritius
1971	Bahrein, Gambia, Oman
1972	Bangladesh, Fiji, Qatar, United Arab Emirates
1973	Democratic People's Republic of Korea, Swaziland
1974	Bahamas, Grenada, Guinea-Bissau
1975	Botswana, Comoros, Mozambique, Tonga
1976	Angola, Cape Verde, Papua New Guinea, Sao Tome and Principe, Suriname
1978	Djibouti
1979	Seychelles
1980	Equatorial Guinea, Saint Lucia, San Marino, Zimbabwe
1981	Dominica
1982	Bhutan
1983	Saint Vincent and the Grenadines, Solomon Islands, Vanuatu
1984	Antigua and Barbuda, Cook Islands, Kiribati, Saint Kitts and Nevis
1985	Brunei Darussalam
1990	Belize, Namibia
1991	Latvia, Lithuania, Marshall Islands, Micronesia (Federated States of), Tokelau [b]
1992	Armenia, Azerbaijan, Bosnia and Herzegovina, Croatia, Georgia, Kazakstan, Kyrgyzstan, Puerto Rico, [b] Republic of Moldova, Slovenia, Tajikistan, Turkmenistan, Uzbekistan
1993	Czech Republic, Eritrea, Estonia, Slovakia, The Former Yugoslav Republic of Macedonia, Tuvalu
1994	Nauru, Niue
1995	Palau
1997	Andorra

[a] Listed according to the year on which they became a party to the Constitution or the year of admission to associate membership.

[b] Associate Member.

outlines of coordinated research, and to train those concerned directly or indirectly with international health and medicine. Expert advisory panels and committees have been a useful and effective means of securing technical information and guidance for WHO's programmes. They comprise large numbers of the world's leading medical scientists and health administrators in fields of interest to WHO. Their views and recommendations, contained in the reports of expert committees or expressed by panel members individually, are used by the Executive Board and Secretariat in preparing WHO programmes.

For many purposes, WHO has directly approached country medical services and individuals in every part of the world. The Organization has set up formal laboratory networks for reference and exchange of information on various subjects, and for coordinated programmes of research. Those for influenza and poliovirus research and for biological standardization are among the best known. The system covers most fields of health and medicine. This association is often based on formal agreements between individual countries and WHO. WHO's assistance also consists in facilitating an exchange of workers, or in providing essential technical supplies. The cooperation of nongovernmental organizations (NGOs), in addition to governmental ones, has been most valuable for obtaining information and ensuring the wide application of any necessary development or investigation. NGOs have supplied technical data, made known the objectives of the Organization, joined in various programmes and assisted in developing interest in international health work.

In order to increase knowledge, a direct or indirect objective in most WHO programmes, WHO has sys-tematically used existing national centres and institutions whose services are made available by the responsible national authorities. Various types of activities are undertaken: general or special surveys of existing conditions; inquiries into a particular problem by a number of investigators in the laboratory, the hospital or the field; analyses of existing circumstances to guide further research; and coordination of such activities in an international health programme. A natural adjunct to providing general technical services for all countries and direct services to individual countries has been the use of international publications. From the outset, WHO found it necessary and desirable to continue and expand the international publications programme that it had taken over from its predecessors.

Whereas WHO's first Director-General had overseen the establishment of the new Organization, Dr Marcolino Gomes Candau, who was elected in 1953 and served until 1973, made his mark in the application and extension of the principles enunciated in the Constitution to the real-life situations prevailing worldwide.

During the 1960s, cholera, plague and yellow fever persisted and remained potentially dangerous. In addition, new diseases or syndromes appeared (e.g. mosquito-borne haemorrhagic fever). Mass campaigns and the development of new methods limited the extent of malaria, yaws, poliomyelitis, yellow fever, tuberculosis and typhus. In the field of virus diseases, new vaccines – such as measles and freeze-dried smallpox vaccines – brought new hope for the future. There were considerable developments in chemotherapy and chemoprophylaxis.

The 1970s witnessed the beginning of a new awareness of the rights, status, and role of women which re-

For many purposes, WHO has directly approached country medical services and individuals in every part of the world.

sulted in greater independence for women and their increased participation in all aspects of economic, political and social life. However, there was still much to be done to achieve sex equality in most countries. The increasing involvement of women in economic life influenced, in turn, the family lifestyle. The demand for day-care services, preschool care and education facilities increased, and this period saw the emergence of a new type of family and new types of relationship between men and women and between parents and children.

Considerable emphasis was placed on the evaluation of developmental progress in general and social progress in particular, and there was a shift towards the measurement of social development and changes in well-being by non-monetary indicators and away from excessive reliance on such indicators as per capita gross national product. Ways of measuring the impact of health action on the improvement of health status were given increasing priority. Among health status indicators, life expectancy and infant mortality were often selected with other social indicators for the construction of composite indices of social progress. Long delays in data processing which affected the timeliness of information, and the lack of coordination between the health administration and other sectors, limited the usefulness of health-related socioeconomic statistics. There were often no national or international guidelines or standards on data collection procedures, classification schemes and coding rules, with the result that statistics were heterogeneous and incompatible, data on health expenditure being one example.

WHO's third Director-General, Dr Halfdan Mahler, took over in 1973 at a time of profound changes in international political and economic relationships. His mandate (until 1988) encompassed the next significant phase for the Organization, typified by a new awareness of health as an essential part of human development.

In 1974, the Sixth Special Session of the United Nations General Assembly adopted the Declaration and the Programme of Action for the establishment of a new international economic order. In the same year, the UN General Assembly approved the Charter of Economic Rights and Duties of States, and 1974 was designated as World Population Year.

1975 was the International Women's Year. Special international conferences relating to the environment included the Human Settlements Conference, held in 1976, the Water Conference and the Desertification Conference, both held in 1977.

The public and the mass media showed a growing interest in the organization of health-related matters, and at the international level, the debate took place not only in health organizations such as WHO, but also within groupings of countries representing all shades of social and economic development and political opinion (e.g. the OAU, groupings of Latin American countries, the CMEA countries, the European Economic Community, and the OECD). Health development was also given increasing emphasis in the policies of a number of organizations and programmes of the United Nations system, such as UNICEF, UNDP, the World Bank, UNFPA, UNEP, ILO and UNESCO.

The concept of health development, as distinct from the provision of medical care, was a product of recent policy thinking. Through WHO in particular, countries elaborated a number of fundamental principles for health development. One was that governments have responsibility for the health of their people, and at the

The concept of health development, as distinct from the provision of medical care, was a product of recent policy thinking. Through WHO in particular, countries elaborated a number of fundamental principles for health development.

A landmark in the development of health policy was the International Conference on Primary Health Care which took place in 1978 in Alma-Ata.

same time people should have the right as well as the duty, individually and collectively, to participate in the development of their own health. Governments and the health professions also have the duty of providing the public with the information and social framework that will enable them to assume greater responsibility for their own health. These principles led to the further principle of individual, community and national self-determination and self-reliance in health matters, self-reliance not being synonymous with self-sufficiency.

The distribution of resources affecting health came under close scrutiny. This led to the widespread acceptance of the need for a more equitable distribution of health resources within and among countries. Increasing emphasis was laid on preventive measures well integrated with curative, rehabilitative and environmental measures. Biomedical and health services research underwent critical analysis, and policies were aimed at orienting such research more closely to the solution of problems that are highly relevant to people's priority needs (socially relevant research). Within WHO, two special programmes were set up in response to this trend: in 1972, the Special Programme of Research, Development and Research Training in Human Reproduction; and in 1975 the Special Programme for Research and Training in Tropical Diseases. Health technology underwent the same kind of critical analysis, and the concept of appropriate technology for health emerged. This was understood to mean a technology that is scientifically sound, adapted to local needs, acceptable to the community, maintained as far as possible by the people themselves in keeping with the principle of self-reliance, and capable of being applied with resources

that the community and the country could afford. This technology had to be applied through well-defined programmes delivered through a countrywide system incorporating the above concepts and based on primary health care.

From Alma-Ata to 1998

A landmark in the development of health policy was the International Conference on Primary Health Care which took place in 1978 in Alma-Ata, attended by delegations from 134 governments and by representatives of UN system organizations, other agencies and NGOs.

The Conference declared that the health status of hundreds of millions of people in the world was unacceptable and called for a new approach to health and health care to shrink the gap between the "haves" and "have-nots", to achieve a more equitable distribution of health resources, and to attain a level of health for all the citizens of the world that would permit them to lead a socially and economically productive life. The Conference further affirmed that the primary health care approach was essential to an acceptable level of health throughout the world and acknowledged that this could be attained through a fuller and better use of the world's resources.

Thus, in endorsing the report of the International Conference on Primary Health Care in 1979, the World Health Assembly and the United Nations General Assembly reaffirmed that health was a powerful lever for socioeconomic development and peace, and that the goal of health for all by the year 2000, which was essential for raising the quality of life, could be attained through the primary health care approach. In 1981, the World Health Assembly adopted the Global Strategy for Health for All by the Year 2000, inviting Member States to formulate, or strengthen and implement, their strategies for health for all accordingly and to monitor their progress and evaluate their effectiveness, using appropriate indicators to this end.

Since the foundation of the World Health Organization there has been an evolution of international health manpower policies, which has both reflected and heightened national health leaders' awareness of key manpower issues. Political pressure, and societies' demand for medical education, brought for some years an almost unrestricted expansion of training capacity; manpower production developed a momentum of its own, increasing demand and ignoring needs. Soon countries had too many health professionals who could only function within a relatively narrow range of skills and were unable, or unwilling, to practise the kind of health care that most people required or to go to the places where they were needed. In 1979, WHO recommended that governments take action to ensure the availability of adequate numbers of appropriate types of health personnel, recognizing that this would involve the reorientation of existing health workers, the development of new categories of workers in health and related sectors, and training of all manpower to serve the community. The potential role of traditional medical practitioners, birth attendants and voluntary health workers, was also evoked.

The Action Programme on Essential Drugs was established in 1981 to promote the development of national drug policies and essential drug lists. These two activities were given a strong boost by a major conference of experts in Nairobi on the rational use of drugs, a concept which placed essential drugs in the context of a comprehensive approach to the selec-

tion, procurement, prescription and use of the most essential drugs and gave impetus to the need for full professional involvement, quality control, reliable information and other elements of sound national drug policies (Box 3).

Box 3. The WHO Model List of essential drugs

In the 1970s, whereas the developed countries were faced with problems of overconsumption and misuse of drugs, in the developing countries essential drugs were not available in sufficient quantities, were too costly, and were sometimes of questionable quality.

There was a need to reorient WHO's activities in this area so as to develop a global approach relating priorities in the matter of drugs to health priorities in general. All the parties concerned shared a common responsibility and should cooperate fairly, and all the partners must also abide by certain rules.

It was considered necessary that countries should formulate their own national drug policies, setting their own priorities as regards research, production, control and distribution of pharmaceuticals. It was clear that those policies would differ in different countries, depending on many factors. For countries that had difficulty in obtaining essential drugs it was also important that WHO should be able to give advice and information and assist with the training of personnel responsible for drug control.

Accordingly, the World Health Assembly requested WHO to advise Member States on the selection and procurement, at reasonable cost, of essential drugs of established quality corresponding to their national health needs. The first WHO Model List was published in 1977. This list contained 208 pharmaceutical products and received a mixed reception from both the pharmaceutical industry and the health professions.

The List has since been revised nine times. Its definition as a "common core" of essential drugs for basic needs, drugs which "satisfy the health care needs of the majority of the population and should therefore be available at all times in adequate amounts and in the appropriate dosage forms" remains as valid today as it was 20 years ago. Over the years a total of 166 new products have been added while 68 have been deleted, demonstrating the dynamic nature of the ongoing review which focuses both on changing global health needs and therapeutic options. As of 1997, there were 306 products on the List.

The success of the Model List lies in its effectiveness as a tool for drug supplies, for education and for highlighting lacunae in therapeutic needs, thereby speeding up availability of new drug treatments. It should always be considered in the context of national drug policies which address not only drug use, but also procurement and supply strategies, drug financing, drug donations and drug education for health professionals and consumers alike.

The developing

countries were

experiencing an

epidemiological

transition, with rapid

ageing of the popula-

tion together with an

increasing incidence

of noncommunicable

diseases linked to

changes in lifestyle.

The period 1985-1990 was characterized by dramatic changes in both the political and the economic situations. On the positive side, there was a widespread move towards democratization of political systems and greater participation of people in determining their own future. Human rights, equity and social justice increasingly became basic concerns in the political decision-making process. The expression of individual and ethnic rights, however, led to increased violence and local conflicts and strife in some countries such as Afghanistan. Economic policy also changed drastically and there was an increasing trend towards recognizing the importance of health as a basic element of development. However, the least developed countries faced difficulties even in maintaining basic minimum services in the social sector, including health. Structural adjustment programmes reduced public expenditure and accelerated the expansion of the private sector (the drug market, private clinics, etc.).

And yet, the period witnessed perceptible improvements in health care coverage and health status, though such progress was uneven, differing in various parts of the world, among population groups within countries and in different age groups. While commitment to the aims of health for all remained firm and Member States generally adopted the primary health care approach as described in the Declaration of Alma-Ata for the development of their health care systems, the implementation of strategies to achieve those aims had in many cases slowed down. This slowing down resulted not only from economic factors but also from the rigidity of health systems, weak infrastructure, the constraints on achieving real participation by all related sectors and the inadequacy of efforts to promote health and prevent specific health problems.

At the same time, the developing countries were experiencing an epidemiological transition, with rapid ageing of the population together with an increasing incidence of noncommunicable diseases linked to changes in lifestyle. The growing prevalence of cancer, cardiovascular disease, diabetes and other chronic conditions in addition to the long-standing problems of communicable diseases such as cholera, malaria and tuberculosis imposed a double burden on health care systems in these countries. There were also worrying trends in mortality from accidents and suicide in young adults, particularly in the developed countries. In addition, the pandemic of HIV infection and AIDS imposed a particularly heavy new burden on developing countries. All these realities had to be taken into account in implementing public health action geared to achieving the goal of health for all through primary health care.

The election of Dr Hiroshi Nakajima as Director-General of WHO in 1988 came at a time of global political and economic upheaval unprecedented since the end of the Second World War. Local civil strife and armed conflict became more widespread, drawing WHO increasingly into participation in humanitarian emergency activities, and involvement in issues of human rights (Box 4). The end of the Cold War stimulated a major realignment of global political and economic relationships. In many countries, these global changes were accompanied by greater emphasis on market-based economies and democratic reforms which stressed individual rights and responsibilities for health, food, housing, education and political representation. At the same time, the decline in the pace of economic growth, the growing debt burden in many countries and economic structural adjustment resulted in fewer resources for international development activities and for national funding for health and social sector programmes. Confronting these serious limitations, national authorities worldwide were increasingly preoccupied with health sector financing, particularly the sharply rising costs of medical care which threatened the sustainability of cost-effective primary health care interventions.

These dramatic global changes were accompanied by other transitions that significantly affected health status and disease patterns, such as growing environmental health problems resulting from natural resources degradation and pollution, and improper use and disposal of hazardous materials; significant demographic changes caused by rapid population growth in some countries, unplanned urbanization, and mass migration of refugees due to natural and manmade disasters; and greater expectations regarding the level and quality of health care created by expanding medical technology and health awareness. The spread of the AIDS pandemic and the resurgence of diseases such as tuberculosis and malaria not only threatened to jeopardize hardwon improvements in health status, particularly in terms of life expectancy and infant mortality, but also led to health deterioration in some countries, further inhibiting economic development.

In spite of financial constraints being a major obstacle to supporting Member States in implementing and sustaining their health services, WHO was able to adjust to 12 consecutive years of no real growth in the regular budget through the use of extrabudgetary resources, which increased from about one-fifth of the budget in 1970 to slightly more than half in 1990. Paradoxically these extrabudgetary programmes created a fi-

Box 4. Health and human rights

WHO's Constitution states that "The enjoyment of the highest attainable standard of health is one of the fundamental rights of every human being without distinction of race, religion, political, economic or social condition". On two separate occasions, in 1970 and 1977, the World Health Assembly has proclaimed that "health is a human right", and the same affirmation was made by the International Conference on Primary Health Care, held in 1978 in Alma-Ata under the joint auspices of WHO and UNICEF.

The 50th anniversary of the entry into force of WHO's Constitution coincides with the 50th anniversary of the adoption of the Universal Declaration of Human Rights. The right to a standard of living adequate for health and well-being is enshrined in Article 25 of the Declaration. It is fitting that the two anniversaries will be commemorated in a combined, integrated manner in 1998 by WHO, and that "health as a human right" is one of the 10 themes to be emphasized during WHO's 50th anniversary events.

The Task Force on Health in Development, established pursuant to a resolution adopted by the World Health Assembly in 1992, was mandated to recommend appropriate arrangements for the protection of basic health as a human right and, in consultation with all partners concerned, to initiate a process of education and consensus-building to ensure that health status is protected in the development process. WHO identifies human rights and the closely related domain of ethics as over-arching principles that should be taken into account in all relevant WHO programmes and activities.

Steps are now being taken to intensify WHO's role in the human rights sector, in conjunction with its many governmental and nongovernmental partners. This newly invigorated approach by WHO to the field of human rights should enable the Organization to give clear recognition to an infrequently cited paragraph of the Preamble to the Constitution, which proclaims that "The health of all peoples is fundamental to the attainment of peace and security".

nancial drain on regular budget programmes which subsidized the extrabudgetary administrative activities. Moreover, while these extrabudgetary resources usually supported important health interventions, competing policy and budgetary considerations often arose between decisions of the Executive Board, the World Health Assembly and regional committees, and those of the donor-dominated management structures of the extrabudgetary programmes.

Concerned with the need to respond to these profound changes, the

The years since 1992

have witnessed a

deep commitment by

the WHO Secretariat

to undertake the

profound institutional

reforms required by

Member States to

ensure that the

Organization is ready

to assume its role

at the dawn of the

21st century.

Executive Board decided in 1992 to undertake a review of the extent to which WHO could make a more effective contribution to global health work and in Member States. It found that, although health for all remained valid as a guiding principle, the Organization and Member States had not been able to finance and implement their programmes at a pace which would ensure the achievement of the targets. The Organization was at a pivotal decision point, and must either redouble its efforts and concentrate its resources on achieving health-for-all goals or revise those goals to achievable levels in the light of changing world conditions.

The association of health for all with the year 2000 had been a motivational concept for the past 15 years. However, it had come to be seen as limiting, sometimes misunderstood and proposing a time-frame which was not universally attainable. More realistic operational targets and indicators were needed to guide future international health work by WHO and Member States. Operational targets such as eradication of poliomyelitis or dracunculiasis, and extension of primary health care, should define minimum acceptable levels of health status or services, consonant with the principle of equity. Thus, the year 2000 could represent only the first milestone in the continuum towards health for all.

The years since 1992 have witnessed a deep commitment by the WHO Secretariat to undertake the profound institutional reforms required by Member States to ensure that the Organization is ready to assume its role at the dawn of the 21st century, and to respond more effectively and efficiently to changing needs in countries.

WHO must now take full advantage of the opportunities provided by the globalization of the economy, technological innovations and the information explosion, which through the impending knowledge revolution can enable individuals wherever they may be to achieve their health potential.

How WHO works and what it does

The international norms and standards developed by WHO have served public health by unifying diagnostic and therapeutic procedures, improving the compatibility of research data, containing the spread of disease, and ensuring the quality of food, drinking-water, and pharmaceutical products. At the same time, WHO also operates as a goal-oriented organization, working to achieve time-limited objectives decided upon by its governing bodies and advisory groups.

WHO sets the standards

Since 1948, the Organization has carried out a wide range of normative activities. Some were inherited from the international health bodies which preceded WHO (the *International classification of diseases* and the *International health regulations*). Some relate to WHO's directing functions (e.g. the list of International Nonproprietary Names for pharmaceutical substances, the Guidelines for drinking-water quality, the Codex Alimentarius, the Code of Marketing of Breast-milk Substitutes). WHO's coordinating functions can be illustrated by its historically significant work in the fields of biological standardization and vaccine research.

Classification is fundamental to the quantitative study of any phenomenon. It is recognized as the basis of all scientific generalization and is therefore an essential element in statistical methodology. Uniform definitions and uniform systems of classification are prerequisites in the advancement of scientific knowledge. In the study of illness and death, therefore, a standard classification of disease and injury for statistical purposes is essential.

The **International statistical classification of diseases and related health problems** (ICD), with its associated rules and guidelines for information collection, coding and tabulation, is the standard international statistical tool for the study of causes of mortality and morbidity. The main purpose of the ICD is to permit the comparison of causes of mortality and morbidity between countries at the same point in time, and within and between countries over time, thus enabling the provision of comparable statistics for decision-making in disease prevention and the provision of care at different levels, and facilitating the obtaining of epidemiological data for research purposes.

The statistical study of disease began with the work of John Graunt on the London Bills of Mortality in the early 17th century. While over three centuries have contributed something to the scientific accuracy of disease classification, there are many who doubt the usefulness of attempts to compile statistics of disease, or even causes of death, because of the difficulties of classification. To these, one can quote Professor Major Greenwood: "The scientific purist, who will wait for medical statistics until they are nosologically exact, is no wiser than Horace's rustic waiting for the river to flow away".

The first attempt to classify diseases systematically was made in the 18th century, published under the title *Nosologia Methodica*. At the beginning of the 19th century, the classification of disease in most general use was the *Synopsis Nosologiae*

Methodicae published in 1785. In 1839, the General Register Office of England and Wales, found in William Farr – its first medical statistician – a man who not only made the best possible use of the imperfect classifications of disease available at the time, but who laboured to secure better classifications and international uniformity in their use. The utility of such a classification of causes of death was recognized internationally in 1853. Numerous attempts were made thereafter to establish a universally acceptable classification but the general arrangement proposed by Farr, including the principle of classifying diseases by anatomical site, survived as the basis of the *International list of causes of death*.

The Health Organization of the League of Nations also took an active interest in vital statistics and appointed a commission of statistical experts to study the classification of diseases and causes of death, as well as other problems in the field of medical statistics. A monograph was prepared that listed the expansion in the rubrics of the 1920 *International list of causes of death* that would be required if the classification was to be used in the tabulation of statistics of morbidity. This study was published in 1928.

After WHO was created, it assumed responsibility for continuing the regular revisions of the *International list of diseases and causes of death*, starting with the Sixth Revision in 1948. The classification was subsequently revised in 1955 and 1965. The Ninth Revision in 1975 saw the introduction of a system for the dual classification of diseases according to both their etiology and manifestations, as well as a classification of the morphology of tumours. It was during the currency of the Ninth Revision (1979-1992) that the use of the classification was extended from the

After WHO was created, it assumed responsibility for continuing the regular revisions of the International list of diseases and causes of death.

traditional applications of statistics of underlying causes of mortality and the indexing of hospital medical records to include medical insurance schemes, the recording of adverse effects in drug monitoring as well as reasons for encounter in primary care and resource allocation in health care. This enormous growth in the use of the ICD was largely due to the availability of personal computers which enabled users to operate systems which had previously only been feasible on mainframe computers.

Fourteen years instead of the usual 10 were allowed for the preparation of the Tenth Revision of the ICD, in order to enable an in-depth review to be made of the structure and content of the classification in the light of both national and international public health requirements. The main innovation in the Tenth Revision, which came into effect on 1 January 1993, is the use of an alphanumeric coding scheme of one letter followed by three numbers at the four-character level. This had the effect of more than doubling the size of the coding frame in comparison with the Ninth Revision, the greatly increased clinical detail being contained in 12 420 rubrics compared with some 6700 in ICD-9.

WHO, through its network of 10 collaborating centres for the classification of diseases, each based on a particular language or geographical area, has now established a mechanism for the Tenth Revision which enables the classification to be updated periodically according to need.

In parallel with the development of the Tenth Revision of the ICD, a "family" of fully-compatible disease and health-related classifications has arisen to meet the needs of specialist groups for greater clinical detail than that provided by the four-character classification. Such specialty-based adaptations already exist for oncology, psychiatry, neurology, dentistry and stomatology, paediatrics and dermatology, while others are planned for rheumatology and orthopaedics, and external causes of injuries.

One of the first responsibilities of WHO was to unify the separate international sanitation treaties in a single code. WHO adopted the *International sanitary regulations* in 1951, which replaced the previous set of treaties among Member States. The *International sanitary regulations* were amended a number of times in the 1950s and 1960s, and renamed the ***International health regulations*** (IHR) in 1969. The IHR were amended in 1981 to remove smallpox from the list of diseases subject to the Regulations. Today, the IHR represent the only international health agreement on communicable diseases that is binding on Member States.

The purpose of the IHR is to help prevent the international spread of diseases and, in the context of international trade, to do so with the minimum of inconvenience to the passenger. This requires international collaboration in the detection and reduction or elimination of the sources from which infection spreads rather than attempts to prevent the introduction of diseases by legalistic barriers that over the years have proved to be ineffective. Ultimately, however, the risk of an infective agent becoming established in a country is determined by the quality of the national epidemiological services and, in particular, by the day-to-day national health and disease surveillance activities and the ability to implement prompt and effective control measures.

No regulations can be expected to foresee every disease eventuality and, in certain situations, diseases and conditions other than those covered by the IHR may be of concern to na-

> The purpose of the IHR is to help prevent the international spread of diseases and, in the context of international trade, to do so with the minimum of inconvenience to the passenger.

tional health authorities and the travelling public. The IHR cannot refer specifically to diseases that were not known at the time the Regulations were last revised. This is the case with AIDS. Nevertheless, any requirements for an HIV antibody test certificate ("AIDS-free certificate") is contrary to the Regulations, since Article 81 states that "no health document, other than those provided for in these Regulations, shall be required in international traffic".

The success of WHO in globalizing disease control programmes might suggest that the defects of international law have not hobbled its effectiveness in improving health care worldwide. However, despite having the authority to do so, WHO has been reluctant to use international law, and its effectiveness has been questioned. A 1975 WHO publication stated that the IHR have not functioned satisfactorily at times of serious disease outbreaks. More recently, WHO's efforts with the IHR have been called a failure, and noncompliance with these regulations has increased in connection with reporting disease outbreaks.

WHO's reluctance to apply international law has been attributed to its organizational culture, which is dominated by scientists, doctors and medical experts. The global threat posed by these infections represents in many ways a test case for international public health law. The effectiveness of international law depends on the consent of States, which means that sovereignty and its exercise determine the fate of international legal rules. In adopting a legal strategy for its emerging infectious disease action plan, WHO has to convince its Member States to take certain actions in response to disease emergence.

International Nonproprietary Names for pharmaceutical substances (INNs) are also referred to as common or generic names. As a result of the rapid industrial expansion and development of a large number of synthetic drug substances which became available internationally, the World Health Assembly in 1950 recognized the need to develop one standard name worldwide to identify newly developed pharmaceutical substances. A single internationally recognized name for an active drug substance is vital for safe prescribing and dispensing, and for ease of communication among scientists and health professionals. In contrast to the tradenames, INNs are intended to be used as public property without constraint, i.e. nobody should own any proprietary rights, thus the inclusion of "nonproprietary" in the designation INN. WHO collaborates closely with national nomenclature commissions to select a single name with worldwide acceptability for each active substance that is to be marketed as a pharmaceutical. To date some 6900 names have been selected. The selection of an INN follows established rules so that the name itself communicates to medical and pharmaceutical health professionals the therapeutic or pharmacological group to which the active drug substance belongs. Newly selected INNs are published first as proposed and, provided no objection was raised within a permissible period of four months, again as a recommended INN in *WHO drug information*. The list gives the names in Latin, English, French and Spanish. The cumulative list which is published periodically includes in addition the Russian version and more detailed information, such as references to pharmacopoeial monographs and international and national names that are identical or different to INNs. A CD-ROM version is in preparation.

The International standards for drinking-water quality were first published by WHO in 1958 as an aid to

A single internationally recognized name for an active drug substance is vital for safe prescribing and dispensing.

No matter where

they live, consumers

should enjoy adequate

protection against

the risks of

foodborne diseases.

the improvement of water quality and treatment. The second edition appeared in 1963 and the third one in 1971. These publications were used as guidance by many countries in the formulation of national standards. Consequently their name was changed to **WHO Guidelines for drinking-water quality** with a first edition in 1984, and the second edition in 1993. The Guidelines now consist of three volumes, containing (*i*) recommendations; (*ii*) health criteria and other supporting information; and (*iii*) surveillance and control of community supplies.

The Joint FAO/WHO **Codex Alimentarius** Commission was established in 1962 to protect the health of the consumer and, at the same time, to ensure fair practices in food trade. Codex has been working since and has elaborated a number of food standards, guidelines and recommendations. However, while member governments of Codex have been asked to accept these standards, it has been left for governments to decide whether they should or should not implement them. It has established more than 200 food standards, over 40 codes of hygienic and technological practice and more than 3000 maximum residue limits for pesticides and veterinary drugs in foods, as well as maximum limits for over 700 food additives and contaminants, and has contributed to harmonizing food standards worldwide.

No matter where they live, consumers should enjoy adequate protection against the risks of foodborne diseases. This can be achieved, without restricting international trade, if all countries harmonize their regulations by using international standards as a basis for their sanitary measures. Codex is also in the process of elaborating general standards covering food additives, contaminants and toxins to provide a wider basis for protecting

consumers' health. Following the Uruguay Round of Multilateral Trade Negotiations in 1994, countries agreed to reduce tariff barriers for many agricultural commodities so as to encourage free trade. As a result, non-tariff barriers became a real concern because they could undermine the promotion of international trade if put into practice in an arbitrary or discriminatory way *(Box 5)*.

When the World Health Assembly adopted the **International Code of Marketing of Breast-milk Substitutes** in 1981, it called on governments to translate it into legislation, regulations or other suitable measures, and to involve all concerned parties in its implementation. In pursuit of its aim to contribute to safe and adequate nutrition for infants, the International Code affirms that: governments are responsible for ensuring that objective and consistent information is provided on infant and young child feeding; that there should be no advertising or other form of promotion to the general public of breast-milk substitutes or other products within the scope of the Code; and that health workers should encourage and protect breast-feeding. 158 Member States have since reported to WHO on a wide range of approaches they are using to give effect to the International Code, such as adopting new legislation and regulations; reviewing and updating existing laws; preparing and updating guidelines (e.g. for health workers, manufacturers and distributors); negotiating and updating agreements with health workers and infant-food manufacturers; and establishing committees to monitor and evaluate the impact of national measures.

The significance of **biological standardization** for global health programmes was recognized in the early years of the 20th century by the League of Nations and its Commis-

Box 5. Links between health and trade

Trade in services is a rapidly growing activity accounting for an increasing share of national product in both developing and industrialized countries. The World Trade Organization (WTO) has organized multilateral negotiations to liberalize trade in services, resulting in the General Agreement on Trade in Services (GATS).

"Services" are generally described as being distinct from physical commodities, being intangible, nontransferable economic goods. For trade purposes, GATS defines services in terms of the ways in which they can be supplied; e.g. across a border (in the health field, an example would be telemedicine), or through people who are service suppliers (such as health professionals working outside their home country).

Relatively few countries have made commitments in the health sector under GATS. Some 27% of WTO Members (half industrial and half developing countries) agreed to open up hospital services to foreign enterprises, and 35% (in similar proportions) did so for medical and dental services. Some 19% (mostly industrial countries) scheduled the services of health personnel other than physicians.

It is much too early to assess the impact of the Agreement on trade in health services. However, there is a growing awareness of its potential for both industrial and developing countries. In the general context of rising health care costs coupled with a growing trend to reduce public spending in the social sectors, the advantages of exporting health sector skills and technology, or of attracting higher-spending foreign customers to health facilities, are obvious.

But how can objectives of profitability and resource generation be reconciled with that of improving the population's health status? WHO has identified three interim policy objectives to further that goal: equitable access to care (i.e. equal utilization of health services for the same need, with users contributing according to their economic capacity); quality of care (this refers to the standard of the health care system); and efficient use of resources (i.e. a given output is produced at minimum cost, or maximum output is produced at a given cost).

However, some health professionals tend to think of international trade as an area of little relevance for public health activity. Yet even as early as 1949 the World Health Assembly called the attention of the Director-General to the need for eliminating quarantine restrictions of doubtful medical value which interfere with international trade and travel. But not until 1995 did an international trade agreement come into force to respond to the concern that as other trade barriers came down, sanitary and phytosanitary measures might be used for protectionist purposes. It therefore encourages countries to apply harmonized measures based on international standards, guidelines and recommendations which, in turn, reinforces WHO's norms. For example, the agreement stipulates that in the case of food safety the international references are those of the Codex Alimentarius Commission – which implements the Joint FAO/WHO Food Standards Programme.

Nor is WHO called upon solely for its norms. Its expertise is becoming increasingly valuable in a particularly sensitive area of trade relations, that of settling disputes. In a dispute between the European Union and the United States in 1997, WHO experts provided scientific evidence on risk assessment procedures used to determine potential risk to human health, a key element for the findings of WTO's dispute settlement panel. As expanding trade raises the likelihood of litigation, WHO may well in the future be increasingly called upon to advise as the only international source of impartial scientific expertise in health matters.

sion on Biological Standardization. This work was subsequently taken over by WHO and its Expert Committee on Biological Standardization. The importance given by WHO to re-establishing international activities in biological standardization in the post-war era is indicated by the fact that this was one of its earliest actions. Since then, WHO has recommended procedures for ensuring the safety and efficacy of biological medicinal products, which include vaccines, plasma products and diagnostic agents. It does this by establishing WHO international biological reference materials, primary standards that ensure the comparability of the activities of biologicals worldwide, and by drawing up requirements and guidelines for ensuring the safety and potency of specific biologicals. These are developed following extensive global consultation and serve as guidance for national health authorities. The rapid expansion of the biologicals field, together with the development of novel biotechnologies, not only in developed countries but also in a number of developing countries, raises new and specific challenges for product safety and efficacy. There is thus an increasing need for international standards for ensuring the quality of biological products and for developing a coordinated international approach to all aspects of regulation and standard setting in this area.

From the earliest days of WHO, formal laboratory networks were set up by the Organization for reference, exchange of information and coordination of research programmes, particularly in the area of **vaccine research** (e.g. for influenza and poliovirus). The global investment in basic research, begun about 50 years ago, is now paying rich dividends in the availability of new vaccines. The pace of innovation is expected to increase well into the next century and beyond.

WHO policy trends

General programmes of work and principles

Within the framework of WHO's Constitution, general programmes of work lay down medium-term objectives for a specified period (4-6 years) *(Table 2)*, while programme budgets set out immediate objectives for activities to be undertaken during a biennium (formerly one year).

In 1950, the First general programme of work stated five basic principles: all countries and territories should take part in the Organization's work; assistance in the development of health services should be supplied only at the request of the government

Table 2. WHO's general programmes of work

	Adopted	Period covered
First	1950	1952-1956
Second	1955	1957-1961
Third	1960	1962-1966
Fourth	1965	1967-1972
Fifth	1971	1973-1977
Sixth	1976	1978-1983
Seventh	1982	1984-1989
Eighth	1987	1990-1995
Ninth	1994	1996-2001

concerned; the services afforded should foster national and local self-reliance and initiative, and should be adapted to the environment; WHO should stimulate and coordinate current research; services should be available to all Member States.

Different emphasis was given at different times to WHO's role and functions in response to the world health situation. Functions have traditionally been grouped into two categories: direction and coordination of international health work, and technical cooperation with countries.

The **international directing and coordinating function** started with the establishment of international norms and standards inherited from the preceding international organizations. The early work included drugs and biological substances for prophylactic or therapeutic use, the *International statistical classification of diseases, injuries and causes of death* and the *International health regulations (see above)*.

Technical cooperation, on the other hand, was a new task assigned to WHO, which no preceding organizations had undertaken. In 1950, the First general programme of work stated that regional offices should be responsible for this activity, with headquarters providing technical guidance and coordination. The importance of fostering self-reliance of

The global investment in basic research, begun about 50 years ago, is now paying rich dividends in the availability of new vaccines.

the country was stressed from the outset, and repeated in every successive general programme of work. When WHO's involvement is finished, the country should be able to continue on its own.

By 1960, the distinction between the two major functions had become artificial. By 1975, a study on the interrelationships between the central technical services of WHO and programmes of direct assistance to Member States led to the recognition that an integrated approach to the development of programmes was needed, all programme activities at all levels being mutually supportive and parts of a whole, with more responsibility being given to WHO's country offices. This led to a significant evolution in the concept of WHO's technical cooperation. Formerly, WHO activities in countries tended to be based on the traditional concept of technical aid or assistance, implying a donor-to-recipient relationship without mutual exchange. This was replaced by a new concept of technical cooperation characterized by equal partnership among the cooperating parties. Towards the end of the 1970s, there was a shift in the WHO regular budget towards technical cooperation: the proportion allocated increased from 51% in 1977 to 60% in 1980. In the 1970s and 1980s, WHO increasingly promoted technical cooperation among developing countries. In the 1990s the Organization made efforts to ensure that its regional and global levels acted in complete coordination.

Criteria for activities and priorities

Within this framework, WHO's activities were aimed at yielding results that could be demonstrable to governments. The activities therefore followed a careful analysis with countries of their needs in support of their strategies. WHO introduced a planning process in the field of health during the late 1950s, based on modern science and technology. This was emphasized particularly in the Fifth general programme of work, which identified four principal programme objectives: the strengthening of health services; the development of health manpower; disease prevention and control; and the promotion of environmental health. The Sixth summarized the criteria for WHO's involvement as: the problem has been clearly defined; the problem is of major public health and socioeconomic importance; the potential for the solution of the problem has been demonstrated; there is a strong rationale for WHO's involvement; and WHO's non-involvement would cause serious adverse health repercussions.

The programme also emphasized the need to have specified targets, and sometimes output indicators, for each programme objective and stipulated that the progress of the work towards those targets was to be assessed by the regional committees, the Executive Board and the World Health Assembly.

The Seventh and Eighth general programmes of work were somewhat more elaborate, indicating the main thrust of each programme. Following the Alma-Ata Conference and the subsequent launching of the global health-for-all strategy, the WHO Secretariat produced a "medium-term programme" for each programme in respect of the periods covered by the Sixth, Seventh and Eighth general programmes of work, so as to facilitate the preparation of the programme budgets to reflect directly the objectives and targets that were set. The annual programme and budget estimates became the biennial programme budget as from 1976-1977 to allow for flexibility in implementation. To eliminate certain weak-

In the 1970s and 1980s, WHO increasingly promoted technical cooperation among developing countries.

nesses that had been observed (focus on resources allocated and activities planned, rather than on products or outputs; lack of flexibility to cope with changing situations and actual performance; and fragmentation of programmes instead of their integration), the Ninth general programme of work simplified its contents, reduced the number of programmes and set 25 numerical targets to be attained by countries by 2001.

Programme orientation and targets

Strengthening national health services. The First general programme of work stressed the need to integrate specialized health service activities in a general health programme (or basic health services). The Fifth general programme of work emphasized the need for maximum coverage of health programmes, particularly of the potentially underprivileged, as was the need for programmes planned in advance, instead of assistance to single services of limited scope. This led to the adoption in 1975 of the new approach of primary health care for the promotion of national health services. To counter the perception that the development and strengthening of the health system infrastructure is a "tedious and bureaucratic job", in comparison with specific activities which appear "more glamorous and more important" the Eighth general programme of work emphasized the strengthening of health infrastructure. Education and training of the various categories of health personnel was given high priority from the beginning, both from the quantitative and qualitative points of view, to cope with the changing needs of the community and with the evolving health technologies.

Promoting and protecting health. The Fifth, Sixth and Seventh

general programmes of work emphasized protecting mother and child health, including family planning, and health of workers and elderly people. The Seventh stressed action against undernutrition and nutritional deficiencies, but also against nutritional excess and imbalance.

The Fifth noted that a dark side of industrialization and urbanization was the emergence of factors detrimental to health, e.g. pollution, road accidents and stressful city life, and that the previous concept of environmental sanitation had evolved into that of environmental health.

The Eighth general programme of work noted steady progress in the efforts to address environmental and social issues affecting health, and promoting and protecting the health of specific population groups such as the elderly. It also stressed that the scope of general health protection and promotion extends beyond prevention and control of diseases by medical technology; it is an evolving concept that encompasses fostering lifestyles and other social, economic, environmental and personal factors conducive to health.

The Ninth general programme of work envisages that WHO continues its support to the implementation of strategies agreed upon at the United Nations Conference on Environment and Development in 1992 to achieve ecologically-sustainable development and to prevent and control environmental health risks.

Preventing and controlling specific health problems. The diseases of great public health concern in the early days of WHO included those affecting maternal and child health, malnutrition, tuberculosis, malaria, venereal diseases, endemic treponematosis, smallpox, plague, cholera and yellow fever. The Organization has adapted itself continually to the changing world situation. Starting

The scope of general health protection and promotion extends beyond prevention and control of diseases by medical technology.

from international quarantine and epidemiological intelligence of communicable diseases, which WHO inherited from its predecessors, the scope of epidemiological surveillance has gradually been extended since the 1970s to cover environmental hazards, noncommunicable diseases and other existing and emerging health problems.

Two major policy decisions were taken in the 1950s, namely, on malaria eradication in 1955 and on smallpox eradication in 1958. The malaria eradication programme could not achieve its goal in spite of remarkable initial gains. Countries' failure in integrating the programme into the general health services, as well as the development of vector resistance to insecticide and parasite resistance to chemotherapy, are considered to be the main factors involved. The strategy was subsequently modified, with renewed emphasis on control programmes as and where needed. Some progress occurred in the 1970s and early 1980s, but the malaria situation has worsened since then.

The smallpox eradication programme, on the other hand, was the most brilliant success in WHO's work. After its initiation by the World Health Assembly in 1958, the programme was intensified in 1967, and coordinated efforts of an unprecedented nature began on a worldwide scale. Eradication was achieved in 1977, and the experience gained has been used for programmes of eradication, elimination or control of other communicable diseases.

Recognizing that substantial improvements have occurred in controlling many communicable diseases, due to a greater coverage by, and access to, affordable simple technology to cope with specific problems, such as by immunization programmes, the Ninth general programme of work envisages that poliomyelitis and dra-cunculiasis will be eradicated, measles will no longer be an important public health problem, and leprosy, neonatal tetanus, and iodine and vitamin A deficiencies will be eliminated. On the other hand, the threat from new and re-emerging diseases such as HIV infection, tuberculosis and cholera remains serious.

Mental health and occupational health were included in WHO's programme at an early stage of its development. The growing importance of noncommunicable diseases also in some developing countries as public health problems was soon noted. The Third general programme of work stated that WHO should be prepared to assist countries to control cardiovascular diseases and cancer. The Fifth expressed an increased concern over noncommunicable diseases, disabilities caused by disease and accidents, and behavioural problems as causative factors. Since the 1970s, WHO has been increasingly involved in the prevention and control of noncommunicable diseases, besides supporting and coordinating research on them.

WHO has always responded to countries' requests for emergency assistance. The Ninth general programme of work stresses that WHO should also facilitate the transition from emergency relief to rehabilitation and development.

Medical and health research. The First general programme of work stated that WHO should not as a rule carry out direct medical or scientific research as such, but should endeavour to stimulate and coordinate work done in these fields. During the first 10 years of its existence, WHO conducted some research as an integral part of its programme activities, but there was no special effort to promote and coordinate medical research on a large scale. The need to promote research into determinants of health

> Smallpox eradication was achieved in 1977, and the experience gained has been used for programmes of eradication, elimination or control of other communicable diseases.

WHO focused its

attention on

well-defined priority

areas for health

research, such as

human reproduction

and tropical diseases.

– i.e. the interrelation of economic, social and health development – has also been recognized since the 1960s. Following a study in 1958 on WHO's role in research, an intensified medical research programme was started in 1960. The Advisory Committee on Medical Research was established in 1959 to provide the Director-General with the necessary scientific advice in relation to the research programme; in 1986 it was renamed the Advisory Committee on Health Research.

Important developments in the research programme included the establishment of the International Agency for Research on Cancer in 1965.

On the other hand, a major initiative for interdisciplinary research in epidemiology and communication sciences launched in 1965 was not successful. Subsequently, WHO focused its attention on well-defined priority areas for health research, such as human reproduction and tropical diseases.

WHO's role in research has since been to identify research priorities, strengthen national capabilities and promote international coordination and rapid transfer of information. Research on health systems based on primary health care has been given priority since the 1980s.

Management of WHO's own work. The Seventh general programme of work emphasized the application of a managerial process for WHO's programme development and the optimal use of WHO's resources, to be supported by permanent monitoring and evaluation of programme implementation. The Ninth general programme of work stipulates WHO's managerial requirements in a more rigorous manner than earlier general programmes of work.

Gathering vital information

Statistical services

Activities in health statistics and epidemiological surveillance were inherited from WHO's precursors and reflected in the Constitution, which requires the Organization to establish and maintain such administrative and technical services as may be required, including epidemiological and statistical services. Related obligations of Member States are that each Member shall communicate promptly to the Organization important laws, regulations, official reports and statistics pertaining to health which have been published in the State concerned and that each Member shall provide statistical and epidemiological reports in a manner to be determined by the World Health Assembly.

WHO has traditionally issued several statistical publications on the basis of information provided by Member States. The League of Nations had already published an *Annual epidemiological report* from 1922 to 1938, and this was continued in the *Annual epidemiological and vital statistics* first published in 1951, covering the period 1939-1946. The second edition, covering the years 1947-1949, was considerably enlarged and developed so as to comply with the expressed wishes of national statistical and public health administrations. The *World health statistics annual*, first published in 1962, is the continuation of the series.

The *Epidemiological and vital statistics report*, a monthly supplement for the *Weekly epidemiological record*, was started in 1947. The purpose of this supplement was to provide teaching institutions, certain health administrations and statistical services with a homogeneous periodical freed from episodic data which were of comparatively little interest to them. Each issue contained articles and tables. By 1968, this monthly publication changed its name to *World health statistics report*. The periodicity remained unchanged until the appearance of the *World health statistics quarterly* in 1979.

The need was very soon felt for technical assistance to strengthen national capacity in health statistics, since the countries giving satisfactory information, both on the occurrence of death and on its causes, were very few. Development of vital statistics and civil registration was given priority, and WHO proceeded to advise and assist Member States in improving their epidemiological and statistical data collection and reporting to WHO.

The 1960s saw the advent of computer technology in the health field. A computer was installed at WHO headquarters in 1966 and a considerable part of the statistical work was computerized during the 1970s. Statistical data processing was expedited and the computer made it practicable to store time series in an easily retrievable form, including the data received by WHO from Member States since 1950.

With the rapid development of automation in the industrialized countries, a new approach to health information was advocated, so as to develop comprehensive computer-based management information systems. Unsuccessful attempts were made to develop national health information systems. The main reasons for the failure were the overemphasis on computerization and a lack of clear recognition of the importance of the prerequisites to such computerization: of adequate quality of source data and ability to collect and prepare input to an automated system, and of capacity among health managers and decision-makers to utilize the output information to improve health care.

The movement towards national health information systems, however, was not entirely in vain. By the mid-1970s health planners and managers had begun to realize that the usual epidemiological and statistical reports they received did not suffice. Some information had to be obtained from other sectors concerning matters closely related to health (economic development, unemployment, educational status and literacy, food supply, etc.). All the relevant data had to be assembled from these various sources and then analysed and digested by the health decision-maker. Thus the managerial purpose of the generation of information was recognized more clearly, and this was reflected in the reorientation of WHO's work in this area during the 1980s.

At the request of the Executive Board in 1994, WHO reoriented its reporting style in response to global change and to the expressed need for an annual report on the status of world health, which should at the same time be a report on WHO's activities – *The World Health Report*. Its objective was to provide, through a self-contained, concise but comprehensive annual publication, a review of the global health situation and needs, and of problems faced by health systems, in order to recommend where priority should be given to international health action and to the Organization's activities in that context. Its target readership was new to WHO: non-medical professionals such as policy-makers and planners for development, heads of donor agencies and other international funding institutions, policy-makers in health (e.g. ministers of health, social welfare, etc.), financial experts who decide on the allocation of funds, and the educated public as well as opinion-makers in the media and elsewhere.

WHO reoriented its reporting style in response to global change and to the expressed need for an annual report on the status of world health, which should at the same time be a report on WHO's activities – *The World Health Report.*

Disease surveillance

Since its creation the Organization has given high priority to the timely dissemination of epidemiological information, e.g. on the occurrence of certain communicable diseases which are of international interest. Information received has been processed and feedback provided to all countries without delay through the *Weekly epidemiological record* (now available on Internet).

WHO is also using electronic links to monitor disease through a mechanism to investigate rumours of outbreaks. The information is made available on the *Disease outbreak news* web page. Information is shared through electronic communication links between WHO headquarters, regional offices, country representatives and other groups involved in disease surveillance.

Several agencies are cooperating in a project to link with collaborating centres, laboratories and other institutions electronically by means of local telephone services, radio-to-telephone or radio-to-satellite, in order to share restricted information on priority diseases almost immediately so that countries are better prepared for disease outbreaks and better able to respond to them effectively.

WHO has an influenza surveillance network of specialized laboratories which detect influenza viruses that could trigger a pandemic. FluNet is a prototype World Wide Web site for the electronic submission of influenza data from participating national laboratories. Only designated users can submit data, but the results – graphics, maps and tables of influenza activity on a global scale – are available to the general public. As new data arrive and are verified, the maps and tables are revised to give users an up-to-date overview of the influenza situation. FluNet has speeded up the sharing of information on influenza patterns and virus strains and is becoming an essential tool in preparedness for and prevention of influenza pandemics.

Health legislation

In 1948, the *International digest of health legislation* took over from the section *Lois et règlements sanitaires* of the *Bulletin mensuel de l'Office international d'hygiène publique*.

During WHO's first 10 years, the comparative legislative surveys in the *Digest* bore witness to the enactment of legislation in the traditional areas of quarantine and epidemic information, nomenclature, international standardization, statistics, public health administration, mental health, and maternal and child health. The quarterly *International digest of health legislation* remains the cornerstone of the worldwide transfer of information on health and environmental legislation, and related ethical issues. In 1951, the World Health Assembly adopted the *International sanitary regulations*, revised in 1969 to become the *International health regulations (see above)*.

In the 1960s, the scope of the issues addressed broadened considerably in view of technical and scientific advances and the need to protect the population against unsafe products and working and living conditions. From 1970 to 1980, the scope was further extended to address issues such as abortion, drug abuse, environmental protection, and legislative action to combat smoking.

1977 marked a decisive turning-point in WHO's health legislation activities, which formerly were primarily centred on the transfer of information. The global health legislation programme was to ensure its full concordance with the goal of health for all and the primary health care ap-

WHO has an influenza surveillance network of specialized laboratories which detect influenza viruses that could trigger a pandemic.

proach, embodied in the 1978 Declaration of Alma-Ata. Since 1980, WHO's aim has been to work with Member States, using an integrated approach that combines technical cooperation and information transfer in the strengthening of national health legislation. Thus the 1980s saw a major change in emphasis in WHO's legislative work, shifting from the disease-specific, hospital-based and technology-oriented approach to an approach geared to the promotion of universal access to basic health services.

From 1990 onwards, legislation bears witness to the decline of political ideologies, with power vested in people through more representative structures. This extended the scope of legislative functions to include a greater use of enabling and normative roles, coupled with a revival of the principles of ethics, equity and human rights in public health. WHO has been particularly active in legislation and guidelines addressing research on human subjects, vaccine trials, patients' rights, reproductive technologies, genetics, euthanasia and organ transplantation.

Increased international movement of persons and goods and the ever-increasing emphasis on global health has led to an unprecedented growth of international health legislation, with closer international cooperation by intergovernmental organizations and in the elaboration of common standards and guiding principles, a movement amplified during the period 1992-1995 by the recent United Nations summits.

More specifically in 1997, WHO extended its cooperation with the Health Care Committee of the Russian Parliament with a view to drafting a law on the structure of health care in the Russian Federation. A number of legislative strategies for the realization of the right to health were examined at the International Conference on Human Rights, Bioethics and Health held in cooperation with CIOMS. WHO also collaborated in a workshop on the rights of patients organized by the Research Centre for European Health Law, and an international colloquium on patients' rights as a health-for-all objective, organized by the International Association for Law, Ethics and Science and the Turkish Medical Association.

Of the many areas which WHO must address through a legislative strategy (ranging from health as a human right to the biological determinants of health and the need to safeguard medical confidentiality in the face of the ongoing information and communication revolution) the issue of rapid advances in science and technology is of particular significance. The benefits as well as the potential risks of new technologies must be evaluated in terms of the integrity, dignity and health of the individual. Seeking a balance is not easy, and the problems created fall within the fields of both medical ethics and health law. Policy-makers will need to intervene in accordance with the value system of each country and culture.

Informing the world

The WHO Constitution asserts that "informed opinion and active cooperation on the part of the public are of the utmost importance in the improvement of health". From the start, WHO has used all existing means of communication to convey information around the globe (print, telegraph, photographs, magnetic sound recording and television). In 50 years, WHO has built up extensive networks providing regular input to its comprehensive data banks on health and disease. Communicating the information generated by those networks is one of WHO's essential functions.

In 50 years, WHO has built up extensive networks providing regular input to its comprehensive data banks on health and disease.

The exciting and rapid developments in communication and the dissemination of information that have taken place during that half-century have had a profound impact on how WHO does its work. In 1977 the first personal computers went on sale to the general public, and are now commonplace in many parts of the world. They enable the daily use by millions of people worldwide of the Internet (originally a network of computers in government, academic and scientific institutions developed in the 1960s in the United States to enable researchers to share information). The number of Internet users is predicted to reach 700 million by the year 2000. By connecting to WHO's site on the World Wide Web, Internet surfers can find out about the work of WHO's programmes relating to all aspects of health and disease, and have access to the database of WHO's library. Abstracts from WHO's journals are available, as is the complete text of many WHO newsletters and documents. The Internet user can choose from the hundreds of books in WHO's publications catalogue and send in an order, or can consult any of the resolutions and decisions of the WHO governing bodies dating back to 1948. WHO has also produced several CD-ROMs that contain either encyclopaedic collections of data or compilations of journal issues.

Communication is not merely a one-way process. WHO's computers are host to over 60 e-mail discussion groups on a whole range of health concerns and aspects of the Organization's work. These e-mail lists exist so that information can be shared and ideas exchanged openly in an informal manner.

A strong working *library* was recognized as essential to the technical work of WHO as early as 1946. By 1947 the library collection was begun and a monthly *Library news* was distributed free of charge. In its early years, the library supplied thousands of books, journals, photostats and microfilms to Member governments to replace collections damaged during the Second World War and to furnish core sets of medical literature to countries. In the early 1970s, the WHO Medline Centre operated from the library, providing searches from Medline, and photocopies of articles to people working in developing countries. In 1986 the library moved from a manual to an automated library information system and all library functions were automated simultaneously. From the mid-1980s onwards the library moved ahead with its electronic library initiative. Library services were offered 24 hours a day, CD-ROM databases were introduced, and an optical disk system replaced paper for full-text storage of WHO technical documents.

The WHO library acts as a central purchasing agent to obtain books, journals and information material for libraries worldwide, enabling libraries with a lack of foreign currency to order material under the WHO revolving fund. It also runs an international exchange of free books and journals in 72 countries (comprising 219 libraries). Document delivery is provided under an agreement with the National Library of Medicine in Washington and the Library of the British Medical Association.

In 1997, WHO's reference librarians answered an estimated 17 000 queries from around the globe dealing with the work of WHO that came in by letter, fax, e-mail, telephone and in person. The indexing and cataloguing of recently-acquired non-WHO publications are being outsourced to a commercial firm, and procedures for online input of these data to the library database have been established.

While dissemination of information by electronic means has become a vital part of what WHO does, the Organization is equally concerned to ensure that information on health and disease is also transmitted in more conventional forms. WHO's ***publishing activities*** cover books and journals on a variety of topics, often in six official languages *(Box 6)*, such as manuals on preventing and controlling disease, recommendations on international standards and procedures, guidance on health service management, training materials for health workers, and reports of expert groups. Arrangements are often made with other institutions or with commercial publishers for translation and publication in national languages.

A commitment to the dissemination of information also means helping others to disseminate it too. The *Bulletin of the World Health Organization* regularly publishes research papers from developing countries, but WHO is aware that the results of much health research in developing countries do not come to the notice of scientists elsewhere because of the limited English writing skills of the researchers. This can be remedied by holding scientific writing workshops in developing countries to guide health researchers in presenting the results of their work for publication. A survey of the impact of workshops already held in Latin America has shown that, after attending the workshops, health researchers published more papers than before and were more confident in their ability to prepare scientific papers for national and international journals.

For WHO's voice to be heard, the publishing effort must also make an impact within the global publishing industry. This impact was achieved by the development of a commercial capability for publications that has put WHO at the forefront of commercial success in terms of sales income within the UN system. Commercial capability was primarily achieved by outsourcing country-level sales and marketing to WHO sales agents, who are generally among the most important scientific, technical and medical booksellers in their countries.

Accessibility and commercial goals could not be achieved without an efficient delivery system. The delivery system was gradually developed using modern technology. WHO's master mailing list manages over 300 000 addresses, tracks dissemination patterns and provides geographical and reader category profiles to achieve specific goals. This system has recently been improved, by specifically developed technology to ensure rapid invoicing, so that significant increases in sales occurred without the need to sizeably increase staff, thanks to the productivity gains achieved.

Sales in 1997 were worth around $4 million,[a] recording more than a decade of uninterrupted sales growth for WHO publications. Sales income has doubled since 1986, the WHO sales agent network has grown to cover more than 100 Member States (with more than a dozen new agents or clients on account appointed in 1997), and the distribution function is now more than 90% self-financed through sales income. WHO publications were displayed at major book fairs and scientific congresses throughout the world, the Frankfurt Book Fair, the International Conference on Health Promotion (Indonesia), the IFGO World Congress on Gynaecology and Obstetrics (Denmark) and the World Congress of Gerontology (Australia).

Large numbers of books are distributed free while many others are sold at reduced prices in developing

> Sales in 1997 were worth around $4 million, recording more than a decade of uninterrupted sales growth for WHO publications.

---

[a] Throughout the report, the sign $ denotes United States dollars.

Box 6. WHO's language services

Recognizing that the extension *to all peoples* of the benefits of medical, psychological and related knowledge is essential to the fullest attainment of health, WHO seeks to communicate the best available health information to all Member States in the most effective way. To ensure equity of access to health information in a polyglot, multicultural world, WHO must communicate essential health information in different languages.

WHO's translators – a judicious mix of fixed-term, temporary and free-lance staff – work on a wide range of material, especially scientific and technical information, and policy documents for the deliberations of the governing bodies.

The rules of procedure of the World Health Assembly and Executive Board provide that Arabic, Chinese, English, French, Russian and Spanish shall be the official languages. Regional committees have their own distinctive pattern of languages. In 1948, the Executive Board decided that publications should appear in English and French. Spanish was added in 1954. Russian became a language of publication in 1960. Arabic and Chinese were included shortly before the Alma-Ata Conference in 1978.

Recognizing that equity of access to health information cannot be ensured by six official languages that are unknown to many millions of intended readers,[a] WHO has sought to encourage translations into national and regional languages outside the Organization, in collaboration with country and regional offices. By 1997, translations of WHO technical books and documents in over 60 target languages had been published with some 100 translated WHO books published annually by publishers and scientific institutions, ministries and professional associations in countries, at no additional cost to WHO.

While the principles of parity of official languages and equity of access to health information have been consistently affirmed, the means of communication of WHO's language services have kept pace with the development of information and communication technologies. Thus, WHO's wealth of expertise in technical terminology, built up over 50 years, is no longer archived on index cards and disseminated in printed bulletins, but is maintained and disseminated in the form of a computerized terminology database.

A just-completed study of the translation process as part of WHO's documentation chain has yielded recommendations that, when implemented, will result in efficiency savings. The integrated management of the multilingual flow is to be achieved through a computerized job tracking system, while an electronic document processing system will make possible for the first time an electronic repository for all WHO documents and publications in all languages.

At the same time, technology is of little help without the human values of scientific training, linguistic talent, and respect for the author and the reader, as appears daily in the work of WHO's language services. Since any information pertaining to human health must meet the highest standards, WHO translators must also render ideas from one language into another with understanding and accuracy of meaning, context and style. At WHO, translation talent serves health workers in countries throughout the world.

---

[a] For example, it is likely that many of the 476 million speakers of Hindi, 207 million speakers of Bengali, 187 million speakers of Portuguese, 126 million speakers each of Japanese and German, 170 million speakers of Malay and Indonesian – particularly primary or intermediate-level health workers – are unable to read or work in one of WHO's official languages.

countries. In addition, hundreds of documents for general or limited circulation are issued every year by WHO's technical programmes, giving detailed reports on the latest developments in health and health care. Accessibility through free distribution, primarily in developing countries, was improved in 1997 by the expansion of the WHO depository library network to 158 and the growth of the public reference point network to 915 participants. Even so the total number of publications distributed free was kept at zero-growth.

Three issues are foreseen as priorities in the next century. How will technology continue to influence dissemination policies and procedures? How will WHO be able to maintain services to developing countries? How can the Organization cope with the ever-increasing demand for publications and information in an environment of static staffing and shrinking financial resources? Demand from developing countries is increasing, and servicing that demand is labour-intensive. To satisfy it, innovative ways to achieve economies must be found.

WHO management

Since 1950, WHO's successive general programmes of work have emphasized the need for the Organization to be effective and efficient and able to yield results which can be demonstrable to governments. In 1965, the importance of introducing evaluation criteria into programme planning was stressed and in 1971 the use of modern scientific and technical methods in programme management was recommended. In 1994, the harsh political climate led to the rigorous stipulation of managerial requirements for WHO, to an extent never yet experienced in earlier general programmes of work. WHO keeps under constant review administrative procedures to ascertain consistency with the Organization's objectives, determining compliance with established rules and regulations, ascertaining the reliability of internally-developed financial and management data, reviewing the economical and efficient use of the Organization's resources and the extent to which assets are safeguarded from loss, as well as assessing measures taken to prevent fraud, waste and malfeasance.

The *financial situation* of the regular budget for 1997 was difficult owing to a serious shortfall in the collection of contributions, which considerably weakened WHO's financial position. Consequently, programme implementation was unstable and required very close monitoring. During the course of 1997, a modernized computer programme for the regional office administration and finance information system was introduced in three regional offices. Extrabudgetary contributions continued to increase. As in previous years governments were the main source of such voluntary donations, but significant sums were also received from multilateral development agencies, foundations and nongovernmental organizations.

Providing an adequate and efficient level of logistics support for the smooth and effective functioning of WHO's technical programmes is the primary concern of the *general administration*. This has required ongoing adjustment in response to the reduction in resources. In order to maintain acceptable levels of service, the scope of several outsourced contracts has been increased. Furthermore, with the recent deregulation in the global telecommunications market, important economies will be realized through the renegotiation of WHO's communications contract. With a view to taking full advantage of new and emerging technologies, video conferencing has been introduced as a further means of communication, and multimedia technology is under study for the production of documents.

WHO's *supply services* have adapted their role from a purely demand-led procurement entity to become a more active and efficient partner of WHO's technical programmes, thus responding better to country needs. For example, important quantities of vaccines and injection materials to meet the cyclical epidemics of meningitis are kept in stock ready for immediate shipment, and various medical kits have been developed and are available for use during emergencies. Increased bulk purchasing should lead to further economies.

Since 1950, WHO's successive general programmes of work have emphasized the need for the Organization to be effective and efficient and able to yield results which can be demonstrable to governments.

> **Box 7. Staff allegiance to WHO**
>
> All staff members of WHO subscribe to the following oath or declaration: "I solemnly swear (undertake, affirm, promise) to exercise in all loyalty, discretion, and conscience the functions entrusted to me as an international civil servant of the World Health Organization, to discharge those functions and regulate my conduct with the interests of the World Health Organization only in view, and not to seek or accept instructions in regard to the performance of my duties from any government or other authority external to the Organization."
>
> *WHO Staff Regulations, article 1.10*

All staff members

of WHO are

international civil

servants. Their

responsibilities are

not national but

exclusively

international.

All ***staff members*** of WHO are international civil servants. Their responsibilities are not national but exclusively international. By accepting appointment, they pledge themselves to discharge their functions and to regulate their conduct with the interests of the World Health Organization only in view. In addition to displaying the highest level of technical competence and integrity, they must also be sensitive to cultural differences in order to be effective in a multicultural environment *(Box 7)*.

The staff have traditionally had the right of association for the purpose of developing staff activities and making proposals and representations to the Organization concerning personnel policy and conditions of service, and since 1976 the Executive Board has invited a representative of the staff to present a statement reflecting staff views on such matters.

During 1997, work continued on implementing the reforms in the Organization's personnel policy initiated in 1996. In keeping with recent trends in both the public and private sectors, personnel management has been redirected to become less process- and more service-oriented, with greater emphasis on the role of human resources management as a support service and facilitator for the technical programmes in the achievement of their goals.

In 1997 there was a 50% increase in the number of short-term consultancy contracts, and a 28% increase in short-term professional contracts, compared with the same period in 1996. While this was partly due to the considerable reduction in the number of posts in 1995, it also reflects a general tendency to rely more on short-term professionals and consultants to provide highly specialized services for specific activities of limited duration. While the total number of staff in the professional category decreased in 1997, the proportion of women rose slightly (by 0.6%) to just over 27%.

Chapter 2
Measuring health

In view of major limitations imposed by the lack of suitable measurements that can capture the meaning of health as defined in the WHO Constitution ("Health is a state of complete physical, mental and social well-being and not merely the absence of disease or infirmity") this assessment of health trends uses conventional indicators such as life expectancy, mortality and morbidity. Efforts are under way, however, to develop indicators of positive health such as health expectancy and its variants, but problems of standardization of definitions and comparability of values derived inhibit their usage for trend assessment at this stage.

The Global Strategy for Health for All by the Year 2000 (HFA2000) set the following guiding targets:

- life expectancy at birth above 60 years;
- infant mortality rate below 50 per 1000 live births;
- under-5 mortality rate below 70 per 1000 live births.

In 1997, nearly 3.8 billion people (64% of the global population) lived in at least 106 countries that had reached those values. In 1975, there were at least 1.2 billion (30% of the global population) living in 69 countries. At least 102 countries (60% of the global population) reached all these values in 1995. The percentage of the global population living in countries which have reached these values since 1955, and which are expected to reach them by 2025, are shown in *Fig. 1*. There is, however, increasing evidence that as national average values are beginning to converge, internal disparities among population groups are widening.

Life expectancy at birth has increased globally by 17 years, from 48 in 1955 to 65 in 1995, and is projected to reach a level of 73 years by 2025, when it is expected that there will be no country with a life expectancy at

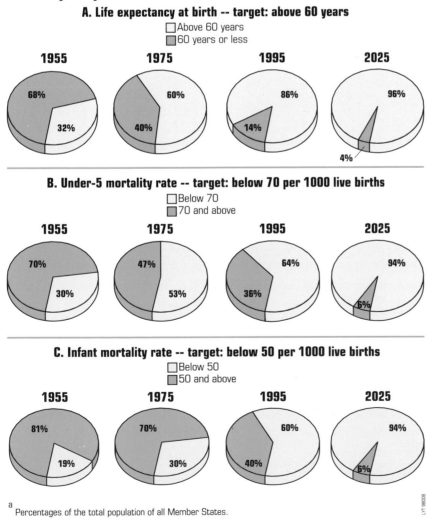

Fig. 1. Progress in achieving global targets for health for all by the year 2000 [a]

A. Life expectancy at birth -- target: above 60 years
- Above 60 years
- 60 years or less

| 1955 | 1975 | 1995 | 2025 |

B. Under-5 mortality rate -- target: below 70 per 1000 live births
- Below 70
- 70 and above

C. Infant mortality rate -- target: below 50 per 1000 live births
- Below 50
- 50 and above

[a] Percentages of the total population of all Member States.

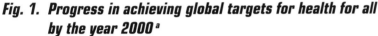

LYT 98008

Fig. 2. Survival curves, 1955-2025

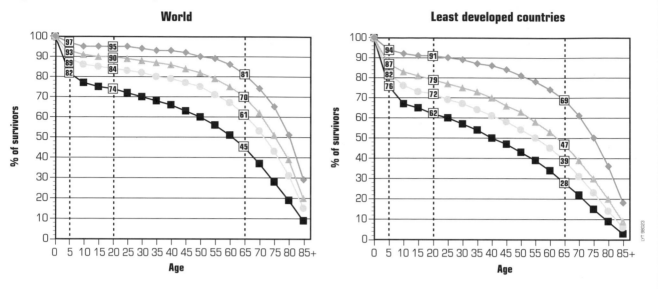

World

Least developed countries

Legend:
- 1955
- 1975
- 1995
- 2025

birth below 50. Even for the least developed countries (LDCs), the increase was about 15 years (from 37 in 1955 to 52 in 1995). The increase is expected to be 13 years between 1995 and 2025, when life expectancy for these countries will reach 65. In all, more than 5 billion people now live in 120 countries where life expectancy at birth is above 60. About 890 million people live in 26 countries where life expectancy at birth increased by 10 years or more between 1975 and 1995. About 1 billion people live in 56 countries where a similar increase is expected between 1995 and 2025. Such spectacular progress is not shared by all, however. More than 50 million people are still living in countries with a life expectancy at birth below 45. About 300 million people live in 16 countries which experienced a decrease in life expectancy at birth between 1975 and 1995. The range in national values for life expectancy at birth is expected to decrease from 43 years in 1955 to 31 in 2025.

Some of the population who are likely to be alive by the end of the 21st century are already born and alive today. Their *survival rates* have

been increasing significantly since 1955. As shown in *Fig. 2*, the overall trend is that global survival rates – the chances of surviving 5, 20, 65 or 80 years – have improved during the period 1955-1995. The same is true of the equivalent survival rates in the LDCs, but the percentages are considerably lower than the global percentages. For every 100 babies born in 1995, globally 70 are expected to live to at least 65 years, but in the LDCs only 47 are expected to do so. Globally for every 100 persons aged 20 in 1995, about 70 are forecast to survive at least 50 years (to age 70). Only 50 are likely to survive to this age in the LDCs.

Mortality trends

In its search for a simple and meaningful measure of health, WHO proposed in its second Report on the World Health Situation (in 1963), the ***proportional mortality ratio*** – the number of deaths at age 50 and above as a percentage of deaths at all ages – as a possible indicator. Applying this measure to study historical trends, globally the proportional mortality ratio increased from 34% in 1955 to 45% in 1975, and 58% in 1995; it is expected to be around 80% in 2025. Here again disparities are striking – in 1955, the LDCs had a value of 20% compared with 27% for other developing countries and 75% for the developed market economies; in 1995, the LDCs had a value of 26%, other developing countries 56% and the developed market economies 91%.

Overall ***mortality adjusted for age and sex*** composition of the population declined globally from 1860 deaths per 100 000 population in 1955 to 910 deaths per 100 000 in 1995 – a 50% reduction – and is projected to fall further to 610 deaths per 100 000 in 2025; for the LDCs, however, the standardized death rate fell by more than 40% from 1955 to 1995 and should be about 950 deaths per 100 000 in 2025. There was also a reduction globally of 67% from 1955 to 1995 in death rates among children under 5 and of 66% among those aged 5-19. Among those aged 20-64, the reduction was about 50%. In respect of those aged 20-64, death rates declined by 56% for females but only 49% for males. Here too, while age- and sex-specific mortality has been falling, the pace of decline is not uniform.

Fig. 3 shows the number of deaths at different ages and their distribution expressed as a percentage of total deaths. The general trend in the percentage of deaths occurring in the various age groups, both for the developed market economies and for the LDCs, is downward, except in the age group 65 and above. Overall, the number of deaths worldwide was the same in 1995 as in 1955 but with a significant decline of about 50% among children under 5, and of about 30% in the age group 5-19. There was an increase of about 5% in the working population aged 20-64. However, a relatively small reduction of 6% was experienced by the female population

in the reproductive age group 15-49. A comparison of the age distribution of total deaths worldwide and their trends reveal a changing pattern both for the developed market economies and the LDCs. Less than 2% of total deaths in the developed market economies in 1995 occurred among the population aged below 20, and about 1% is projected for 2025. In the LDCs however, the decreasing trend in the proportion of deaths among children, and a rapid increase in the proportion of deaths among older people, are noticeable. In the case of children, the proportion was nearly 50% in 1955, had decreased to 41%

Fig. 3.   *Age structure of deaths, 1955-2025*[a]

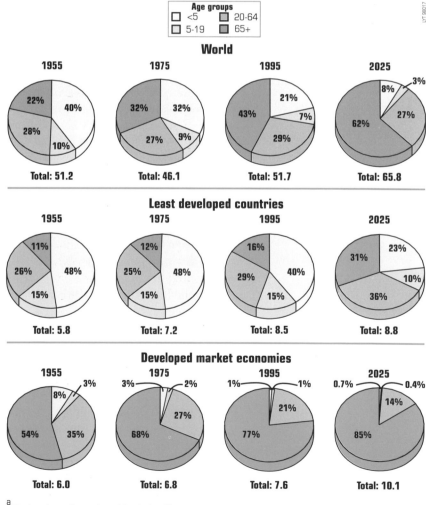

At least in respect

of mortality,

gender difference

seems to favour

the female population

at all ages.

by 1995, and is expected to be 23% in 2025 – about half of what it was in 1955. Unfortunately, the proportion of deaths among adults – the working-age population – has been increasing from about 25% in 1975 to 29% in 1995, and is expected to be almost 36% in 2025.

Worldwide, there have also been differential patterns in *age- and sex-specific death rates* since 1955. The death rate per 100 000 population declined between 1955 and 1995 from 5280 to 1720 among children under 5; from 620 to 210 among older children and adolescents aged 5-19; from 1040 to 500 among adults aged 20-64; and from 7550 to 6040 among older people aged 65 and above.

The relative death rate among females compared with males (the ratio of age-specific death rates for females to that of males) increased from 96% in 1955 to 99% in 1995 for children under 5, but decreased from 102% to 97% for older children and adolescents aged 5-19, from 79% to 68% for adults aged 20-64 and from 85% to 81% for older people aged 65 and above. Even for the age group 15-49, the ratio of death rates among women of childbearing age to men aged 15-49 declined from 84% to 73%. At least in respect of mortality, gender difference seems to favour the female population at all ages, although the relative decline in rates among children under 5 has not been so rapid as for other age groups.

The death rate among women of childbearing age decreased from 620 per 100 000 in 1955 to 230 per 100 000 in 1995, and is likely to reach 140 per 100 000 by 2025. Globally, about 585 000 women die each year of pregnancy-related causes, most of which are preventable. The *maternal mortality ratio*, representing the risk of pregnancy-related deaths associated with each pregnancy, was estimated at 430 maternal deaths per 100 000 live births in 1990 globally, but it varies widely among and within countries. For every 100 000 live births there were about 13 maternal deaths in the developed market economies, but more than 1050 in the LDCs. In other words, one woman dies of pregnancy-related causes for every 100 babies born alive. Less is known about the incidence and prevalence of pregnancy-related morbidity and disabilities. Although the immediate causes of maternal mortality and morbidity are inadequate care of the mother during pregnancy and delivery, other factors include women's subordinate status, poor health and inadequate nutrition.

Under-5 mortality rates decreased from 210 per 1000 live births in 1955 to 121 in 1975, and to 78 per 1000 in 1995 – a decrease of 42% between 1955 and 1975 and of 36% between 1975 and 1995, when the child survival initiative was launched. It is expected to decline further to 37 per 1000 live births by 2025.

In 1995, at least 105 countries (with 50% of global live births and 50% of children under 5 worldwide) have an estimated under-5 mortality below 70 per 1000 live births. In 1955, this was the case for 40 countries (18% of global live births) and in 1975 for 75 countries (37% of global live births). The pace of progress in under-5 mortality reduction during 1975-1995 was not so fast as during 1955-1975. It is expected to accelerate during 1995-2025 with 151 countries (89% of global live births) having an under-5 mortality rate below 70 per 1000 by the year 2025. In 1955 there were only three countries with an under-5 mortality rate below 20 per 1000 live births; by 2025 at least 84 countries are expected to have such a low rate. While all countries improved their under-5 mortality, at least 82 countries (with about two-thirds of live births worldwide) registered significant decreases in under-5 mortality – of at least 40 per 1000 live births – between 1975 and 1995.

In the developed market economies, the under-5 mortality rate declined by 52% during 1955-1975 and by 57% during 1975-1995. It is expected to reach a level of 7 per 1000 live births by 2025 from the present level of 8 per 1000 live births. For the developing world, under-5 mortality declined by 45% during 1955-1975 and by 37% during 1975-1995 and is expected to reach by 2025 a level of 40 from the present level of 87 per 1000 live births. However, even in countries that have made notable progress, child mortality is still unacceptably high. The LDCs in particular continue to struggle to reduce mortality rates; under-5 mortality decreased from about 280 to about 150 per 1000 live births between 1955 and 1995. Seven countries – six of which are in Africa – still have under-5 mortality rates greater than 200 per 1000 live births in 1995.

Infant mortality has continued to decline in recent decades. Globally, the ***infant mortality rate*** (IMR) fell from 148 per 1000 live births in 1955 to 90 per 1000 in 1975, and to 59 per 1000 in 1995 – a decrease of 39% from 1955 to 1975, and a further 34% decrease from 1975 to 1995. The IMR is projected to reach a value of 29 per 1000 live births in 2025.

Overall, the number of countries with an IMR below 50 per 1000 live births increased from 23 countries in 1955 to 70 in 1975, and to 102 (34% of global live births) in 1995. It is expected that by 2025 there will be at least 151 countries (43% of global live births) with an IMR below 50 per 1000. In 1955, the ratio of the highest value of IMR to the lowest value was 13 to 1; in 1975 it was 25 to 1; and in 1995, the ratio was 42 to 1.

For the developed market economies, the IMR declined by 58% be-

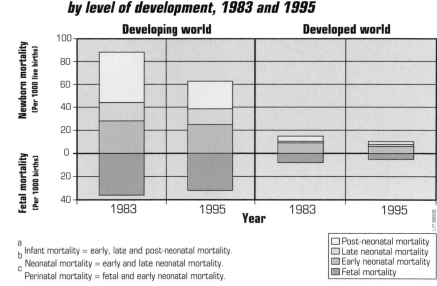

Fig. 4. Infant,[a] neonatal[b] and perinatal[c] mortality, by level of development, 1983 and 1995

a Infant mortality = early, late and post-neonatal mortality.
b Neonatal mortality = early and late neonatal mortality.
c Perinatal mortality = fetal and early neonatal mortality.

tween 1955 and 1975 and by a further 57% between 1975 and 1995. The present level is of 6 per 1000 live births and it is expected to reach by the year 2025 a level of 5. The developing world experienced a decline in the IMR of 41% during 1955-1975 and of 36% during 1975-1995, and it is expected to decline further to reach a level of 32 by the year 2025 from the present level of 62 per 1000 live births. In the LDCs, the IMR changed only from 186 to 104 per 1000 between 1955 and 1995 – about 75% of the decline experienced by developing countries other than LDCs. In 1995, there were 24 countries – 20 of them in Africa – where one in every 10 liveborns died within a year of birth. By 2025 the IMR is expected to decline to 50 per 1000 – still double the average of 25 per 1000 live births for developing countries other than LDCs.

While infant mortality declined markedly during the early 1980s and late 1990s, most of this improvement was among older infants. The death toll during the perinatal period (stillbirths and during the first week of life) has fallen only slightly from 64

Fig. 5. Global causes of death, 1997[a]

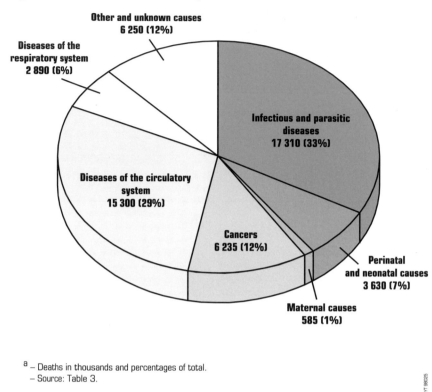

Other and unknown causes
6 250 (12%)

Diseases of the respiratory system
2 890 (6%)

Diseases of the circulatory system
15 300 (29%)

Infectious and parasitic diseases
17 310 (33%)

Cancers
6 235 (12%)

Perinatal and neonatal causes
3 630 (7%)

Maternal causes
585 (1%)

[a] – Deaths in thousands and percentages of total.
– Source: Table 3.

Fig. 6. Causes of death: distribution of deaths by main causes, by level of development, 1985, 1990 and 1997

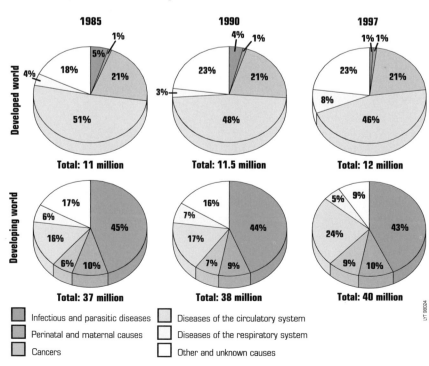

1985

Developed world

1%
5%
18%
4%
51%
21%

Total: 11 million

1990

4% 1%
23%
3%
48%
21%

Total: 11.5 million

1997

1% 1%
23%
8%
46%
21%

Total: 12 million

Developing world

17%
6%
16%
6%
10%
45%

Total: 37 million

16%
7%
17%
7%
9%
44%

Total: 38 million

5% 9%
24%
9%
10%
43%

Total: 40 million

■ Infectious and parasitic diseases
■ Perinatal and maternal causes
□ Cancers
□ Diseases of the circulatory system
□ Diseases of the respiratory system
□ Other and unknown causes

to 57 deaths per 1000 live births. It is also estimated that mortality during the neonatal period (the first 28 days of life) has declined from 40 to 36 deaths per 1000 live births during 1983-1995 *(Fig. 4)*. In all, there have been about 4 million stillbirths, 3.2 million deaths during the first week of life and 1.6 million deaths among newborns living more than a week but dying within 28 days after birth. There are about 9 million deaths of which 7.5 million are perinatal deaths and 4.8 million neonatal deaths annually worldwide.

Disease trends

Based on available information, WHO estimates that, of more than 50 million deaths worldwide in 1997, about one-third were due to infectious and parasitic diseases such as acute lower respiratory diseases, tuberculosis, diarrhoea, HIV/AIDS and malaria; 29% were due to circulatory diseases such as coronary heart disease and cerebrovascular diseases; and about 12% were due to cancers *(Fig. 5)*. While deaths due to circulatory diseases declined from 51% to 46% of total deaths in the developed world during the period 1985-1997, they increased from 16% to 24% of total deaths in the developing world *(Fig. 6)*. Cancer deaths increased from 6% to 9% of total deaths in the developing world but they formed a constant proportion of 21% of total deaths in the developed world. Infectious and parasitic diseases decreased from 5% to 1% of total deaths in the developed world and from 45% to 43% of total deaths in the developing world. This confirms earlier findings that noncommunicable diseases are emerging as a major killer in the developing countries as well. An approximate distribution of deaths by cause is given in *Table 3*. *Table 4* gives the leading causes.

Table 3. Global health situation: mortality, morbidity and disability, selected causes for which data are available, all ages, 1997 estimates[a]

Diseases/conditions (based on ICD-10)	Deaths	New (incidence)	All (prevalence)	Persons with severe activity limitation[b]
		Number (000)		
	Deaths	Cases		Persons with severe activity limitation[b]
ALL CAUSES	52 200			
Certain infectious and parasitic diseases (selected), of which:	**17 310**			
Acute lower respiratory infection (ALRI)	3 745	395 000[c]	...	...
Tuberculosis	2 910	7 250	16 300	8 420
Diarrhoea (including dysentery)	2 455	4 000 000[c]	...	...
HIV/AIDS	2 300	5 800	30 600	
Malaria	1 500-2 700	300 000-500 000	...	...
Measles	960	31 075	...	...
Hepatitis B	605	67 730	...	...
Whooping cough (pertussis)	410	45 050	...	...
Neonatal tetanus	275	415	...	...
Dengue fever/dengue haemorrhagic fever	140	3 100	...	...
Noma/cancrum oris	110	140	770	30
Trypanosomiasis, African (sleeping sickness)	100	150	400	200
Leishmaniases	80	2 000	12 000	...
Leishmaniasis, visceral (kala-azar)	80	500	2 500	
Leishmaniasis, cutaneous and mucocutaneous	...	1 500	9 500	
Amoebiasis (Entamoeba histolytica)	70	48 000	...	...
Hookworm diseases (ancylostomiasis and necatoriasis)	65	...	151 000[d]	...
Rabies (dog-mediated)	60	60[e]	...	...
Ascariasis (roundworm)	60	...	250 000[f]	...
Meningococcal meningitis (see also bacterial meningitis)	50	...	500	60
Onchocerciasis (river blindness)	45	...	17 655	770
Trypanosomiasis, American (Chagas disease)	45	300	18 000	...
Yellow fever	30	200	...	...
Schistosomiasis	20	...	200 000	120 000
Japanese encephalitis	10	45	...	...
Trematode infections (foodborne)	10	...	40 000	...
Trichuriasis (whipworm)	10	...	45 530[g]	...
Cholera (1996 notifications)	10	145	...	...
Leprosy	2	570	1 150	3 000
Poliomyelitis, acute	1.8	35	...	10 600
Plague (1995 notifications)	0.14	2.9	...	...
Giardiasis	...	500	...	...
Endemic treponematoses	...	460	2 600	260
Dracunculiasis (guinea-worm infection)	...	70	70	...
Hepatitis C	...	...	170 000	...
Trachoma	...	...	152 420	5 600
Lymphatic filariasis	...	...	119 100	119 100
Sexually transmitted diseases (selected), of which:				
Trichomoniasis	...	170 000	113 000	...
Chlamydial infections, including lymphogranuloma (venereum)	...	89 000	85 000	...
Gonococcal infection (gonorrhoea)	...	62 000	23 000	...
Anogenital warts	...	30 000	...	...
Anogenital herpes	...	20 000	...	...
Syphilis	...	12 000	28 000	...
Chancroid	...	2 000	2 000	...
Others (including emerging diseases e.g. influenza, Ebola, Lassa)	630	...	...	...
Malignant neoplasms (cancers) – all sites	**6 235**	**9 240**	**57 455**	
Trachea, bronchus and lung	1 050	1 190	4 465	...
Stomach	765	925	3 715	...
Colon and rectum	525	890	6 185	...

Diseases/conditions (based on ICD-10)	Deaths	Number (000)		Persons with severe activity limitation [b]
		Cases		
		New (incidence)	All (prevalence)	
Liver	505	510	1 415	...
Breast (female)	385	895	7 995	...
Oesophagus	355	370	1 135	...
Mouth and pharynx	260	420	2 810	...
Prostate	235	460	3 505	...
Lymphomas [h]	225	375	2 740	...
Leukaemia	215	260	1 565	...
Cervix	195	425	3 955	...
Bladder	140	300	2 330	...
Ovary	120	185	1 655	...
Kidney	100	170	1 255	...
Body of the uterus	65	160	1 425	...
Melanoma of skin	40	120	915	...
Other malignant neoplasms	1 055	1 585	10 390	...
Diseases of the blood and bloodforming organs and certain disorders involving the immune mechanism (selected), of which:	**240**			
Thalassaemias and sickle cell disorder	240	290	2 320	...
Haemophilia	...	15	420	...
Anaemia, of which:	...	...	1 987 300	...
Iron deficiency anaemia	...	...	1 788 600	...
Endocrine, nutritional and metabolic diseases (selected), of which:	**370**			
Malnutrition including protein-energy malnutrition (PEM)	370 [i]	...	170 000 [i]	...
Diabetes mellitus	...	10 540	142 540	...
Iodine deficiencies (disorders of thyroid gland), of which:	...	...	...	...
Goitre	...	...	844 700	...
Cretinoids	...	...	49 600	49 600
Cretinism	...	...	16 500	16 500
Mental and behavioural disorders (selected), of which:	**200**			
Dementia	200	2 610	29 000	15 950
Mood (affective) disorders	...	122 865	340 000	146 000
Schizophrenic disorders	...	4 500	45 000	27 000
Anxiety disorders	...	...	400 000	...
Mental retardation (all types)	...	...	60 000	36 000
Diseases of the nervous system (selected), of which:	**220**			
Bacterial meningitis (excluding neonatal meningitis)	135	...	1 200	160
Parkinson disease	60	305	3 765	2 635
Multiple sclerosis	25	105	2 505	750
Epilepsy	...	2 000	40 000	10 000
Diseases of the circulatory system (selected), of which:	**15 300**			
Ischaemic (coronary) heart disease	7 200	...	...	...
Cerebrovascular disease	4 600	...	9 000	...
Other heart diseases (e.g. peri-, endo-, and myocarditis and cardiomyopathy)	3 000	...	...	...
Rheumatic fever and rheumatic heart disease	500	...	12 000	...
Hypertensive disease	...	...	690 600	...
Diseases of the respiratory system (selected), of which:	**2 890**			
Chronic obstructive pulmonary disease (COPD)	2 890	...	600 000	...
Asthma	...	...	155 000	...

Diseases/conditions (based on ICD-10)	Number (000)			
	Deaths	Cases		Persons with severe activity limitation [b]
		New (incidence)	All (prevalence)	
Diseases of the musculoskeletal system and connective tissue (selected), of which:				
Neck and back disorders	...	...	1 039 200	...
Arthritis and arthrosis, of which:	...	...	...	...
Osteoarthritis	...	...	189 500	...
Rheumatoid arthritis	...	...	165 000	...
Pregnancy, childbirth and the puerperium (selected), of which:	**585**	**76 300**		
Haemorrhage	145	14 000	...	...
Indirect obstetric causes	115	13 200	...	...
Sepsis	90	11 800	...	...
Abortion	75	19 700	...	...
Hypertensive disorders in pregnancy	75	6 900	...	...
Obstructed labour	45	7 200	...	...
Other direct obstetric causes	40	3 500	...	...
Certain conditions originating in the perinatal period (selected), of which:	**3 630** [k]			
Prematurity	1 120	...	...	...
Birth asphyxia	920	...	...	...
Congenital anomalies	495	3 600	...	...
Neonatal sepsis and meningitis	440	...	...	...
Birth trauma	430	...	...	...
Other causes	225	...	...	...
External causes (selected), of which:	**1 165**			
Suicide	835	...	...	...
Occupational injuries due to accidents at work	330	250 000	...	25 000
Occupational diseases	...	217 000	...	20 000
Other and unknown causes	**4 055**			
Visual disability (blindness and low vision), of which:				**179 200**
Blindness (total):	...	...	44 800	44 800
Onchocerciasis-related	...	45	290	290
Cataract-related	...	...	19 340	19 340
Glaucoma-related	...	...	6 400	6 400
Trachoma-related	...	...	5 600	5 600
Vitamin A deficiency-xerophthalmia (children under 5)	...	...	2 740	2 740
Other	...	...	10 430	10 430
Hearing loss (41 or more decibels)			**123 000**	**123 000**

[a] No adjustments have been made for comorbidity. Caution should be exercised when using these data for comparative purposes as estimation procedures may have been refined from one *World Health Report* to the next.

[b] Permanent and long-term.

[c] Incidence figure refers to episodes.

[d] Number of infected persons is 1.25 billion.

[e] In addition, approximately 50 million doses of vaccine are used for post-exposure prophylaxis.

[f] Number of infected persons is 1.38 billion.

[g] Number of infected persons is 1 billion.

[h] Includes Non-Hodgkin lymphoma, multiple myeloma and Hodgkin disease.

[i] This excludes 4.8 million malnutrition-associated deaths among children under 5.

[j] Figure refers to children under 5.

[k] This excludes neo- and perinatal deaths due to neonatal pneumonia, neonatal tetanus and neonatal diarrhoea.

... Data not available or not applicable.

Table 4. Global health situation: leading causes of mortality, morbidity and disability, selected causes for which data are available, all ages, 1997 estimates[a]

Diseases/conditions (based on ICD-10)	Deaths Rank	Deaths Number (000)	Cases New (incidence) (000)	Cases Rank (prevalence)	Cases All (prevalence) (000)	Persons with severe activity limitation Rank	Persons with severe activity limitation Number (000)
Ischaemic (coronary) heart disease	1	7 200	...		...		...
Cerebrovascular disease	2	4 600	...		9 000		...
Acute lower respiratory infection	3	3 745	395 000		...		...
Tuberculosis	4	2 910	7 250		16 300		8 420
COPD	5	2 890	...	5	600 000		...
Diarrhoea (including dysentery)	6	2 455	4 000 000	1	...		...
HIV/AIDS	7	2 300	5 800		30 600		...
Malaria	8	1 500–2 700	300 000–500 000	2	...		...
Prematurity	9	1 120	...		4 465		...
Cancer of trachea, bronchus and lung	10	1 050	1 190		...		...
Measles	11	960	31 075		...		...
Birth asphyxia	12	920	...		...		...
Occupational injuries		330	250 000	4	...	9	25 000
Occupational diseases		...	217 000	5	...	10	20 000
Trichomoniasis		...	170 000	6	...		...
Mood (affective) disorders		...	122 865	7	340 000	1	146 000
Chlamydial infections		...	89 000	8	...		...
Hepatitis B		605	67 730	9	85 000		...
Gonococcal infection (gonorrhoea)		...	62 000	10	...		...
Amoebiasis (Entamoeba histolytica)		70	48 000	11	23 000		...
Whooping cough (pertussis)		410	45 050	12	...		...
Iron deficiency anaemia		...	...	1	1 788 600		...
Neck and back disorders		...	...	2	1 039 200		...
Goitre		...	...	3	844 700		...
Hypertensive disease		...	...	4	690 600		...
Anxiety disorders		...	...	6	400 000		...
Arthritis and arthrosis		...	...	7	354 500		...
Ascariasis (roundworm)		60	...	9	250 000		...
Schistosomiasis		20	...	10	200 000	3	120 000
Hepatitis C		...	...	11	170 000		...
Malnutrition including PEM		370	...	12	170 000		...
Hearing loss (41 or more decibels)		...	...		123 000	2	123 000
Lymphatic filariasis		...	...		119 100	4	119 100
Cretinoids		...	...		49 600	5	49 600
Mental retardation (all types)		...	4 500		60 000	7	36 000
Schizophrenic disorders		...	...		45 000	8	27 000
Cataract-related blindness		...	...		19 340	11	19 340
Cretinism		...	...		16 500	12	16 500

Leading selected causes of mortality

	Rank	Deaths Number (000)
Ischaemic (coronary) heart disease	1	7 200
Cerebrovascular disease	2	4 600
Acute lower respiratory infection	3	3 745
Tuberculosis	4	2 910
COPD	5	2 890
Diarrhoea (including dysentery)	6	2 455
HIV/AIDS	7	2 300
Malaria	8	1 500–2 700
Prematurity	9	1 120
Cancer of trachea, bronchus and lung	10	1 050
Measles	11	960
Birth asphyxia	12	920

Leading selected causes of morbidity

	Rank New (incidence)	Cases New (incidence) (000)	Rank All (prevalence)	Cases All (prevalence) (000)
Diarrhoea (including dysentery)	1	4 000 000		
Malaria	2	300 000–500 000		
Acute lower respiratory infection	3	395 000		
Occupational injuries	4	250 000		
Occupational diseases	5	217 000		
Trichomoniasis	6	170 000		
Mood (affective) disorders	7	122 865	8	340 000
Chlamydial infections	8	89 000		
Hepatitis B	9	67 730		
Gonococcal infection	10	62 000		
Amoebiasis	11	48 000		
Whooping cough (pertussis)	12	45 050		
Iron deficiency anaemia			1	1 788 600
Neck and back disorders			2	1 039 200
Goitre			3	844 700
Hypertensive disease			4	690 600
COPD			5	600 000
Anxiety disorders			6	400 000
Arthritis and arthrosis			7	354 500
Ascariasis (roundworm)			9	250 000
Schistosomiasis			10	200 000
Hepatitis C			11	170 000
Malnutrition including PEM			12	170 000

Persons with severe activity limitation (permanent and long-term)

Leading selected causes	Rank	Number (000)
Mood (affective) disorders	1	146 000
Hearing loss (41 or more decibels)	2	123 000
Schistosomiasis	3	120 000
Lymphatic filariasis	4	119 100
Cretinoids	5	49 600
Mental retardation (all types)	6	36 000
Schizophrenic disorders	7	27 000
Occupational injuries	8	25 000
Occupational diseases	9	20 000
Cataract-related blindness	10	19 340
Cretinism	11	16 500

[a] Source: Table 3.

WHO has been assessing the health situation and publishing the findings through the Report on the World Health Situation at regular intervals since 1954. The first of these reports recognized, among others, malaria, tuberculosis, poliomyelitis and yaws, as well as respiratory cancer and circulatory diseases, as being of concern. Subsequent reports gradually expanded this list to a wide spectrum of diseases and disorders requiring attention. *Table* 5 shows the diseases/disorders/conditions perceived as problems during the first 30 years of WHO. Some have been eliminated and a few others are under control and have been targeted for eradication or elimination by the end of this century. An overview of progress in controlling them is provided below.

Infectious disease control

During the past few decades, substantial progress has been made in controlling some major infectious diseases. But while some have disappeared or are almost eliminated as public health problems, others remain daunting threats.

WHO's Expanded Programme on Immunization (EPI) was launched in 1974. As a result, by 1995 over 80% of the world's children had been immunized against diphtheria, tetanus, whooping cough, poliomyelitis, measles and tuberculosis, compared to less than 5% in 1974.

Global eradication of **smallpox** was declared in 1980 at the end of an eradication campaign which began in 1967, with the systematic vaccination of entire populations in over 30 endemic countries. The tropical disease **yaws**, which mainly affects the skin and bones, has virtually disappeared. Between 1950, when the first yaws campaign was launched in Haiti, and 1965, 46 million patients in 49 coun-

tries were successfully treated with penicillin, and the disease is no longer a significant problem in most of the world.

Although **cholera** was mainly confined to Asia in the first half of the 20th century through improvements in sanitation elsewhere, the latest in a series of pandemics recorded since the early 19th century has been affecting much of the world since the 1960s, with epidemics ranging from South-East Asia to the Eastern Mediterranean, West Africa and parts of Latin America. Epidemics have become more widespread and more frequent in Africa since the 1970s. A new strain, *Vibrio cholerae* O139, was identified in India in 1992. Cholera is endemic in some 80 countries and is of concern to all regions of the world.

The global threat of **plague** has declined in the last four decades, largely due to the impact of antibiotics and insecticides and other control measures, but cyclical epidemics still occur and some countries in Africa, the Americas and Asia report cases almost every year. There is evidence of plague in rodents spreading in parts of the United States.

Improvements in standards of sanitation and hygiene in recent decades have also made outbreaks of **relapsing fever** transmitted by lice rare today. They are most likely to occur in unhygienic and crowded conditions arising from wars or natural disasters.

The largest **yellow fever** epidemic ever recorded was in Ethiopia in 1960-1962, causing about 30 000 deaths. There are now about 30 000 deaths globally every year among about 200 000 annual cases, a decline largely due to immunization. However, since the late 1980s there has been a dramatic resurgence of yellow fever in Africa and the Americas. It is endemic in 34 countries of Africa, including 14 of the world's poorest, and in most of these, immunization

Substantial progress has been made in controlling some major infectious diseases.

Table 5. Importance of selected diseases and conditions over time according to the Report on the World Health Situation

Disease	Report 1 1954-56	Report 2 1957-60	Report 3 1961-64	Report 4 1965-68	Report 5 1969-72	Report 6 1973-77	Report 7 1978-84	Report 8 1985-89
Infectious diseases								
Malaria	●					●	●	●
Tuberculosis	●	●	●	●	●	●	●	●
Cholera	●	●	●	●	●		●	
Poliomyelitis	●	●	●	●			●	●
Yaws	●	●	●					
Hepatitis, infectious	●		●					●
Relapsing fever	●				●			
Plague	●				●			
Yellow fever	●							●
Trachoma	●	●		●				
Onchocerciasis	●			●			●	
Leprosy	●	●	●	●	●	●		●
Smallpox	●	●	●	●	●	●		
Schistosomiasis	●		●	●	●		●	●
Sexually transmitted diseases		●		●	●	●	●	●
Influenza		●		●				
Filariasis			●	●		●		
Dysentery			●	●				
Trypanosomiasis, African			●			●		●
Trypanosomiasis, American			●	●	●			●
Ascariasis				●				
Ancylostomiasis				●				
Trichuriasis				●				
Diarrhoea				●		●	●	●
Meningitis				●	●		●	
Acute respiratory disease					●			●
Diphtheria						●		
Viral haemorrhagic fever						●		
Endemic treponematoses						●		●
Measles							●	●
Tetanus							●	●
Dracunculiasis							●	●
AIDS							●	●
Pneumonia								●
Dengue haemorrhagic fever								●
Pertussis								●
Rabies								●
Japanese encephalitis								●
Leishmaniasis								●
Chronic conditions								
Cancer	●	●	●	●	●	●	●	●
Circulatory diseases	●	●	●	●	●	●	●	●
Endocrine, nutritional and metabolic diseases	●			●	●	●	●	●
Accidents		●	●			●		
Mental disorders					●	●	●	●
Others								
Handicap						●		
Tobacco-related disorders								●
Alcohol-related disorders								●
Occupational injuries								●
Agrochemical-related hazards								●

programmes are weak. Outbreaks occurred in several countries in West Africa in 1994-1995, and in 1995 Peru experienced the largest yellow fever outbreak reported from any country in the Americas since 1950. The present situation is reflected in *Map 1*.

Recent environmental changes closely linked to water resources development, and increases in population densities, have led to the spread of **schistosomiasis** to previously low-endemic or non-endemic areas, and the disease remains endemic in 74 developing countries. Most of the transmission occurs in Africa, where there is an urgent need for a renewed commitment to control on the part of endemic countries and donors.

The **onchocerciasis** control programme which began in West Africa in 1974 has since protected an estimated 36 million people from the disease. The African Programme for Onchocerciasis Control began in January 1996 and covers 19 additional countries. The Onchocerciasis Elimination Programme in the Americas was stated in 1991 in six Latin American countries and aims to eliminate severe pathological manifestations of the disease and to reduce morbidity in the Americas through the distribution of ivermectin. It is expected that the global elimination of onchocerciasis as a public health problem will be achieved before 2008.

Prevalence of the parasitic **Chagas disease** (which exists only in the Americas from Mexico to Argentina) is currently estimated at 16-18 million in 21 endemic countries. The disease is being targeted for elimination of transmission by the year 2010 in the southern cone countries of Latin America.

There has been an important recrudescence of **sleeping sickness** (African trypanosomiasis), particularly in central Africa, where reported

Map 1. Yellow fever, 1997

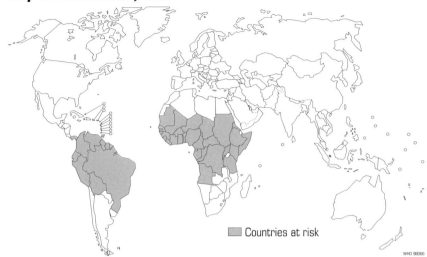

Countries at risk

WHO 98066

cases have more than doubled over the past few years. In 1997, the World Health Assembly acknowledged the danger of epidemics in a number of African countries. Ideally by the year 2000, at least 70% of all people at risk should be reached through medical surveillance, and prevalence of the disease should be reduced to a degree at which it is no longer a public health problem.

The first effective injectable vaccines against **poliomyelitis** were

Map 2. Reported measles incidence rate, 1996

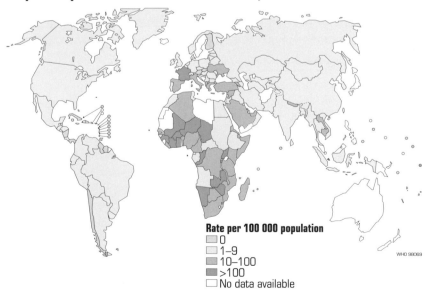

Rate per 100 000 population
0
1–9
10–100
>100
No data available

WHO 98069

Box 8.   Lymphatic filariasis

A WHO plan to treat more than 1 billion people – a fifth of the world population – with a dose of medicine could lead to the elimination within about 20 years of lymphatic filariasis, one of the most painful and unpleasant of all tropical diseases – and simultaneously reduce the burden of other parasitic infections.

Lymphatic filariasis, a bloodborne disease transmitted by mosquitos, causes elephantiasis and male genital damage. It is a major social and economic scourge in the tropics and subtropics of Africa, Asia, the Western Pacific and parts of the Americas, affecting over 120 million people in 73 countries. More than 1.1 billion people live in areas where there is a risk of infection.

In 1997, the World Health Assembly adopted a resolution calling for the global elimination of the disease as a public health problem, in view of rapid advances during the previous decade in diagnosis, clinical understanding, treatment and control, the successes of recent control programmes, and increasing political commitment.

The mainstay of WHO's elimination strategy is the use of simple, safe, inexpensive, conveniently delivered drugs that kill the parasite. An additional benefit is the simultaneous effectiveness of these medications against other well-entrenched diseases such as intestinal worms, lice and scabies.

The available drugs are albendazole, diethylcarbamazine (DEC) and ivermectin. Once-yearly administration of single doses of these drugs, given in 2-drug combinations, will reduce parasite blood counts by 99% for a year or more. Dramatic reductions in transmission have been documented in highly endemic areas even in the first year.

The success of the strategy has been made possible by the commitment of pharmaceutical companies.

SmithKline Beecham plc, which has already supported the development of drugs and programmes for controlling other tropical diseases, has agreed to donate to WHO for its programme on control of tropical diseases sufficient quantities of albendazole for as long as is necessary in order to eliminate the disease. The firm has also agreed to provide funds and human resources to help support the global elimination programme.

At the same time, Merck & Co., Inc., through Merck Research Laboratories, has recognized that ivermectin is especially needed as part of the combination for treating lymphatic filariasis in Africa because of its overlap with onchocerciasis and loiasis, diseases for which community-wide exposure to the alternative drug DEC may be unsafe. Merck is making ivermectin available for research programmes, some of which may be countrywide in scope, that will be carried out with WHO.

Further support has come from the Arab Fund for Economic and Social Development, which will provide funding for filariasis elimination in those of its member countries affected by the disease. The World Bank has strongly endorsed this new global elimination programme.

With encouragement and support from WHO, 13 countries have now revised their national filariasis control strategies and plans of action to take advantage of the new tools and approaches available. Seven of these countries have already initiated national programmes. In India, the largest, 40 million people were being targeted to receive single-dose treatment on National Filariasis Day early in 1998. WHO will support all endemic countries with the necessary technical advice and assistance for developing implementation plans for treatment, monitoring, evaluation and operational research.

introduced in 1955; since then the disease has gradually been eliminated in much of the world. Reported cases worldwide have declined by over 90% since the campaign for global eradication by the year 2000 was launched in 1988. Polioviruses have disappeared from the Americas, and the Western Pacific Region is rapidly becoming polio-free. The Indian subcontinent remains heavily affected and the disease is still endemic in western and central Africa and some countries in the Eastern Mediterranean Region.

In 1966, WHO estimated that there were 10.5 million **leprosy** patients in the world with 1.8 million registered for treatment. WHO developed and promoted multidrug therapy, which it began to recommend in 1981. Since then, over 8.4 million patients have been cured and the global leprosy burden reduced from 5.4 million registered cases in 1985 to 0.9 million in 1997. Most cases today are in South-East Asia, with relatively small numbers in Africa, the Americas, the Western Pacific and Eastern Mediterranean. WHO's goal is to eliminate leprosy as a public health problem by the year 2000, i.e. to reduce global prevalence to less than 1 per 10 000 population.

Progress towards the elimination of *dracunculiasis* (guinea-worm disease) in the past decade has been spectacular, with the number of cases falling worldwide from an estimated 3.2 million in 1986 to 70 000 in 1997. The disease affects those living in the most rural parts of 18 countries located in Africa south of the Sahara and Yemen. Twenty-one formerly endemic countries have been certified as free of dracunculiasis transmission.

The outlook for *filariasis* control and elimination is such that an international task force for disease eradication identified filariasis as one of only six currently eradicable or potentially eradicable diseases, and in 1997 the World Health Assembly called for the elimination of lymphatic filariasis as a public health problem globally *(Box 8)*. The disease is of concern in Africa, the Eastern Mediterranean, and South-East Asia.

For the blinding disease *trachoma* the target is elimination by 2020 through long-lasting antibiotics. About 6 million people currently alive in Africa and Asia have been irreversibly blinded by it; another 152 million suffer from the disease and need treatment.

Measles remains the leading killer among vaccine-preventable diseases of children, and is still a concern in all six WHO regions. Despite excellent progress in recent years, particularly in the Americas, where there is hope of eliminating it by the year 2000, measles still kills about 1 mil-

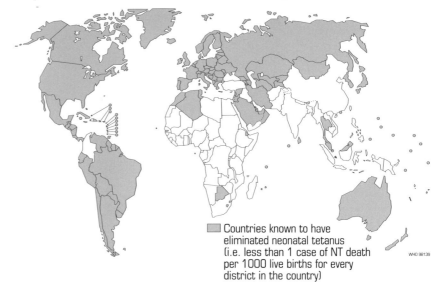

Map 3. Neonatal tetanus elimination status, 1997

Countries known to have eliminated neonatal tetanus (i.e. less than 1 case of NT death per 1000 live births for every district in the country)

WHO 98139

lion children a year. In some countries, mostly in Africa, measles vaccine coverage is below 50%, which means that the disease will continue to be epidemic there *(Map 2)*.

Tetanus of the newborn is the third killer of children after measles and pertusis among the six EPI vaccine-preventable diseases and is a concern in all WHO regions except Europe. Between 800 000 and 1 million newborns a year died from tetanus in the early 1980s. An estimated 730 000 such deaths are now prevented every year, particularly by targeting elimination efforts to high-risk areas. In 1997, there were an estimated 275 000 deaths. WHO estimates that in 1995, about 90% of neonatal tetanus cases occurred in only 25 countries. The current status of elimination of neonatal tetanus is shown in *Map 3*.

Once also a target for eradication, *malaria* remains a major threat. In 1954 there were 2.5 million deaths annually and 250 million cases worldwide; now there are 1.5-2.7 million deaths and 300-500 million cases, 90% of them in tropical Africa, and the disease is endemic in 100 coun-

Map 4. Hepatitis B prevalence, 1997 estimates

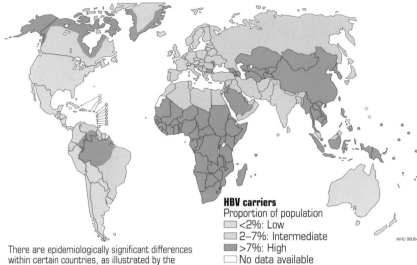

HBV carriers
Proportion of population
- ☐ <2%: Low
- ☐ 2–7%: Intermediate
- ■ >7%: High
- ☐ No data available

WHO 98064

There are epidemiologically significant differences within certain countries, as illustrated by the Amazon Basin and the Arctic Rim.

tries. The aim of the current Global Malaria Strategy is to reduce mortality by at least 20% compared to 1995 in at least 75% of affected countries by the year 2000. In 1997, WHO accelerated malaria control activities in 24 endemic countries in Africa. By the end of 1997, the objective of 90% of the affected countries having a national control plan in place was achieved.

Complacency towards *tuberculosis* in the last three decades led control programmes to be run down in many countries. The result has been a powerful resurgence of the disease, now estimated to kill around 3 million people a year, with 7.3 million new cases annually. WHO declared tuberculosis a global emergency in 1993. About 3 million cases a year occur in South-East Asia, and nearly 2 million in sub-Saharan Africa, with 340 000 in Europe. One-third of the incidence in the last five years can be attributed to HIV, which weakens the immune system and makes a person infected with the tubercle bacillus 30 times more likely to become ill with tuberculosis. Strains of the bacillus resistant to one or more drugs may have

infected up to 50 million people. WHO is promoting directly-observed treatment, short-course (DOTS) as the treatment strategy for detection and cure.

Epidemic *meningitis* is a recurrent problem in the "meningitis belt" of Africa stretching from Senegal to Ethiopia and including all or part of at least 15 countries with an estimated population of 300 million people.

Increasing urbanization during the last decades has led to a corresponding increase in the prevalence of *dengue and dengue haemorrhagic fever*. These conditions are reported from over 100 countries in all WHO regions except Europe. Dengue fever, and in particular life-threatening dengue haemorrhagic fever (DHF), often occurs in massive epidemics. In 1996, severe dengue epidemics were reported from 27 countries in the Americas and in South-East Asia, and dengue and DHF outbreaks were reported from Brazil, Cuba, India and Sri Lanka. As yet there is no vaccine or drug available for the control of dengue and DHF, and therefore WHO's strategy continues to be based on prevention of transmission by controlling the vector.

There is also a disturbing increase in the number of *leishmaniasis* infections. The disease is related to economic development and environmental changes which increase exposure to the sandfly vector. More recently the combination of visceral leishmaniasis and AIDS has risen in parts of the Americas, Eastern Mediterranean and South-East Asia with the spread of the AIDS pandemic. In anticipation of a worsening situation WHO has set up a surveillance system, with 10 countries already able to detect any major epidemiological change.

The *hepatitis B* virus infection (HBV) is a global problem, with 66% of the world's population living in areas where there are high levels of infection (*Map 4*). More than 2 billion people worldwide have evidence of past or current HBV infection and 350 million are chronic carriers of the virus, which is harboured in the liver. The virus causes 60-80% of all primary liver cancer, which is one of the three top causes of cancer deaths in East and South-East Asia, the Pacific Basin and sub-Saharan Africa.

Vaccination is the most effective way of preventing HBV transmission. The hepatitis B vaccine is the first and currently the only vaccine against a major human cancer. Following WHO recommendations, 90 countries have now integrated it into their national immunization programmes. By this means, the target is to reduce new HBV carriers in children by 80% by the year 2001. For many countries, however, the major impediment to the universal introduction of the vaccine has been its cost. Even at $ 0.50 per dose, a three-dose series of vaccinations is more expensive than the combined cost of the other six EPI vaccines. WHO and UNICEF have developed a support strategy to help the poorest and neediest countries to procure the vaccine. Implementation of this strategy, and the achievement of high HBV coverage, could effectively eliminate transmission of the disease by the year 2025.

First identified in 1989, the **hepatitis C** virus (HCV) has now become a major public health problem (*Map 5*). The incidence of HCV infection worldwide is not well known, but from a review of published prevalence studies on HCV, WHO estimates that 3% of the world population is infected with HCV and around 170 million individuals are chronic carriers at risk of developing liver cirrhosis and liver cancer. In many countries particular population subgroups such as volunteer blood donors have a very high prevalence of HCV infec-

Map 5. Hepatitis C, 1998 estimates

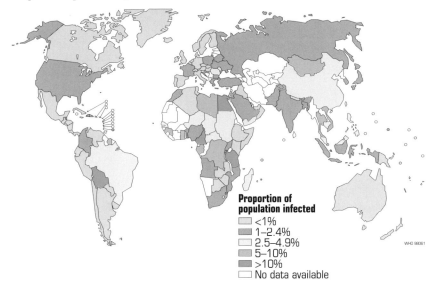

Proportion of population infected
- ☐ <1%
- ■ 1–2.4%
- ☐ 2.5–4.9%
- ▨ 5–10%
- ■ >10%
- ☐ No data available

WHO 98061

tion, especially in the developing world. In the United States an estimated 4 million people have contracted the disease, four times more than HIV infection; approximately 30 000 new acute infections and 8000-10 000 deaths occur each year; it has also become the leading reason for liver transplantation. In France, 500 000-650 000 persons are infected, 3% of whom contracted the disease through blood transfusion. Australia also reports a prevalence of HCV infection far greater than that of HIV infection. In Canada, at least half of hepatitis C cases are associated with the use of injectable drugs but the actual proportion may be much greater; it is also the leading reason for liver transplantation.

Although HCV infection is not so easily transmitted as hepatitis B or HIV infections, its tendency to induce chronic liver disease in 50-80% of cases, leading to serious long-term clinical sequelae, places it among the pathogens of major public health concern. HCV is also characterized by genetic diversity enabling it to escape the host's immune system. In addition, the natural course of the disease is

Cancer of the breast,

colon and prostate

have emerged in

several countries

in which they were

hardly known

20-30 years ago.

uncertain, vaccine development is difficult, response to therapy is poor, and societal and medical costs can be high.

WHO called a meeting of experts in April 1998 to achieve a clearer understanding of the natural history of the disease and to develop appropriate approaches to diagnosis and monitoring, therapeutic intervention and prevention of transmission.

Noncommunicable disease control

The increased life expectancy recorded in recent decades, together with changes in lifestyle stemming from socioeconomic development, paradoxically have favoured noncommunicable diseases, especially circulatory disorders, cancer and some forms of mental illness. **Pellagra**, a dietary disorder among populations consuming maize or sorghum and little else, was a public health problem in the 1960s and 1970s in parts of Africa and Asia. Major outbreaks of this deficiency disease rarely occur today because of fortification of cereal products and nutrition education, but there have been several outbreaks in the past 20 years in refugee and displaced populations dependent on food aid where the cereal in rations has been unfortified maize.

Coronary heart disease and stroke account for at least 12 million deaths a year, cancer kills 6 million, and 2.8 million deaths are due to chronic obstructive pulmonary disease (COPD). These and other noncommunicable diseases now cause 39% of all deaths in developing countries, where they affect younger people than in industrialized countries – an alarming trend. The epidemiological transition, with its double burden of infectious and chronic diseases, is common to many

developing countries, where 64% of deaths due to circulatory diseases, 60% of cancer deaths and 66% of COPD deaths now occur.

In contrast, some industrialized countries – Australia, Canada, Finland, New Zealand and the United Sates in particular – have shown dramatic reductions in mortality from *circulatory diseases* in the last two or three decades. These have been achieved by reducing risk factors such as hypertension and tobacco use and by introducing beneficial changes in diet, together with improvements in treatment. A project in North Karelia, Finland, shows that the effects are sustainable over a 20-year period. Here, a 65% reduction in coronary heart disease mortality in middle-aged adults was achieved by ensuring decreases in three main risk factors: cholesterol, hypertension and smoking. Noncommunicable disease prevention in Finland contributed most to the six-year increase in life expectancy over the last 25 years, during which time the number of people on disability pensions because of cardiovascular disease fell by about 25%. In Poland, changes in the pricing of meat and dairy products have clearly affected coronary heart disease death rates. In the United Kingdom, deaths from heart disease are reported to have fallen to second place as the most common cause, being replaced by cancer.

In many parts of the world, dramatic shifts in *cancer* occurrence are being observed. In several newly industrialized regions cancer has become, unexpectedly quickly, one of the leading causes of death. Cancer of the breast, colon and prostate have emerged in several countries in which they were hardly known 20-30 years ago. In western European countries and North America, more than 30% of tumours are associated with dietary habits.

Of more than 9 million cancer cases newly diagnosed in 1997 worldwide, 52% occurred in the developing countries. For all countries, lung cancer was the most common in men, followed in developed regions by prostate cancer, colorectal cancer and stomach cancer. In developing regions, stomach cancer is second, followed by liver cancer and cancer of the oesophagus. In women, breast cancer is the most common in affluent populations, followed by colorectal cancer, lung cancer and stomach cancer. In developing areas, breast cancer is also the most common, but cervical cancer is almost as common; stomach cancer and colorectal cancer are third and fourth respectively. The most remarkable changes in the rankings compared to 10 years ago are the steep upward trend of prostate cancer (partly due to the introduction of early detection programmes); the increase in breast cancer, especially in developing countries; and the increase in lung cancer worldwide. Much of the upward trend in the last few decades in rich countries has been due to tobacco smoking, a trend likely to be mirrored in coming years in developing countries, where smoking will also increase COPD deaths.

Population ageing, unhealthy diets, obesity and a sedentary lifestyle are the main factors that explain the alarming upward trend in recent years in *diabetes mellitus*. There are about 143 million sufferers and this number is projected to rise to almost 300 million by the year 2025.

Along with increased longevity and socioeconomic development has come an increase in some forms of *mental disorder* in the last two or three decades. Depression, schizophrenia and dementia rates have been rising, partly because more people are living to an age where the risk of developing these disorders is greater.

Depression is also now being seen at younger ages and more frequently in countries as different as Lebanon, and the United States. On the basis of population ageing, it is projected that the number of persons with schizophrenia will increase by 45% between 1985 and the year 2000. Social and environmental factors play a role too, particularly in explaining increases in alcohol and drug abuse, suicide, violence and other behavioural problems.

Emerging and re-emerging diseases

The last 20 years have seen the emergence of at least 20 new disease-causing organisms around the world. Of these the human immunodeficiency virus (HIV) which causes *AIDS* has had by far the most profound global impact. An unknown disease before 1981, AIDS has caused an estimated 11.7 million deaths since the epidemic began.

Some of the other new diseases include *Legionnaires' disease*, a form of potentially fatal pneumonia caused by bacteria which contaminate water and air-conditioning systems, and the deadly *Ebola haemorrhagic fever*, which has been confined to countries in tropical Africa. Both were first identified in 1976, in the United States and the Democratic Republic of the Congo respectively, and sporadic outbreaks of both diseases have since occurred elsewhere. WHO has played a leading role in the investigation and control of Ebola outbreaks. Recent years have seen the reappearance of *Rift Valley fever*, caused by a virus first isolated in 1931 in the Rift Valley of Kenya but which has also appeared in Egypt. At the end of 1997, WHO investigated a large outbreak of the disease in north-eastern Kenya and neighbouring Somalia.

There have also been sporadic outbreaks of *monkeypox*, a disease

AIDS has caused

an estimated

11.7 million deaths

since the epidemic

began.

Box 9. Creutzfeldt-Jakob disease (CJD)

Since the announcement in March 1996 of the occurrence of a new clinico-pathological variant of Creutzfeldt-Jakob disease (nvCJD) in the United Kingdom, evidence has demonstrated that nvCJD is almost certainly caused by the bovine spongiform encephalopathy (BSE) agent.

Because products potentially contaminated by BSE were widely exported, the risk of nvCJD is worldwide. Furthermore, the results of new research raise the possibility of secondary iatrogenic spread of the disease, emphasizing the need for accurate case detection.

In May 1996 the WHO Consultation on clinical and neuropathological characteristics of nv CJD and other human and animal transmissible spongiform encephalopathies recommended that global CJD surveillance should be established. Experience gained from implementing this recommendation has led to the redefinition of a "suspected case" and a "case" to improve ascertainment, particularly in developing countries with low autopsy rates.

The average incubation period of nvCJD is unknown and estimates vary from 10 to more than 20 years. This makes prediction of the future number of cases difficult, but a potentially large epidemic with tens of thousands of cases, or more, is possible. The identification of effective treatment is therefore of paramount importance, and a WHO consultation in February 1998 stressed the pressing need for further research into the molecular properties of the CJD agent, to help identify effective means of treating the disease.

clinically similar to smallpox, in Africa in the last 20 years. The smallpox vaccine protected against both diseases, but as vaccination stopped after smallpox eradication in 1980, children born since then are likely to be more susceptible to monkeypox than their elders. The largest outbreak ever recorded occurred in the Democratic Republic of the Congo in 1996-1997, involving more than 500 people, and was investigated by WHO specialists. While the natural host of some other infectious diseases remains unknown, there is strong evidence associating the new variant of *Creutzfeldt-Jakob disease* (nvCJD), a degenerative brain condition, with the consumption of beef and other products from cattle suffering from or infected by the agent causing bovine spongiform encephalopathy *(Box 9)*. Because there may be a latent period of many years between infection and the

appearance of symptoms of nvCJD, it is impossible to estimate the scale of a potential epidemic based on the relatively small number of cases so far identified in the United Kingdom. WHO has convened expert group meetings on the disease.

Three *influenza* pandemics have occurred in this century – in 1918, 1957 and 1968. The WHO network for global influenza surveillance, which comprises 110 national influenza centres, maintains constant vigilance for evidence of the next pandemic *(Box 10)*. These surveillance activities first identified human infection with a new influenza virus called A(H5N1) in Hong Kong. Initial fears that the outbreak heralded the start of a new pandemic were proved to be unfounded by investigations involving close collaboration between WHO and the Chinese Government.

Health expectancy

For a long time, knowledge of life expectancy at different ages, the infant mortality rate and the distribution of the causes of death according to the principal disease headings was sufficient to assess the health status of populations and to determine national public health priorities. However, during the last 20 years the need for a new type of indicator has arisen as a result of changes such as the lengthening of life expectancy due to the fall in mortality at older ages, and the issue of quality of the years lived, at very old ages in particular. The former indicators remains indispensable, as important mortality inequalities still remain between countries and between the different groups making up populations. As not much is known about the limits of human longevity, health expectancy indicators – which provide information on the population's functional state and

Box 10. Influenza – Preparing for a 21st century pandemic

WHO's global surveillance activities first identified human infection with a new influenza virus called A(H5N1) in Hong Kong in mid-1997 at one of the Organization's collaborating centres. The possibility that the outbreak heralded a global influenza pandemic did not materialize during the first 10 months after the emergence of the virus among humans, but the threat of a virus more easily transmitted between humans remains.

Sooner or later, however, such a pandemic will occur – and history shows that it must be taken with the utmost seriousness. The WHO Network for Global Influenza Surveillance, which involves 110 national influenza centres, therefore maintains constant vigilance.

New influenza viruses to which nobody is immune cross the barrier from animals to humans at unpredictable times. These events can result in local epidemics, but a few lead to global pandemics. Influenza was first described by Hippocrates in 412 BC and about 30 possible pandemics have been documented in the last 400 years. Three have occurred in this century – in 1918, 1957 and 1968.

The 1918 pandemic of what was known as Spanish Flu was by far the most devastating, killing more than 20 million people worldwide between 1918 and 1920. The virus responsible is believed to have originated in swine. The pandemic occurred because the new virus was easily transmitted from person to person.

Birds and poultry in particular are other sources of influenza viruses, and the A(H5N1) virus in Hong Kong infected chickens from a source or reservoir in nature that is still to be identified, before emerging in humans. Significant person-to-person transmission of this virus does not seem to have taken place. However, as a precautionary measure during the outbreak, the Hong Kong authorities destroyed poultry flocks to eliminate the risk of further transmission, and a team of experts organized by WHO took over 1800 samples from birds and animals of 16 species to identify the natural reservoir of the virus and the extent of its spread in the animal population.

WHO has for many years played a leading role as a watchdog on the look-out for a pandemic, active in global influenza surveillance and in vaccine preparation. Every February, experts review results from WHO's influenza network and make a recommendation on the antigenic composition of the next year's influenza vaccine. WHO transmits this recommendation to health authorities and vaccine manufacturers.

Although the date of the next influenza pandemic cannot be predicted, the certainty of its eventual arrival means that pandemic emergency response plans have to be prepared in advance. WHO has created a Task Force of Experts on Influenza whose members include the directors of four main collaborating centres in Australia, Japan, the United Kingdom and the United States, WHO staff and representatives from three of the 110 national influenza centres which collaborate with WHO on surveillance.

The Task Force is developing a plan for the global management and control of a pandemic. The plan includes the promotion of high-growth seed virus for vaccine and the facilitation of vaccine production and international distribution and the dissemination of information, and logistic and other support, to national health authorities. It calls for each of these authorities to develop its own emergency response to a pandemic.

The A(H5N1) outbreak in Hong Kong was the first one in which WHO pandemic planning was used, with the step-by-step collection of information necessary to decide whether or not a new vaccine was required. The outbreak also provided the opportunity to adjust the plan in line with experience. In this way the scientific information necessary to make rational decisions on influenza control is being steadily accumulated.

on its vitality (levels of activity and participation) as well as on its quality of life (level of felt or perceived health) – are well adapted to the new conditions.

In recent years, the number of calculations of health expectancy (disability-free life expectancy, life expectancy in good perceived health, etc.) has increased. They are used in order to assess whether the lengthening of life expectancy is accompanied or not by an increase in time lived in bad health. The concept of life expectancy has thus been extended to morbidity and disability.

The notion of health expectancy was first put forward in the United

Fig. 7. Evolution of life expectancy and life expectancy without severe disability, selected countries, males at age 65

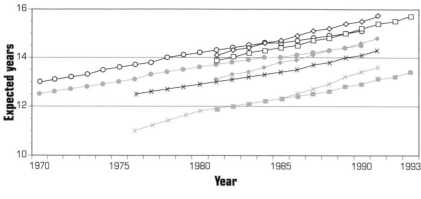

Australia
— ■ — Severe disability-free life expectancy
— □ — Life expectancy

France
— ◆ — Severe disability-free life expectancy
— ◇ — Life expectancy

United States of America
— ● — Severe disability-free life expectancy
— ○ — Life expectancy

United Kingdom
— ✕ — Severe disability-free life expectancy
— ✕ — Life expectancy

States in 1964 and a first method of calculation was proposed in 1971. In 1984, a group of experts in the epidemiology of ageing proposed to WHO a general model of health transition for computing health expectancy. This model, which distinguished between total survival, disability-free survival and survival without disabling chronic disease, led to the calculation of life expectancy, disability-free life expectancy and life expectancy without chronic disease.

Thanks to this model the evolution of mortality, morbidity and disability can be assessed simultaneously. From the evolution of discrepancies between the three indicators the possible occurrence of different health scenarios can be estimated – pandemic of chronic diseases and disabilities, compression of morbidity, contradictory evolutions including the scenario of dynamic equilibrium, or postponement of diseases, disabilities and mortality to older ages. However, combining those different dimensions

to provide a unitary index requires social consensus.

Since 1989, most researchers working on the development of these calculations have joined an international research network called REVES (*Réseau Espérance de Vie en Santé/* International Network on Health Expectancy and the Disability Process). Today, a first estimate of health expectancy (generally a disability-free life expectancy) is available for 48 countries. These indicators do not make international direct comparisons possible, owing to the specific characteristic of national health surveys which provide the major part of the information used in the calculations. Most authors however now distinguish between life expectancy without severe disability and life expectancy without disability, all levels combined.

Based on available information, *Fig. 7* shows that life expectancy without severe disability at age 65 in men progresses roughly in parallel with total life expectancy for the countries selected.

In the countries examined, the increase in life expectancy is not accompanied by an increase in the time spent with severe disability. The results indicate at worst a pandemic of light and moderate, but not of severe disabilities. They tend to confirm the theory of dynamic equilibrium which partly explains the increase in life expectancy by a slowing down in the rate of progression of chronic diseases. Thus, although the decline in mortality can lead to an increase in the prevalence of disabilities, these disabilities are less severe.

Chapter 3
Health across the life span

Childhood diseases

such as diphtheria,

scarlet fever and

rheumatic heart

disease were in

steady decline well

before vaccines

and antibiotics

became widely

available.

This chapter looks at trends and developments in health throughout the life span, dealing with four specific age groups – infants and small children; older children and adolescents; adults up to the age of 65; and older people, with a special focus on women's health.

Infants and small children

Viewed globally, the improvements in infant and child health in the past 50 years have been nothing less than spectacular, and appear likely to continue into the next century. For example, 210 of every 1000 babies born in 1955 died before their fifth birthday – a total of 20.6 million deaths in that year. By 1995 the death rate had fallen to 78 per 1000 (10.6 million deaths) and should decline further to 37 per 1000 by 2025, when it is projected that the total deaths will be 5.1 million.

In measuring the trends of the past 50 years, the reasons for both success and failure have to be understood in order to achieve further progress and to eliminate the gross disparities that persist between and within countries. Three dimensions of health development need to be taken into account: the epidemiological patterns of disease and deficiencies – including the interactions of diseases and deficiencies and the mortality levels; the social, economic and health infrastructure; and the priority strategies and adequacy of the actions taken to address the preventable and treatable causes of death and illness in infancy and childhood.

Overall reductions in under-5 and infant mortality are accelerating in much of the world. However global, regional and even national data often hide variations between and within countries that are important for health policies and programmes both globally and locally. The fate of a child is determined by its biology and its environment. Its risk of dying is influenced biologically by its gender, its natural defences and its nutrition; and by its physical, microbial, social and cultural environments.

The living conditions of families, the prevalence and modes of transmission of infectious disease agents and the nutritional status of the child are among the strongest immediate determinants that set the different levels of under-5 mortality rates around the world. Substantial improvement in at least one, but preferably all three of these elements is required in order to effect a significant overall decline in the rates.

The decline in deaths among the under-5s in the developed countries since the late 1940s is largely attributable to improvements in sanitation, water supply, housing, food supply and distribution and general hygiene. Childhood diseases such as diphtheria, scarlet fever, and rheumatic heart disease were in steady decline well before vaccines and antibiotics became widely available.

A similar decline in specific diseases is occurring now in the developing world, mainly as a consequence of general improvements in sanitation, water supply, education and access to preventive and curative health care in the community. These improvements are similar to those that took place in the developed economies of Europe and North America 50-80 years ago. However, progress has been more rapid due to the historical lessons learned and the advent of new knowledge and technologies that influence prevention, treatment, nutrition and fertility regulation.

Unfortunately, the progress recorded is not the full picture. Many countries – the least developed – have been unable to make or sustain similar progress over the years. In a few countries, child mortality levels are still above 200 per 1000 live births, and in others the levels are declining slowly, at a rate of no more than 1-2% per year.

About 10 million children born in 1997 will die before reaching their fifth birthday. Although this is barely half

the toll of 21 million such deaths in 1955, it remains unacceptably high. In the developing world in 1995, about 7.5 million of these children died from one or, frequently, more than one of five conditions: malaria, malnutrition, measles, acute respiratory infections and diarrhoea (Fig. 8). Other major causes are related to pregnancy and childbirth, sepsis, neonatal tetanus and AIDS. Often it is impossible to know which actually killed the child, because of difficulties in distinguishing the signs and symptoms of some of these diseases from one another. In many of the least developed countries, the odds are still heavily stacked against the child's survival.

The everyday nature of these deaths disguises the complex sequence of events leading to them – the remorseless process of repeated episodes of infections, often sequential, not infrequently concurrent. Each episode is accompanied by loss of appetite and decreased food intake, and each time the illness itself makes increased demands on the child's energy. Local health care facilities, if they exist, may be ill-equipped and poorly supplied, and inadequately staffed, with patterns of care that are rarely optimal and may even be harmful. Often, the child struggles for life in a highly crowded, unhygienic and poorly ventilated environment that facilitates the transmission of respiratory infections and malaria.

The tragedy is that most of these deaths in the under-5s could be prevented and the conditions treated within the resources of most, although not all, countries. The greatest positive impact on child mortality results from a combination of immunization, improved maternal health, family planning, and improved nutrition – interventions that affect nutritional status and prevent or provide effective treatment for the common infectious diseases of childhood.

Fig. 8. Main causes of death among children under age 5, developing world, 1995[a]

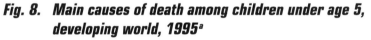
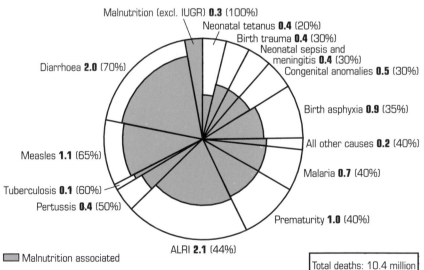

- Malnutrition (excl. IUGR) **0.3** (100%)
- Neonatal tetanus **0.4** (20%)
- Birth trauma **0.4** (30%)
- Neonatal sepsis and meningitis **0.4** (30%)
- Congenital anomalies **0.5** (30%)
- Birth asphyxia **0.9** (35%)
- All other causes **0.2** (40%)
- Malaria **0.7** (40%)
- Prematurity **1.0** (40%)
- ALRI **2.1** (44%)
- Pertussis **0.4** (50%)
- Tuberculosis **0.1** (60%)
- Measles **1.1** (65%)
- Diarrhoea **2.0** (70%)

▨ Malnutrition associated

Total deaths: 10.4 million

Disease clusters

Neonatal and perinatal causes. Neonatal tetanus, birth trauma, neonatal sepsis and meningitis, congenital anomalies, birth asphyxia, prematurity.
Integrated management of childhood illness. Malaria, acute lower respiratory infection (ALRI), measles, diarrhoea, malnutrition.

a
Number of deaths in millions followed by % malnutrition-associated deaths in brackets.

LYT 98002

Infant mortality rates are composed of two biologically and epidemiologically distinct components. The first is neonatal mortality, which is largely influenced by the health and care of the mother before and during pregnancy and during delivery, and the care of the infant in the postpartum period. The second is the postneonatal period, which is largely affected by environmental factors, feeding and other aspects of care. Historically, infant mortality rates are declining from previously high levels, even in the absence of specific technical interventions.

Neonatal mortality refers to deaths of infants between birth and the seventh day of life – the early neonatal period; and from the 8th to the 28th day of life – the late neonatal period.

Perinatal mortality refers to deaths of babies after 22 completed weeks of gestation, during birth and during the first seven days of life – the perinatal period. Fetal death or *stillbirth* is death prior to the complete expulsion or extraction from the mother of the fetus, irrespective of the duration of pregnancy.

About 9 million babies are either born dead or are born alive only to die within their first 28 days of life. While the causes of about 4 million stillbirths occurring worldwide are difficult to assess, research shows that nearly half of all stillborn babies have died as a result of maternal complications during labour and delivery. Many stillborn babies would have been perfectly normal infants if appropriate care had been given at birth. The longer the baby survives, the more likely it is that the death will be due to causes other than those related to pregnancy and delivery. More than two-thirds of the nearly 4.8 million newborn deaths are among fully developed babies born at term and apparently well equipped for life; how-

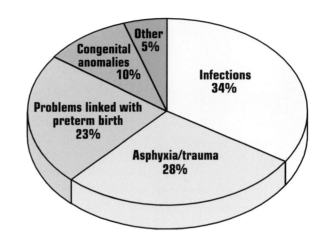

Fig. 9. Causes of neonatal death, 1995

- Other 5%
- Congenital anomalies 10%
- Problems linked with preterm birth 23%
- Infections 34%
- Asphyxia/trauma 28%

ever, at least 4 out of 5 newborn deaths are due to infection, birth asphyxia, birth injury and problems linked to preterm birth *(Fig. 9)*. Congenital anomalies, usually thought to be the main cause of death in babies, account for a relatively small percentage of these deaths. Helping these babies to survive and grow up into healthy adults does not require expensive technology. Good newborn care at birth does not require sophisticated equipment; it calls for a set of simple preventive measures and a little prompt extra care *(Box 11)*. WHO's Mother-Baby package lists straightforward and simple interventions at various stages of pregnancy, and during and after birth, that are known to improve the health and save the lives of mothers and babies.

Controlling childhood diseases through immunization

The world continues to underuse the most cost-effective public health intervention of all – immunization. It is unacceptable that at least 2 million children still die each year from diseases for which vaccines are available at low cost. Immunization has been

Box 11. Essential newborn care

All newborn babies need basic care: cleanliness, warmth, early and exclusive breast-feeding, eye care, immunization, resuscitation when necessary.

Some newborns need special care: sick newborns need early recognition of danger signs, prompt treatment.

Preterm and low birth weight infants need more cleanliness, more warmth, more attention to breast-feeding, more effective recognition and treatment of infections.

It took smallpox

nearly two centuries

to be eradicated.

But after 35-40

years, polio is well

on the way

to eradication.

responsible for the most dramatic changes in child health in the last few decades. Vaccines have prevented death, disease and disablement among hundreds of millions of children.

In 1948, immunization programmes were largely restricted to industrialized countries, and even then were often partially implemented. It was not until the formation of WHO's Expanded Programme on Immunization in 1974, when less than 5% of children were being immunized, that developing countries began to create national schedules and programmes. Now, only around 20% of the world's children remain unimmunized. First smallpox was eradicated. Since then, as coverage for each of the childhood vaccines rose, disease incidence fell. Large outbreaks previously experienced in almost every country are now less frequent and of lower intensity.

From 1981 there was a fourfold increase from approximately 20% to reach the 1990 goal of 80% immunization coverage among infants worldwide with BCG, measles, and the third dose of DPT (diphtheria, pertussis, tetanus) and oral poliovirus vaccines. An estimated 3 million young lives were saved from measles, neonatal tetanus and pertussis in 1990 alone. By 1995, over 80% of the world's children had been immunized against diphtheria, tetanus, whooping cough, poliomyelitis, measles and tuberculosis. During 1995, in addition to the 500 million routine immunization contacts with children under 1 year of age, a record 300 million children throughout the world – almost half of those under the age of 5 – were immunized during mass campaigns against polio.

Despite these successes, children are still slipping through the safety net. For example, even though globally 80% of children are immunized against measles, vaccination cover-

age is variable. There are frequently pockets of low coverage, especially among the urban poor, where children are in frequent contact with each other and easily transmit disease. Many years have elapsed between the invention of vaccines and their widespread use today in immunization programmes. Fortunately, the interval between successful field trials and large-scale application is shortening. It took smallpox nearly two centuries to be eradicated. But after 35-40 years, polio is well on the way to eradication, and it is only about 30 years since measles immunization began (Box 12).

Large epidemics of *poliomyelitis* occurred regularly in the 1950s in all industrialized countries, causing panic among parents and crippling thousands of children every summer. Following the development and widespread routine use of anti-polio vaccines, the disease rapidly disappeared in industrialized countries and was eliminated as a public health problem there in the early 1960s. However, epidemic poliomyelitis continued to be a major public health problem in most developing countries. The incidence of paralytic polio in the developing world began to decrease only after routine immunization of infants with oral polio vaccine (OPV) in the late 1970s.

Virtually all endemic countries in the world have now begun to implement the WHO-recommended strategies to eradicate polio – supplementary mass immunization with OPV and surveillance for acute flaccid paralysis. Polio has been eradicated from the Americas since 1991, and is on the verge of eradication in Europe and the Western Pacific. The major reservoirs of wild virus transmission are in South Asia and sub-Saharan Africa, although eradication activities are progressing in virtually all endemic countries of these regions.

During national immunization days in 1997, supplemental OPV was provided to almost two-thirds of the world's children under 5, that is to more than 400 million children. To monitor progress towards eradication, establishing and improving surveillance for acute flaccid paralysis has now become an urgent priority. The development of systems for the surveillance of flaccid paralysis often lags behind the implementation of national immunization days, and major efforts are needed in many countries to increase the quality of such surveillance.

Countries with the lowest immunization coverage are nearly always countries with internal conflicts. Infrastructures are weakened or destroyed, resulting in large numbers of children remaining unimmunized and in outbreaks of vaccine-preventable diseases. Intense efforts to accelerate polio eradication in such circumstances include using such techniques as "days of tranquillity" when fighting stops to allow immunization to take place. Polio-free countries and areas are increasingly at risk of reinfection from countries which remain endemic; should this occur, it will delay the global eradication goal. The full benefits of global eradication will be realized only when polio has been eradicated from the most remote areas of all countries. Eradication by the year 2000 or soon thereafter remains feasible, provided that adequate additional funding is made available and the current momentum of polio eradication activities can be maintained.

By 1996, estimated ***measles*** morbidity and mortality worldwide had fallen by 78% and 88%, respectively compared to the pre-vaccine era. During the 1990s, the widespread use of innovative measles control strategies in the Americas and countries as diverse as Mongolia, South Africa and

---

Box 12. *Eradicating measles through immunization*

Based on implementation of a combination of measles immunization and surveillance strategies, countries are considered to be in one of three stages:

- ***Control.*** Reduction of incidence and/or prevalence to an acceptable level as a result of deliberate efforts, requiring continued control measures. The objective is to achieve high routine coverage with one dose of measles vaccine among infants to reduce measles morbidity and mortality.
- ***Outbreak prevention.*** Aggressive immunization strategies have prevented forecasted measles outbreaks.
- ***Elimination.*** Reduction of incidence to zero as a result of deliberate efforts, requiring continued control measures.

In the Americas, WHO has implemented a periodic mass immunization strategy combined with strengthening of surveillance to interrupt measles transmission and eliminate the disease by the year 2000. Other regions and countries have implemented or are considering the implementation of strategies aimed at interrupting measles virus transmission. Recently, the WHO Eastern Mediterranean Region has pledged to eliminate measles by the year 2010, and the European Region is planning to do so by the year 2007. In the future, the sum of all regional efforts towards elimination will result in the global eradication of measles, obviating the need for further control measures.

From 1977 to 1990, the global reported coverage with one dose of measles vaccine administered through routine services increased from approximately 5% to 80%, and then remained stable at that level until 1996.

The results of recently published studies indicate that the current WHO policy of offering vitamin A at the same time as measles vaccine to 9-month-old infants is appropriate, safe and effective. The benefit of administering vitamin A in cases of measles at any age has never been questioned and continues to be recommended by WHO as part of the integrated management of childhood illness.

Despite the widespread availability of safe and effective measles vaccines since 1963, measles still accounts for 10% of the global mortality from all causes among children aged under 5 years. Although measles eradication is technically feasible, programmatic, political and financial obstacles must be overcome before the goal of eradication can be achieved.

---

the United Kingdom demonstrated that high-level measles control and even interruption of transmission is feasible over large geographical areas. The evaluation of these country and regional elimination strategies will provide valuable information for developing a global measles eradication strategy. While the current measles vaccine is one of the safest, most effective and cost-effective vaccines ever developed, plans are in hand to develop a more heat-stable vaccine which could be used in mass campaigns, would not need the cold chain and could be administered without needle and syringe.

Tetanus of the newborn is the third killer of children after measles and pertussis among the six EPI vaccine-preventable diseases. While between 800 000 and 1 million newborns died from tetanus in the early 1980s, an estimated 730 000 such deaths are now prevented every year, particularly by targeting elimination efforts to high-risk areas. In 1997, there were an estimated 275 000 deaths.

Diphtheria is a respiratory infection transmitted through close physical contact, especially in overcrowded and poor socioeconomic conditions. In 1990, a large outbreak of diphtheria occurred in the Russian Federation and by the end of 1994, it had spread to all the newly independent States. At least 90% of all diphtheria cases reported worldwide during 1990-1995 were in these countries. The epidemic appears to be waning after massive immunization. This epidemic serves as a reminder of the danger of not maintaining immunization levels in a community.

Acute respiratory infections and diarrhoea

In the late 1960s, WHO scientists noted exciting developments in the treatment of cholera, in particular the treatment of patients using oral rehydration therapy (ORT), which depended on a solution made by dissolving dried salts in clean water, and avoided using expensive and hard-to-transport intravenous fluids. Field trials determined that it was feasible for peripheral health workers to use ORT

for the treatment of acute diarrhoea in children under 5. They also showed that children treated with ORT and feeding actually gained weight. Research in different countries confirmed the benefits and safety of ORT. Based on this information, WHO promoted the wide use of ORT to reduce mortality from the acute diarrhoea and associated malnutrition that was at the time claiming the lives of over 5 million children per year. In 1978, a new programme was established, combining research with the development of materials and support to establishing programmes in countries. In collaboration with UNICEF and numerous bilateral agencies, WHO assisted over 100 Member States to set up national programmes, define policy, plan activities and train health workers. By the mid-1990s, virtually all health workers were aware of ORT, even if they had not been trained in its use. Fewer dehydrated children were seen at health facilities as families learned to increase fluids and keep feeding children who were suffering from diarrhoea. Exclusive and prolonged breast-feeding was also found to be an effective, feasible intervention to prevent diarrhoea.

In the late 1980s it was shown that acute respiratory infections, mainly pneumonia, were the major killers of children aged under 5. Access to technology or expertise was limited, and many pneumonia cases went untreated. At the same time, children suffering from simple coughs and colds sometimes received antibiotics unnecessarily. Based on a simple approach to pneumonia detection developed in the early 1980s at a collaborating centre in Papua New Guinea, WHO developed and validated guidelines, and established a programme in 1984. The simplified standard case management became the basis of WHO's efforts to reduce

> The simplified standard case management became the basis of WHO's efforts to reduce pneumonia mortality.

pneumonia mortality. Since then, the Organization has developed guidelines, tools and supportive technical documents for clinical management training, programme management and evaluation. Following a general trend towards integration, the programmes for control of diarrhoeal diseases and for acute respiratory infections were merged in 1990.

Integrated management of childhood illness

At the same time, research involving childhood diseases made it clear that single-disease approaches may not be the best for the child. A child does not arrive at the health facility as a "case" of something, but arrives sick, and may have several conditions at once. In some instances, the mother may bring the child in for a problem which may only be a minor manifestation of a dangerous illness. By 1990, it was well documented that most childhood deaths were caused by five conditions: as many as 70% of deaths could be attributed to diarrhoea, pneumonia, measles, malaria and malnutrition. The need for integration at health facilities to rationalize the task of health workers became increasingly evident. In 1992, WHO and UNICEF worked out clinical guidelines that integrated all five conditions. The resulting strategy is called integrated management of childhood illness. Research continues to improve integrated case management and to identify more comprehensive disease prevention activities, including the development and adoption of new vaccines.

In the view of WHO, although the formula for ORS is satisfactory, there may be an even better one. Experience in the field suggests that the process of detecting and managing pneumonia may need to be reviewed;

it may be possible to target antibiotics more effectively to only those children who will really benefit from them. Current efforts are aimed at the first-level health facility, but it is essential to convince the population of the need for urgent medical attention when children are sick.

In addition, complementary strategies for the prevention of some of these diseases are also being promoted and supported. For example, for reducing the incidence of diarrhoea, they include promotion of optimal breast-feeding practices and of the "baby-friendly" hospital initiative, modifying complementary feeding practices, improving water supply and sanitation facilities and promoting personal and domestic hygiene. Adequate breast-feeding in a large number of settings is found to be associated with a 2.5-4-fold lower rate of mortality and less severe cholera and *Shigella* spp. infections. In respect of malaria, they include use of impregnated bednets which, even in the short term, have resulted in a 17-30% reduction in total malaria deaths in young children. For measles, immunization of infants has been an effective intervention for reducing incidence.

Low birth weight and nutritional deficiencies

Low birth weight is defined as a weight at birth of less than 2500 g (i.e. up to and including 2499 g), irrespective of gestational age. It has an adverse effect on child survival and development, and may even be an important risk factor for a number of adult diseases, including non-insulin-dependent diabetes and heart disease. While it is recognized that the etiology of low birth weight is multifactorial, emphasis is given to those maternal factors that are be-

> Research involving childhood diseases made it clear that single-disease approaches may not be the best for the child.

Map 6. Underweight prevalence among preschool children, 1995 estimates

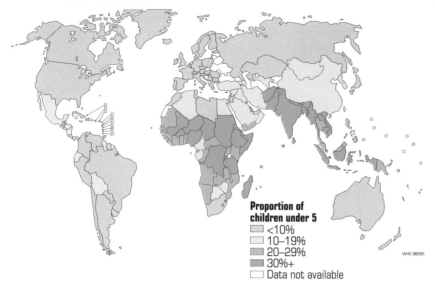

Proportion of
children under 5
□ <10%
□ 10–19%
□ 20–29%
■ 30%+
□ Data not available

WHO 98065

lieved to be of greatest importance in developing countries and that might be amenable to change in the short term. These include poor maternal nutrition, certain infections, pre-eclampsia, arduous work after mid-pregnancy, short birth intervals, and teenage pregnancy. Tobacco and alcohol consumption are additional risk factors.

In infants whose birth weight is very low, the sucking and swallowing reflexes are poorly developed, the retina is easily damaged by high levels of oxygen and there is a risk of intracranial bleeding as a result of birth trauma. Birth weight is influenced by two major factors: duration of gestation and intrauterine growth rate. The preterm infant whose gestation period is less than 37 weeks is physiologically immature and at a higher risk of dying during the neonatal period.

Both during the newborn period and into infancy and childhood, low-birth-weight infants are at much higher risk of mortality and severe morbidity than full-term, full-sized infants. Compared to full-term infants, they have a 3-4 times greater

risk of dying from diarrhoeal diseases, acute respiratory infections and, if not immunized, measles. They are more likely to be malnourished at 1 year. By the age of around 5, the low-birth-weight child, probably having had more cyclic episodes of infection and malnutrition, may be severely stunted (*Map 6*). This growth deficiency will be carried into adult life and translated into reduced work output, and often impaired learning ability.

Globally, WHO estimates that 25 million low-birth-weight infants are born each year, constituting 17% of all live births, nearly 95% of them in the developing world. The incidence of low birth weight varies widely between regions of the world, with levels of 32% in southern Asia (but 9% in eastern Asia), 11-16% in Africa and 10-12% in Latin America and the Caribbean.

The increase in the survival of very low-birth-weight infants in industrialized countries, often with high rates of long-term developmental impairment, has generated an intense scientific and ethical debate about the implications of perinatal interventions which increase survival rate but also result in an increase in severe handicaps. Clearly there is need for further research in some of these areas. But the debate should not deflect attention from what can be done for the vast majority of women and newborns, even the majority of low-birth-weight infants, using simple technologies, good principles of public health and a rational organization of services based on the best knowledge. Perinatal health, together with maternal health and safe motherhood, will be one of the major challenges of the next decade.

Many children in developing countries are subject to multiple risks with, very often, a deterioration of their situation at the weaning period. Born with a low weight, fed with a sub-optimal breast-feeding practice, they are at increased risk of protein-energy malnutrition. ***Breast-feeding*** is one of the most effective, low-cost interventions for neonatal health. Nothing but breast milk is required for the first 4-6 months of life, neither substitutes, nor supplements, nor even water. Even in developed countries breast-feeding lowers the rate of respiratory and gastrointestinal illness to one-fourth that of non-breast-fed infants.

Despite this knowledge, many hospitals and health workers continue to obstruct breast-feeding or fail to recommend it. Putting the infant to the breast just after birth decreases the risk of hypoglycaemia, eliminates the need for prelacteal glucose water and hastens the onset of full lactation. Allowing mother and infant to stay together 24 hours a day, with on-demand feeding, improves health and reduces the risk of disease even in the newborn period. Such a feeding pattern eliminates the epidemics of pathogenic *E. coli* and staphylococcal infections that used to sweep through newborn nurseries and eliminates the fatal necrotizing enterocolitis among very low-birth-weight babies.

WHO estimates that globally, exclusive breast-feeding rates remain low. An estimated 35% of infants are fed only breast milk at some point between birth and four months of age. As awareness of the advantages grows in both developing and developed countries, more Member States are taking steps to protect and promote breast-feeding, and rates are increasing. All too often, however, in countries where malnutrition and mortality are high, these rates remain low. Many countries (especially in Europe) continue to have low breast-feeding rates, although they are slowly improving.

WHO estimates that about one-third of the world's children are affected by ***protein-energy malnutrition***; 76% of these children live in Asia (mainly southern Asia), 21% in Africa and 3% in Latin America. As many as 206 million children in developing countries are stunted (stunting is associated with poor developmental attainment in children and functional impairment in adults). Efforts to accelerate economic development significantly will be unsuccessful until optimal child growth and development are ensured.

Iodine deficiency has been described as the world's single most significant cause of preventable brain damage and mental retardation. Iodine deficiency disorders affect about 14% of the world population, and 834 million people are affected by goitre. Iodine deficiency in the fetus, due to inadequate iodine status of the mother, is associated with a greater incidence of stillbirths, spontaneous abortions, congenital abnormalities, low birth weight, infant and child mortality, and may lead to cretinism. The IQ scores of iodine-deficient children and adults are lower than those of people who are not iodine-deficient. Significant improvement in mental development, school performance and motor development have been demonstrated with iodine supplementation of primary school children.

Childhood obesity and its consequences are emerging as a global problem. Data from 79 developing countries and a number of industrialized countries suggest that, by WHO standards (>+2 standard deviations above the reference median weight for height), about 22 million children aged under 5 are overweight. Obesity affects almost 10% of schoolchildren in industrialized countries and high rates are also emerging in some of the developing ones. Some 30% of obese children become obese adults.

Obesity is also a significant risk factor for a range of serious non-

In most countries of the world, the duration of breast-feeding is declining or shows no change.

communicable diseases and conditions. WHO has initiated a review of associated morbidity and mortality with a view to developing guidelines for Member States on obesity prevention and management. Improved prevention of and therapy for childhood obesity are the most cost-effective approaches to reduce morbidity and mortality due to obesity in adulthood; three potential approaches for the preventive interventions to deal with this problem are reduction in dietary energy intake, increase in the energy spent on activity and reduction in inactivity. Children with potentially lethal complications of obesity such as sleep apnoea require rapid and sustained weight reduction. One possible approach in children is a carbohydrate-free diet under careful monitoring and follow-up. The role of drugs in the treatment of obesity is not clear. Some interventions aimed at both parents and children have been successful (e.g. modifications in diet, lifestyle activities and behaviour).

Other childhood diseases of public health concern

Rheumatic fever and rheumatic heart disease (the most common cardiovascular disease in children and young adults) are examples of how social and economic factors, and later health care and medical technologies, have contributed to and then accelerated the decline of a disease that was epidemic in developed countries a century ago. Limited evidence suggests that there has been little if any decline in the occurrence of rheumatic heart disease in developing countries over the past few decades.

Meningococcal meningitis occurs in all parts of the world. In the 1980s an epidemic wave of meningococcal meningitis spread over vast territories in Asia and Africa. Even in non-epidemic years, at least 1 million cases of bacterial meningitis are estimated to occur and about 135 000 children die. About 300 000 of these cases and 30 000 deaths are due to meningococcal meningitis. In epidemic years the number of cases of meningococcal meningitis may double to 600 000 or more, with 60 000 or more deaths.

Asthma, a disorder of the airways, is one of the most common chronic diseases worldwide, with a prevalence rate among children ranging from 1.5% to over 12%. Rates are generally lower in developing countries but globally both prevalence and hospitalization rates have increased by 40% in the last decade. The long-term prognosis of childhood asthma is now a major concern. It has often been suggested that childhood asthma will "disappear" when the patient reaches adulthood. Epidemiological evidence is less optimistic. It has been estimated that 30-50% of children have asthma that disappears at puberty but often "reappears" in adult life. Between one-third and two-thirds of children with asthma continue to suffer from the disease through puberty and adulthood. Asthma in childhood is an example of a chronic disease which can impair children's socialization, school performance and later life. Self-management and care are essential if the asthmatic child is to lead as normal a life as possible.

Paediatric AIDS is substantially underrecognized and underreported, because of difficulties in establishing the diagnosis of HIV infection in infancy, as well as clinical features overlapping with those of the other severe diseases of childhood. In 1997, about 95% of the estimated number of AIDS deaths in children under 15 occurred in the under-5 age group. Perinatal transmission has been well documented, with 15-35% of children of HIV-positive mothers being in-

The long-term prognosis of childhood asthma is now a major concern.

fected and accounting for the majority of children with AIDS. As almost half of all newly infected adults are now women, WHO projects that if current trends continue, by the year 2000, over 13 million women will have been infected and 4 million will have died of AIDS. Their uninfected infants will constitute a growing group of potential orphans, since most of their HIV-infected mothers will die of AIDS within 5-10 years of their birth. By the year 2000 as many as 10 million children under 10 may be orphaned as a result of maternal AIDS in sub-Saharan Africa alone, and projected infant and child deaths from AIDS may increase child mortality rates by as much as 50% in parts of sub-Saharan Africa. But the most alarming trends of HIV infection are in South-East Asia. In some high-prevalence communities, AIDS is already starting to reverse the long-term effects of child health initiatives. Many women are at particularly high risk of infection because of their low socioeconomic status, their difficult living situations and/or the fact that they do not have access to AIDS prevention information. Paediatric AIDS will increase accordingly.

Emerging public health priorities

Although mortality statistics are becoming more reliable, little is still known concerning morbidity of children in different settings. It is crucial to get accurate data – or at least *estimates of morbidity* – in order to train personnel, to prepare relevant programmes and services and to evaluate their performance. The ongoing epidemiological transition in the developing world makes it even more important to target morbidity in order to be successful in combating childhood diseases through ap-

propriate care, including prevention.

The common infectious diseases of childhood are coming under control through a combination of health promotion, prevention and simplified standard treatment regimens. But at the same time, the healthy growth and development of many children is threatened by very rapid, often disruptive social, cultural and economic changes. The emerging *new morbidity* is mainly of a psychosocial nature with a very low mortality rate, except from suicide. It is of increasing importance worldwide: very common in the developed world, and not rare in the developing one. A more refined approach to disease problems is badly needed, since prevention and care should adapt to this interacting process. Globally, the new morbidity is strongly associated with behavioural problems and is therefore much more difficult to prevent than the diseases that have been known for centuries. Countries in an intermediate state of socioeconomic development are accumulating classical and new morbidity and are facing great difficulties as regards the care of the sick.

In terms of emerging morbidity, AIDS represents the most crucial challenge because of its impact on women, children and families. However, other problems should not be overlooked: substance abuse during pregnancy with its harmful effects on both mother and child, and accidental injuries, by far the first cause of potential years of life lost. Accidental injuries are only one of the ill-effects of violence: if other causes are added such as child abuse and neglect, *violent morbidity* is becoming more of a burden. Child abuse and neglect include four distinct conditions: physical abuse, neglect, emotional abuse and sexual abuse. They occur within and outside family settings, in the latter case sometimes in an insti-

> The healthy growth and development of many children is threatened by very rapid, often disruptive social, cultural and economic changes.

Box 13. Healthy child development

Child development concerns not merely physical health but also the process of change whereby a child learns to handle ever more difficult levels of moving, thinking, speaking, and relating to others. In its first year of life, the infant needs to develop a sense of trust in the world. A consistently nurturing and tension-free environment provides the infant with a sense of security. This critical process is usually achieved by 13 months of age.

Unfortunately the health sector, not always appreciating the life-long impact of the interactions of nutrition, child care and nurturing on cognitive and social development, has done little to foster parenting and child care beyond meeting the survival and physical needs of children. Where child development programmes exist, they usually start at the already late age of 3 or 4 years.

The best child development programmes are aimed at strengthening the capacity of mothers, through home visiting and child stimulation from infancy until the age of 3. Early child stimulation interventions within the first year of life have their greatest impact on the most disadvantaged groups and populations, attenuating the effects of poverty, severe malnutrition, low birth weight and prematurity.

Research shows clearly the intimate linkages between physical growth and psychological development, and the powerful relationships among growth, development, health, and care-giving. The mechanisms that promote physical and mental development are not unidirectional from care-givers to children; in fact it is the interaction between the two that is critical. Better-nourished children tend to be more active and able to explore the environment and elicit more interaction from parents, and may be more effective in demanding and getting food. In addition, the care-giving activities within the home that affect child nutrition and psychosocial development are closely related: a major part of giving care to infants and toddlers is simply feeding.

Many households in conditions of poverty still have the resources to provide adequate diets for children and to use good feeding practices. However, they need the knowledge and skills to do so. Families who are severely constrained economically will also need access to food and dietary supplements. Finally, families need help in improving the interactions between care-giver and child, especially the malnourished child.

In general, progress in child health and development will remain frustratingly slow if the national and international health bodies focus only on the medical model of public health strategies directed at the one in 13 children in the developing world who die before reaching the first year of life. It is the legacy of malnutrition, continuous non-fatal illness, and lack of social and environmental stimulation to development that perpetuates the health and social deficits that are transmitted to the next generation, repeating the statistical pattern of one in 13 dying, but 12 of 13 surviving in misery and with prospects of a blighted future.

tutional or non-institutional setting. Child abuse mortality rates for infants in most countries are estimated at around 7 per 100 000 live births, providing a rough global estimate and indicating only the "tip of the iceberg". Although childhood accidents, injuries and disabilities have been recognized as a major problem, meaningful estimates of their incidence worldwide are not available. Greater medical knowledge and better technology mean that more children survive premature birth, congenital malformation, accidents, injuries and malignant diseases. Their survival is often not free of disability.

Increasing **environmental hazards** add their toll to this new pattern of disease, sometimes aggravating pre-existing ill-health, such as asthma, sometimes directly responsible for acute or chronic impairments (toxic, allergic), e.g. lead poisoning in childhood. With the epidemiological transition, some countries are simultaneously facing the burden of classical infancy and childhood diseases, which is not yet solved, and the burden of this new morbidity. They need specific flexible strategies in planning for health services and in care, delivery and the allocation of scarce resources – both human and material.

With increasing and rapid urbanization, **developmental deprivation** of young children is becoming a major issue (*Box 13*). The urban environment can be particularly hostile to children. Density of human population, accompanied by a lack of basic urban services, results in increasing environmental health risks. Poor housing, lack of parental supervision and even abandonment, early childhood labour and other consequences of urban poverty are endemic and contribute to high morbidity and mortality among children. There are limited recreational facilities. Children, particularly those in single-parent families where the parent often has to work long and irregular hours outside the home, suffer from cultural deprivation and face a conflict of value systems, which further contributes to psychosocial difficulties. A significant proportion of urban households is headed by women who in many cases do not have any close relatives living nearby, and the nature of the areas in which they live does not foster the development of other links as alternative support.

Children are the most vulnerable members of society in times of *armed conflicts*. In the past decade around 2 million children have died as a result of war and many times that number have been displaced from their homes. In such conflicts, deaths of children are up to 24 times greater than in times of peace. At present there may be more than 4 million children in the world who have been disabled because of armed conflict, many by landmines.

The number of adult diseases that have their roots in childhood include those that have a strong nutrition-dietary component. *Deficiency diseases* need to be diagnosed and prevented in childhood. Protein-energy deficiency and specific nutritional deficiencies have been eliminated in many parts of the world but some populations are still much affected. Specific examples with long-term adverse effects are iodine deficiency disorders, vitamin A deficiency (*Box 14*), iron deficiency, fluoride deficiency, and vitamin B_{12} deficiency.

Diseases of affluence are increasing in the industrial world and in affluent groups in developing countries. There is population-based and epidemiological evidence identifying specific dietary components that early-on increase the probability of occurrence of adult disease. In the case of some of these components, particularly in relation to cardiovas-

---

Box 14. The deadly deficiency of vitamin A

Vitamin A deficiency affects as many as 256 million children in more than 75 countries and is the world's most preventable cause of blindness. Of some 2.7 million preschool-age children who have eye damage resulting from this deficiency, an estimated 350 000 go blind every year, and up to 60% die within a few months of becoming blind.

Vitamin A deficiency is also linked with an increase in the severity of infections, particularly measles and diarrhoeal disease. Through synergism with measles infection, vitamin A deficiency contributes to some extent to the estimated 960 000 childhood deaths from measles every year. The effect on mortality is pronounced for diarrhoeal disease, is demonstrable for deaths attributed to measles, and very small or maybe absent for deaths attributed to respiratory disease.

This conclusion is based on a meta-analysis of 10 controlled mortality trials in populations where xerophthalmia (the eye condition caused by vitamin A deficiency) is present. The review by the same authors of 17 studies providing information about morbidity outcomes, including morbidity results from the 10 mortality trials, finds very little evidence to suggest that vitamin A status affects the prevalence of general morbidity in young children.

Deficiency occurs where diets contain insufficient vitamin A for the basic needs of growth and development, for physiological functions, and for periods of added stress due to illness. In areas where vitamin A deficiency occurs, women of childbearing age are at high risk of its consequences because they need more of the vitamin during pregnancy and lactation.

Infants who are born depleted of vitamin A need more of this vitamin than can be supplied through their mother's milk after 4-6 months of nursing if they are to be prevented from developing deficiency.

Improvement in vitamin A status may reduce the chance of infectious diseases progressing to their severe forms. Improving the vitamin A status of deficient children and treating cases of measles with vitamin A can substantially reduce childhood morbidity and mortality.

Supplementation with vitamin A has been shown to be effective in reducing mortality by as much as 23% from these conditions in areas where deficiency is common. The results of studies in Ghana and Brazil indicate that vitamin A supplementation is associated with a decrease in the severity of infectious diseases.

Recent findings have indicated that vitamin A is a key modulator of the immune system. Thus, apart from other benefits, sufficient vitamin A stores could significantly reduce the risk of transmission of HIV from infected mothers to their babies.

---

cular disease, reduced consumption can lower the incidence of disease. The result of scientific research continues to support the role of diet in the development of those diseases most responsible for mortality in the developed world: cardiovascular disease and cancer. Excess intakes of saturated fats, with high blood cholesterol levels, are linked to eventual adult coronary heart disease. Risk factors for cerebrovascular abnormalities include high blood pressure, to which obesity, alcohol consumption, and excess salt intake are major contributors. Obesity is also strongly related to the onset of diabetes. The dynamic relationship between modifications in children's diets and sequential changes in their health as adults is beginning to emerge.

WHO's response

WHO has participated in the achievement of outstanding improvements in child health during the past 50 years. By capitalizing on the successes described in the previous section, WHO can lead the way in giving tomorrow's children a better, healthier future.

One target for that future is that by the year 2025 there should be over 5 million fewer deaths among children under 5 than in 1995, with possible decreases of between 30% and 60% in perinatal and neonatal deaths.

In terms of interventions, the scale of future successes will depend largely on wider application of the WHO/UNICEF integrated management of childhood illness, on better detection and management of pneumonia, on improvements in nutrition, and on the continuation of immunization programmes. Most of all it will be shaped by the knowledge and experience gained in the last half-century.

Historical analysis in developed countries covering this century has shown less dramatic reduction in perinatal and neonatal mortality than in postnatal mortality, probably due to the belief that perinatal and neonatal problems are not amenable to public health interventions. Although low

birth weight has been recognized as a major public health problem, improvement has been slow since many aspects of health are involved. More tangible progress has been made in eliminating neonatal tetanus through maternal immunization and promoting breast-feeding and baby-friendly hospitals. WHO has shown that perinatal and neonatal deaths can be reduced by using an essential set of interventions for the mother during pregnancy and delivery and for the newborn child after birth.

Mortality can be reduced by a further 20-30%, and WHO can achieve this by providing guidance (standards, norms, training material) in the area of newborn health to address other issues such as management of sick newborn and care of moderately preterm/low-birth-weight infants. A milestone was the WHO/UNICEF conference on infant and young child feeding (1979), which stimulated action to promote breast-feeding. Related subsequent action included the Innocenti declaration on the protection, promotion and support of breast-feeding (1990), and the baby-friendly hospital initiative. In 1992, the World Declaration and Plan of Action for Nutrition was adopted, including nine goals for the year 2000 and nine action-oriented strategies for improving nutrition.

WHO initially promoted worldwide awareness of protein-energy malnutrition through publications, cooperation with countries in national nutrition surveys, training of personnel and research. WHO/FAO expert groups elaborated guidelines for nutritional assessment, nutritional requirements, the role of nutrition units, and national nutrition policies and strategies. Applied activities and surveillance were developed in many countries, with significant impact on local or national nutritional activities and status. Particular emphasis was on

Perinatal and neonatal deaths can be reduced by using an essential set of interventions for the mother during pregnancy and delivery and for the newborn child after birth.

preventing micronutrient deficiencies, especially of iodine, iron and vitamin A. Global databases were developed on each of these in the 1990s, and indicators and criteria for monitoring the deficiencies, and programmes to combat them, were defined.

By 1997, over 160 countries had received technical and/or financial support from WHO for developing and implementing their national food and nutrition policies and plans. The WHO global database on national nutrition policies and programmes provides information on the progress of countries. The WHO global database on malnutrition and child growth covers over 80% of the world's under-5 children, and the databank on breast-feeding covers 65 countries (over 60% of the world population). The baby-friendly hospital initiative is being implemented in over 170 countries and over 10 700 hospitals are now designated "baby-friendly". Over 140 countries now have national breast-feeding committees or equivalent. A multicountry study on child growth is being set up in order to develop a new international growth reference for infants and young children.

Strategies to prevent malnutrition in children in the early 21st century include supporting countries in eliminating iodine deficiency and its associated brain damage, vitamin A deficiency and its associated blindness and death, and iron deficiency anaemia with its associated mortality and morbidity; improving infant and young child feeding through promotion of breast-feeding and proper timely complementary feeding; and more effectively addressing the nutritional needs of the ever-growing emergency-affected populations.

In order to avoid unsafe injections which can result in the transmission of bloodborne diseases, WHO and UNICEF are working together to ensure that only auto-destruct syringes are used, together with safety boxes, in mass immunization campaigns. The introduction of monitors on all vials of oral polio vaccine supplied through UNICEF will be extended to include vaccine procured directly from international manufacturers. When the discard point is reached, the end user knows that he should discard the vial. This indicator and the revised policy on the use of open liquid vaccine multidose vials in subsequent immunization sessions will help reduce vaccine wastage. It will also help use the vaccine to the full extent of its true stability even in difficult access areas where the cold chain is not reliable, thus reaching children who otherwise would not have benefited from immunization services. More research is needed to develop completely safe needle-free injection technologies. New jet injectors and the administration of vaccines as solids are two of the directions that are currently being investigated and which will need additional funding in the coming years.

Older children and adolescents

During the past 50 years, the health of most children and young people between the ages of 5 and 19 has improved, at least in some ways. Their standard of living is generally higher, they are at risk of fewer infectious diseases, and they are better educated.

They are the children and adolescents who have survived the first five dangerous years of life and are not yet directly challenged by the health problems of adulthood. Of all the age groups, theirs is the healthiest, and it is one during which the foundations can be laid for a long and healthy life.

During the past 50 years, the health of most children and young people between the ages of 5 and 19 has improved.

Table 6. Health problems and health-related behaviours common among adolescents, developing countries

	Conditions / behaviour			
Specific to adolescents	**Affecting adolescents disproportionately**	**Manifested in adolescence, originating in childhood**	**With major implications for future health**	**Affecting adolescents less than children but more than adults**
• Disorders of secondary sexual development • Difficulties with psychosocial development • Suboptimal adolescent growth spurt	• Maternal mortality and morbidity • STD (including HIV) • Tuberculosis • Schistosomiasis • Intestinal helminths • Mental disorders	• Chagas disease • Rheumatic heart disease • Polio	• STD (including HIV) • Leprosy • Dental disease	• Malnutrition • Malaria • Gastroenteritis • Acute respiratory infections
	• Alcohol abuse • Other substance abuse • Injuries		• Tobacco use • Poor diet • Lack of exercise • Unsafe sexual practices	

Healthy children who become healthy adolescents are more likely to become healthy adults.

As children grow and become adolescents they demonstrate growing autonomy, and their decisions, behaviours and relationships increasingly determine their health and development. Yet while their self-reliance increases with age, older children and adolescents lack the status and resources of adults. This limits the range of health-related options open to them. An important feature that distinguishes them from adults is the initiation of risk behaviour. Adolescence is a time of experimentation. The transition from early childhood to maturity involves many hazards, some of which are increasing, and others that are new.

Some health problems, conditions and behaviours are more prevalent among older children and adolescents than other age groups, and may influence their future health (*Table 6*).

Varying in prevalence from one country to another, these include maternity; sexually transmitted diseases, including HIV; other infectious diseases such as tuberculosis, schistosomiasis and helminth infection; mental health; substance abuse; injuries and suicide attempts.

Many of these are issues in developed and developing countries alike, and thus risk affecting all the adults of tomorrow. For these reasons, the health of this age group deserves more attention than it has received in the past. For while relatively few are likely to die at this age, many more may begin high-risk behaviours that continue into adulthood and ultimately increase their risk of premature death. The most obvious of these is tobacco use. Worldwide, most smokers begin before they are 19. It is also at about this time that other hazardous patterns may be established, such as poor nutrition, and alcohol and drug abuse. However, the

5-19-year period is also a time when health-related knowledge, skills, attitudes and values can be acquired. It is a long and unique period of continuous opportunity for public health intervention.

The 5-19 age group represented almost 30% of the total world population of 5.8 billion in 1997. By 2025, that proportion is projected to become one-quarter of a total population of 8 billion. Many of these youngsters – 25% – will be in Africa. It is expected that around 20% of the total population of the Americas, Asia and Europe will be aged 5-19 in 2020.

Only limited data exist on the **causes of death** for the age group 5-19 by region or for individual countries. The age groups tabulated are 5-14 and 15-24. For every country with reliable data, the death rate for young persons aged 5-19 is the lowest of any age group. While the risk of death is low, the available data show that in most countries, many of the leading causes of death are preventable, especially deaths related to intentional and unintentional injury. The leading cause of death for 5-14-year-olds varies by country and gender.

Age at first marriage is one of the most important factors influencing **adolescent fertility**. Populations with later age at first marriage tend to be more urban, have higher levels of education for women, and use family planning more than populations with younger age at first marriage. The percentage of women marrying before age 20 is declining in most countries in the world. However, early age at first marriage is still common in sub-Saharan Africa, where over 40% of women aged 15-19 have been married in many of the countries. The proportion of births to adolescent women that are unplanned is over one-third in 11 of 20 countries with reported data in sub-Saharan Africa and in 7 of 10 countries with reported data in Latin America and the Caribbean. The range is 9-48% in Asia and 20-52% in Latin America and the Caribbean; and the proportion is very high in the United States (73%).

Adolescents aged 15-19 gave birth to 17 million babies in 1997, and 16 million of these births occurred in developing countries in Asia, Africa, and Latin America and the Caribbean. In sub-Saharan Africa, Latin America and the Caribbean, only modest declines are being reported in age at first birth. All countries in Asia report a decline. More than 30% of women aged 20-24 in Latin America and the Caribbean and 50-60% of women aged 20-24 in most of sub-Saharan Africa have their first birth before age 20. Adolescent fertility increases risks for both the mother and the child. For the adolescent, pregnancy is associated with increased risk of numerous pregnancy-related complications and higher maternal mortality. Adolescent mothers tend to discontinue their education and thus reduce their employment options. Their children are more likely to have a low birth weight, to be premature, injured at birth, or stillborn. The mortality rates of infants born to adolescent mothers are higher than for those of women who give birth at older ages. If projections hold however, by 2025 the adolescent fertility rate will have declined by about 40% in Africa, and 16% in Latin America and the Caribbean, although Africa will continue to have the largest adolescent fertility rate of any region (76 per 1000 women). The rate is expected to increase by 20% in Europe, and 8% in North America. Among the 10 largest countries, the highest rate will be in Ethiopia (96 per 1000 women), and the lowest is expected to continue to be in China (6 per 1000 women). The number of births to women aged

> The percentage of women marrying before age 20 is declining in most countries.

15-19 is expected to decrease from 17 million in 1997 to 16 million in 2025.

The rates of completing three years of *schooling* increased between 1987 and 1993, but some countries still have close to 50% dropping out sooner. While there are now generally higher enrolment rates for young people, some areas remain where enrolment has not yet reached 50%. Most countries have similar enrolment rates for boys and girls. Women currently aged 15-19 are at least two to three times more likely than women currently aged 40-44 to have at least seven years of education. The increase in education level was found in almost all countries in sub-Saharan Africa and in all countries in North Africa and the Eastern Mediterranean, in Latin America and the Caribbean. In the developed countries almost all women aged 15-19 had seven or more years of schooling.

Unhealthy sexuality and its consequences

Sexual debut is taking place at younger ages, despite later marriages. Sexual experience before marriage is becoming more common, as are its consequences including sexually transmitted diseases (STDs) and pregnancy. Men are more likely to have sexual experience prior to marriage than women. The age of initiation of sexual activity is less than 18 in most countries of sub-Saharan Africa and around 20 years in Asia, Latin America and the Caribbean. In the United States, it is 16 years for male students and 17 for female students.

Contraceptive use has increased in most countries over the past 20-25 years, as family planning services have become more readily available, but has decreased in some others. Trends in contraceptive use among currently married adolescent women vary by region. Of 13 countries in sub-Saharan Africa with available data, eight reported increases in use over time, and five had decreases. Of 11 countries in Asia, contraceptive use among currently married women aged 15-19 increased over time dramatically in eight, with little change in India, Nepal, and Pakistan. Eleven out of 14 countries in Latin America and the Caribbean showed an increase in use. Sub-Saharan Africa generally had the lowest, and Latin America and the Caribbean the highest levels of use.

As regards the contraceptive methods used by adolescents, a recent study in the United States found that young female students (aged around 15) prefer to use condoms. However, as female students become older, they are gradually less likely to use condoms and more likely to use birth control pills. While overall contraceptive use does not change, use of birth control pills more than doubles and condom use declines by over 30%. At the same time, current sexual activity increases from almost one-quarter around age 15 to almost half around age 18. This appears to signify a change in priority from protection against STDs, including HIV infection, to protection against unplanned pregnancy. Few students appear to be giving high priority to reducing the risk of both unplanned pregnancy and STD infection by using more than one effective contraceptive method, specifically condoms and birth control pills.

WHO estimates that one in 20 teenagers contracts a *sexually transmitted disease* each year. These include HIV/AIDS, gonorrhoea, syphilis, chlamydial infection and herpes. Young people are less likely to seek care for STDs, especially while they are asymptomatic, and the consequences of the delay or absence of

Sexual debut

is taking place

at younger ages,

despite later

marriages.

care can have permanent health effects including sterility and death. The prevalence patterns for STDs in developing countries are up to 100 times those in developed countries for syphilis, 10-15 times higher for gonorrhoea, and 3 times higher for chlamydial infection. Incidence is also higher in developing countries. Among developing countries the rates in Africa are generally higher than those of Asia and Latin America. Human papilloma virus (HPV) can result in cervical cancer 5-30 years after the initial infection. The risk of getting HPV and cervical cancer in those who had intercourse around age 15 has been shown to be double the risk in those who do so after 20.

In 1997, 590 000 children under 15 became infected with **HIV**, bringing the total of those aged up to 15 infected to 1.1 million. One contributing factor is that 1 million children enter the sex trade every year. In most parts of the world, the majority of new infections are in young people between the ages of 15 and 24, sometimes younger. Girls appear to be especially vulnerable to infection, but Uganda has recently shown encouraging evidence that in some cities infection rates have halved among adolescent girls since 1990. Even there, however, rates remain unacceptably high, with up to 1 pregnant teenager in 10 testing HIV-positive. That rate is six times higher than in boys of the same age. These age and sex patterns are thought to be related to young women having older sexual partners, and the increased susceptibility of the immature female reproductive tract to infection. Because the median incubation period between infection with HIV and onset of AIDS is nearly 10 years, many 20-29-year-olds with AIDS may have been infected during adolescence. Surveillance of selected sexual and injecting-drug-use behaviours among adolescents can provide critical information about their risk of acquiring HIV infection.

Substance abuse and its consequences

Adolescence and young adulthood are the periods most associated with the onset of *illicit drug use* worldwide. A European study on drug abuse in 13 cities found that by age 18 more than 20% had tried cannabis. Solvent use is reported in higher proportions among the under-15s. A study in the United States found that the period of highest risk for cannabis initiation was generally over by age 20, having peaked at 18. Cocaine initiation peaks later, between 21 and 24. Age patterns in Asia and Latin America are slightly different, although inhalant abuse is always concentrated among the youngest age group. In Thailand consumers of solvents are generally 15-19 years old. In Pakistan the age of onset of heroin use is just over 12, but cannabis is more widespread among those under 20. Research suggests that adolescents most prone to drug use are concerned with personal autonomy, are uninterested in conventional goals and receive less parental support and more support from friends. Peer use of the substance is a primary influence, and early onset of use is associated with more intense and wider use of other drugs later. A Brazilian survey of drug use in high school students found that violence in the home was the factor most frequently associated with the use of drugs. Young people who cannot see jobs or a better quality of life in their future sometimes use drugs to counteract extreme despair and frustration. The glamorization of drug use through association with pop music culture, television and film portrayals has been noted in some countries.

In 1996, 400 000 children under 15 became infected with HIV.

The age of initiation to injectables is falling in certain population subgroups, such as street children, including those in inner cities of developed countries. In Pakistan the share of those who started using heroin between 15 and 20 years of age is reported to have doubled to 24% of those surveyed. In the Czech Republic 37% of new problem users are aged between 15 and 19, as are 50% of drug addicts in Bratislava, Slovakia. In Bulgaria the age of initiation has fallen from around 18 in the mid-1970s to 15 for heroin and 12 or younger for volatile substances. This pattern also occurs in the United Kingdom, where a survey found that 50% of 16-year-olds in north-western England had tried illicit drugs, and 20% were considered current users. In the United States, the average age for cannabis initiation is around 14 years, and approximately 2% of high school students have reported that they had injected illegal drugs. Male students are more likely than female students to report this behaviour.

Excessive *alcohol drinking* is likely to lead to traffic accidents, injury-related death and disability, and over time, serious degenerative disease of the liver. At least half of those who report drinking started before the age of 15, and a large portion of these started earlier than 12. In studies of high school students in Ghana, Kenya and Zambia, prevalence of drinking was 70-80%. A study of high school students in the United States showed that during 1990-1995 the proportion who had drunk alcohol on one or more of the past 30 days, declined from 59% to 52%, while the proportion who had five or more drinks of alcohol on at least one occasion on one or more of the 30 days preceding the survey declined from 37% to 33% during the same period.

Various studies report that the majority of smokers began *smoking* by the age of 19; in some cases the majority of smokers had adopted the habit by 12 years of age. More boys tend to smoke than girls. In North America, about 20-30% of young people smoke. Given the health consequences, there is a clear need for smoking cessation initiatives targeted towards young people.

Depression and suicide

Adolescence is not an easy time psychosocially, and adjustment indicators are important. The Health of Youth study carried out in European countries found that depression, or the percentage of those reporting that they felt depressed once a week or more, was more common in boys than in girls, and varied considerably among countries. The first symptoms of mental illness emerge before the age of 25, for half of those who will be affected by it. The effects of unipolar depression and bipolar disorder have recently emerged as important, and can lead to problems in social interaction and to suicide in extreme cases.

Deaths from suicide are underreported because of a tendency to group them as accidental deaths or deaths from undetermined causes. Currently information is collected on suicides and parasuicidal acts (deliberate acts with non-fatal outcomes that attempt to cause or actually cause self-harm). In 10 community survey studies on adolescents published since 1986, the yearly prevalence of parasuicidal acts varied between over 2% and 20%. The differences in rates are due to different definitions and measurement issues. The prevalence of parasuicide is estimated to be 10-20 times higher than that of completed suicides. Three times more women than men attempt suicide, while three times more men than women succeed.

Given the health consequences, there is a clear need for smoking cessation initiatives targeted towards young people.

Injuries

Mortality rates due to injury are higher for men than for women. For example, adolescent men aged 15-19 in South Africa are up to 2.5 times as likely to die from violent injuries as are women in the same age group. In the same country, injuries account for 57% of all deaths among 10-19-year-olds. A similar pattern holds for many developing and developed countries. Unintentional injuries such as those resulting from sports, falls and especially traffic accidents, are important causes of death in Nigeria, Singapore and the United States, for example. Other countries have a higher number of intentional injuries that result in death (e.g. some Latin American countries). Injuries happen less at home and more in sports contexts or school after age 11. Boys tend to have higher rates of injury, and more broken bones, than girls. Women are at risk of violence from men they know, often their husband, partner, or ex-partner. In countries where reliable large-scale studies have been carried out, 20-67% of women report being assaulted by the man with whom they live.

Unhealthy nutrition and its consequences

In developing countries, commonly used measures include **stunting**, which refers to being below the fifth percentile of the WHO height-for-age distribution. Stunting was found to have a prevalence of 27-65% in nine out of 11 studies. It occurs in early childhood, when rapid growth should normally occur. Children who are already stunted when they reach adolescence tend not to improve during adolescence. Furthermore, there appears to be a tendency for smallness to be perpetuated across generations.

Thinness, or being below the fifth percentile of the WHO Body Mass Index (BMI) distribution for age, was only found to be prevalent in three studies. Its prevalence was 23-53% and in seven out of eight studies it was twice as prevalent in boys as in girls. BMI improved in girls throughout adolescence, but improved only in boys who had a low BMI at 10 years of age. This may be due to the delay of maturation caused by malnutrition, which is longer for boys than for girls.

Anaemia was identified as a very common nutritional problem in four out of six studies in which it was assessed (32-55%). While girls lose more iron through menstruation, boys may need more iron per kilogram of weight gained as they develop relatively more muscle during adolescence. It is possible that anaemia is responsible for the higher thinness rates in boys, although iron status does improve for boys as growth slows, and it deteriorates for girls, especially if they become pregnant. The consequences of iron deficiency are more serious for women, and they can include reduced levels of energy and productivity, impaired immune function, and increased maternal morbidity and mortality. Iron deficiency anaemia can be due to lack of iron in the diet, poor absorption of iron from food, or significant blood loss at delivery or because of hookworm infection. This is the most common type of anaemia. Causes of non-iron-deficient anaemia include malaria, thalassaemia, and sickle-cell disease. Iron deficiency has a lower threshold, and as a result is prevalent in 82% of 5-14-year-olds. Anaemia affects about half of the 5-14-year-olds in certain regions. The established and emerging market economies have the lowest prevalence of anaemia, followed by the Caribbean. In all other places, every third child is anaemic. Measures that can improve the situation

> Women are at risk
>
> of violence from
>
> men they know,
>
> often their husband,
>
> partner, or ex-partner.

Tuberculosis

has re-emerged

as a major disease

in young people in

developing countries.

include vitamin A, iron, iodine and folate supplementation or fortification, delaying childbearing, and enhancing early childhood growth (6-18 months).

Eating disorders such as anorexia nervosa, bulimia and overeating are more common in the developed countries, as are inactivity and a sedentary lifestyle. In developing countries, the problems are mainly those of obtaining the right nutrients for optimal growth, while daily life tends to include more physical activity.

The extent to which young people are involved in physical activity is a growing concern in developed countries. ***Obesity*** is increasing, especially in the younger age group. Nutritional problems, especially overconsumption of fats or sugars, are taking their toll. The Health of Youth study found that an average of 74% of 15-year-old boys exercised to the point of being out of breath and sweating more than twice a week outside school. Only 52% of girls exercised twice a week, and between the ages of 11 and 15, girls became less active.

Diseases of concern for young people

Intestinal parasites are endemic in many developing areas. Treatment of helminth infection (trichuriasis, ascariasis) improves school performance. The prevalence of hookworm infection peaks around the age of 15. Because of the potential blood loss it causes, it can exacerbate anaemia in those whose diet contains inadequate iron.

While deaths from ***malaria*** tend to occur before the age of 5, the disease takes its toll on the young working population because of its recurrent nature, and contributes to absence from work and school. Cerebral malaria is becoming more and more common in adolescents, perhaps due

to decreased immunity, increased drug resistance, or the use of counterfeit drugs. Malaria is particularly destructive for young pregnant women as it exacerbates anaemia.

Schistosomiasis is the second most prevalent tropical parasitic disease after malaria. As transmission occurs through contact with water contaminated by infected snails, prevalence is highest in young people because of the contact they have with water sources: women fetching water and men swimming. In some African countries schistosomiasis is so common in young men that it is considered to be a sign of passage into adolescence. In young women, as well as causing anaemia it can result in social stigma which reduces chances of marriage. Detection is essential, since a single-dose treatment exists.

Tuberculosis has re-emerged as a major disease in young people in developing countries. If untreated, it can be fatal, and it tends to be more aggressive in this age group, leading from infection to development of the disease sooner. For example, the incidence of tuberculosis among 15-24-year-olds in the United Republic of Tanzania is 14% of the total number of new cases, and 11% of tuberculosis-related deaths occur in this age group.

Vaccine-preventable diseases

As a result of immunization programmes, about 8 out of 10 school-age children and adolescents worldwide have been immunized against six major infectious diseases of childhood. Immunization schedules for basic vaccines vary among different countries. Many boosters are recommended during the school-age period. For example, boosters for BCG have been suggested in many countries at ages 5-7 and 11-14. A tetanus booster is recommended during adolescence, especially for pregnant women, and oral polio is also usually given once during school age. Recent studies on immunization in adolescents have focused on mass campaigns that target this age group, especially concerning hepatitis B.

Young people at special risk

The International Labour Organization estimates the number of **working children** aged between 5 and 14 at 120 million. The majority of these children are in developing countries (61% in Asia, 32% in Africa, 7% in Latin America). In many of these countries, children are traditionally incorporated into the work of their families as soon as they are capable, mostly on farms.

However, many millions of children are forced to seek employment outside the family. Studies indicate that in about 20% of cases, the child's income may be essential to an impoverished family's survival. The United Nations Economic Commission for Latin America and the Caribbean has reported that without the income of working adolescents aged 13-17 years, the incidence of poverty in that region would rise by 10-20%. Thus, many children can be found in hazardous industries, working long hours without rest, in conditions that are physically or mentally dangerous. They are at risk of occupational death or injury due to poor or non-existent safety standards, inattention, fatigue, poor judgement and inexperience in workplaces that have been designed for adults.

In developing countries, exposure to chemicals, especially pesticides, kills more rural children than the most common childhood diseases combined. Research shows that working children are six times more likely to be admitted to hospital than non-working children.

In the past decade an estimated 2 million children and young people have been killed in **armed conflict**, and three times that number have been seriously injured or permanently disabled. By the year 2000, at least 120 million young people could be vulnerable to the indirect effects of armed conflict. More than half of this estimate is made up by the risk in Africa and South-East Asia.

WHO's response

Regrettably, there are few data in most regions of the world on the health status of young people from the age of 5 to 19 years, on age-specific mortality and the leading causes of death, and on the underlying determinants. The available data are insufficient to assess fully the trends in this age group, but the preceding section highlights some areas that are priorities for WHO and for the response of the international community. Approaches traditionally used to prevent health problems and respond to them when they arise in adults, are not always effective in younger people.

For the past 30 years, WHO has been striving to bring adolescent health and development to the forefront in international public health. The main objective has been to expand the knowledge base for adolescent health and development, to understand the meaning, parameters and status of adolescent physical, psychological and social health, and to elucidate the specific actions that will promote the health and development of young people in all societies. The main results so far have been the dissemination of vital information, and publicizing priority needs.

In 1989, WHO was instrumental in bringing together the health and youth sectors in countries from all regions. Since then, a number of

In the past decade an estimated 2 million children and young people have been killed in armed conflict.

The full range

of interventions

for adolescent health

is not yet developed.

databases on major health issues in young people have been established, including on reproductive health. Considerable effort has been invested in expanding the knowledge base for adolescent health and development. For example, a WHO technical report resulted from a WHO/UNFPA/UNICEF study group which met in 1995 to review the evidence of key interventions used in programming for adolescent health. It described the current extent of experience in countries, and highlighted the essential factors and strategies needed to establish, implement and sustain adolescent health programmes. The report aims to provide substantive guidance and reference material useful for programme development in countries.

In parallel with this and in order to bridge the gap between advocacy and action, WHO has developed a series of methods specially adapted for use in the area of adolescent health. All are based upon the central principle of eliciting knowledge directly from young people and adults on their expressed needs and on solutions to their problems which will work.

The full range of interventions for adolescent health is not yet developed. In recent years, emphasis has been placed on supporting efforts that enable adolescents to build life skills. Counselling has been accepted as an important intervention, but the provision of health services to adolescents has received scant attention. Capacity for monitoring progress at the programme implementation level is limited. Weaknesses are difficult to document, and available information is not systematically used or valued. Frequently the measures of impact, such as reducing adolescent pregnancy or substance use, cannot be firmly established as an outcome of a single intervention. Technical resources to

support new programming initiatives in countries are insufficient.

Questions from countries abound – related to statistics and research findings needed to make the case for programme activities and seeking examples from other countries demonstrating promising approaches to inspire new ideas and confirm current directions. These demands cannot always be met because sound programme support materials and resource people are not readily available.

The increased attention to adolescent health has resulted in a burgeoning of projects in developing countries, often focused on single health issues. When resources are limited, efforts focusing on what is perceived as the single most important health problem affecting adolescents in the area, may seem to be meeting the most pressing need. However, there are good technical as well as practical reasons to deal with several related health issues in an integrated manner.

The need to modify approaches to meet the special needs of adolescents is further illustrated by problems associated with the diagnosis and treatment of tuberculosis. WHO is strongly advocating the expanded use of daily observed treatment of short-course chemotherapy regimens (DOTS), as a means to ensure that individuals diagnosed with the disease complete their treatment. Unfortunately, adolescents are generally considered to comply poorly with therapeutic regimens due to factors such as increased autonomy from family and limited resources available to them. The challenge facing individual clinicians and national tuberculosis programmes alike is to determine how best to improve compliance, and to ensure that adolescent patients do in fact take the medications that they need.

WHO has helped Member States to develop and test a range of epidemiological and qualitative guidelines and methodologies to assess the extent and nature of psychoactive substance use, and to develop effective interventions. A consolidated epidemiological manual has been prepared so that Member States can develop standardized instruments and methodologies for data collection, analysis and dissemination.

WHO has already published a first global status report on tobacco or health and provides continuous support to Member States in strengthening national tobacco control. A first draft of the global report on alcohol and public health was prepared in 1997, and work has started on an international framework convention on tobacco control. The finalization of the international framework convention on tobacco control in the year 2000 is expected to establish effective mechanisms for the implementation of national and international tobacco control.

Health education

The key to promoting health in children of school age and adolescents is education. The best opportunities for positively influencing the health of this age group are found in the school (*Box 15*). A WHO Expert Committee on Comprehensive School Health Education and Promotion noted in 1995 that promoting health through schools could simultaneously reduce common health problems; increase the efficiency of the education system; and thus advance public health, education, social and economic development. As a result of the Committee's work, the WHO Global School Health Initiative made 10 recommendations, of which three are most likely to have a direct effect on health.

Firstly, the school environment must provide safe water and sanitary facilities; protect from infectious dis-

---

Box 15. School health guidelines

The Division of Adolescent and School Health of the United States Centers for Disease Control and Prevention, has developed three sets of guidelines that identify the most effective policies and programmes that schools can implement in order to promote healthy choices related to tobacco, nutrition, and physical activity: *Guidelines for school health programmes to prevent tobacco use and addiction* (published in 1994), *Guidelines for school health programmes to promote lifelong healthy eating*, and *Guidelines for school and community health programmes to promote physical activity* (1996). These guidelines were developed through exhaustive reviews of published research and exemplary practice, as well as collaboration with academic experts and over 50 national, federal, and voluntary organizations involved in child and adolescent health.

The guidelines include specific recommendations to help states, districts, and schools implement health promotion programmes and policies that have been found to be most effective in promoting healthy eating and physical activity patterns, and preventing tobacco use, among youth. Recommendations cover topics such as policy development, curriculum selection, instructional strategies, staff training, family and community involvement, and programme evaluation. The guidelines also cover the scientific rationale for school-based chronic disease prevention programmes, as well as how and why these programmes should be delivered within the framework of a comprehensive school health programme.

Target audiences for the guidelines include parents, classroom and physical education teachers, coaches, food service staff, substance abuse prevention staff, school administrators and board members, curriculum developers, textbook publishers, staff development specialists, staff of teacher training institutions, public health and social services professionals, and community-based sport and recreation professionals.

For further information on School Guidelines contact: DASH Inquires, Division of Adolescent and School Health, National Center for Chronic Disease Prevention and Health Promotion, Centers for Disease Control and Prevention, Mail Stop K-32, 4770 Buford Highway, NE, Atlanta, Georgia, USA, or electronic mail at www.cdc.gov/nccdphp/dash.

---

eases; protect from discrimination, harassment, abuse and violence; and reject the use of tobacco, alcohol and illicit drugs.

Secondly, every school must enable children and adolescents at all levels to learn vital skills. Health education should include topics such as infectious diseases, nutrition, preventive health care and reproductive health and should enable young people to protect the well-being of the families for which they will eventually become responsible and the communities in which they reside. Life skills education should help them make healthy choices and adopt healthy behaviour throughout their lives.

Thirdly, every school should prevent when possible, treat when effective, and refer when necessary, common health problems. Schools should provide safe and nutritious food and micronutrients to combat hunger, prevent disease, and foster growth and development. They should establish prevention programmes to reduce the use of tobacco, alcohol and illicit drugs, and behaviour that promotes the spread of HIV infection. They should when possible identify and treat infections, and oral, vision and hearing problems and psychological problems, and refer those affected for appropriate treatment.

Education is the foundation for the future success of the young, as without basic literacy and numeracy the potential for individual development is drastically reduced. As the 5-19 population increases in developing countries over the next 20-30 years, continuing efforts will be needed to increase enrolment in education. The potential for distinction, necessary in defining a young person as autonomous, can come either through excellence in school, sports and other activities, or through unhealthy risk behaviours. Those deriving self-esteem from the positive activities are less likely to seek status through smoking, drinking and drugs.

Delaying the initiation of drinking alcohol, smoking and pregnancy at least until closer to the end of the teenage years should be encouraged through education, parental guidance, health promotion and legislation. More physical exercise and improved nutrition should also be promoted in this age group. In areas where there are high prevalences of

malnutrition, anaemia and helminth infection in children, fortification of foods with iron and micronutrients and anti-helminth treatment should be a priority.

The health of 5-19-year-olds can be protected by restricting their access to tobacco, especially cigarettes. Legislation should be passed to ban the sale of tobacco products to children, and school-based training programmes on the prevention of tobacco use should be more widely introduced. The most successful anti-smoking programmes are those which are oriented to the developmental needs of adolescents, emphasizing the physical and social consequences of smoking and preparing adolescents to resist the social pressure they face from their peers and others.

Fostering respect between young men and women is another priority, essential in shaping the lives of the young and developing strong family units. Family structure is central to their present and future health, and family communication is a determinant of healthy choices. It is particularly important to increase knowledge among adolescents about the value of condoms in giving dual protection from unplanned pregnancies and from sexually transmitted diseases, including HIV. These educational efforts must be made well before they reach the age of 15.

Adults

The expansion of the adult population is one of the most important of the demographic changes now occurring. Those aged between 20 and 64 years represent just over half of all the people in the world, and are expected to account for 58% by 2025. At the same time, the proportion of older people needing support from working-age adults is forecast to increase from about 12% in 1995 to about 17% in 2025.

The young and old of all societies look to adults to provide and care for them. In their working years, adults produce and deliver almost all the essential goods and services that the world consumes. By working, adults earn the means to support their children and their aged relatives. The better the health of the adult population, the greater is its ability to play this vital role, and the better is the health of society as a whole.

This is particularly true of women, whose health critically affects that of their children and of future generations. Women's health receives special attention in both this section and the following section on the health of older people.

Adults aged 20-64 are the chief beneficiaries of the improvements in life expectancy that have occurred in the past 50 years. Between 1955 and 1995, death rates among them declined by 50%. Most people who have reached the age of 20 have a very good chance of surviving beyond the age of 65. In 1955, only 61% of 20-year-olds could expect to reach 65; in 1995 78% could, and by 2025, 85% will.

Leading causes of death

However, this optimistic picture should not obscure the fact that in 1997, there were about 15.4 million deaths among those aged 20-64. All of these deaths can be described as premature. Apart from the human losses to families and dependants, they also constitute a huge loss of economic productivity. The majority of them are preventable. For society's well-being, prevention must be the priority.

Most of these deaths are due to chronic noncommunicable diseases – circulatory diseases, cancers, chronic obstructive pulmonary disease, and diabetes – for which there are well-known risk factors. The most important are tobacco smoking and unhealthy diet. Obesity is becoming one of the most important contributors to ill-health. Heavy alcohol consumption increases the risk of developing some cancers and mental disorders, injuries and cirrhosis of the liver.

Among communicable diseases, tuberculosis, HIV/AIDS, and acute lower respiratory infections are the leading killers.

All of these diseases, infectious and noninfectious, are also major causes of illness and disability. Most of the estimated 1 million yearly deaths due to external causes (such as suicide or occupational injuries) involve adults. Pregnancy-related causes kill 585 000 women a year. Huge numbers of women suffer from domestic and other forms of violence ranging from rape to genital mutilation.

Circulatory diseases

Diseases of the heart and circulation – cardiovascular and cerebrovascular – are for most adults the biggest risks to life. They account for at least 15 million deaths, or around 30% of the annual total, every year. Many who die of circulatory diseases are under the age of 65. Many millions more are disabled by them.

Circulatory diseases are responsible for more than 5 out of 12 million deaths in developed countries, and are rapidly emerging as a major public health concern in most developing countries. They already account for 10 million out of 40 million deaths in the developing world. The most important circulatory diseases are high blood pressure (hypertension), coronary heart disease and cerebrovascular disease. Worldwide, there are more deaths from coronary heart disease (7.2 million) than stroke (4.6 million).

In 1997, there were about 15.4 million deaths among those aged 20-64.

Box 16. Stroke - Destiny or challenge?

Over the past 35-40 years a decline in stroke mortality has been observed in 25 countries, most substantially in Japan, North America, and western Europe, with an acceleration in this decline in the mid-1970s. In contrast, stroke mortality has increased in eastern European countries. There is evidence that stroke is increasing in many developing countries, especially in those where hypertension has become a major public health problem.

Although the reasons for the recent decline in stroke mortality are not fully understood, there is some evidence that both improvements in case-fatality rates (survival after stroke) and in attack rates (the occurrence of the event itself) have caused the improvements in stroke mortality. The limited available evidence suggests that a decline in case-fatality may be related to decreased severity of the disease, with the acute event becoming more mild. Improved management in the acute phase may also have contributed. Declining stroke rates have been attributed in part to improved hypertension control, and increasing stroke incidence has conversely been considered a likely effect of deteriorating lifestyle factors in the population.

The widespread belief that the total burden of stroke is diminishing is mistaken however, because the total number of persons in the older population is increasing as is the proportion of people surviving an acute stroke with disabilities. Stroke will present a formidable humanitarian and economic problem if effective prevention and control measures are not implemented.

Control of hypertension and smoking cessation are most important for stroke prevention. Even modest blood pressure reduction in hypertensive people could reduce stroke events worldwide by half. Further efforts to improve hypertension control are warranted in almost all populations. This requires both more effective drug treatment and non-pharmacological measures to prevent and control high blood pressure.

In many industrialized countries *coronary heart disease* death rates peaked in the 1960s and early 1970s and have since declined dramatically. In Australia, New Zealand and the United States, for example, deaths from coronary heart disease have fallen by more than 50% since the mid-1960s. But this condition is now becoming more frequent in developing countries as their populations age and adopt unhealthy habits and behaviours. The major risk factors are high blood pressure, cigarette smoking, unhealthy diet, lack of physical activity and diabetes.

Cigarette smoking is the most readily preventable risk factor. It causes 17% of all cardiovascular deaths, mostly in people over 65, and accounts for 23% of all cardiovascular morbidity in people under 45. Another important risk factor, high blood cholesterol levels, can be reduced by modifying the diet or by medicaments.

Among circulatory diseases, stroke and other *cerebrovascular diseases* are the second most common cause of death, accounting for more than 4.6 million deaths worldwide. Morbidity and mortality occur mainly in the over-65 age group. High blood pressure, affecting about 20% of the adult population, both in the developed and developing world, is the most important risk factor for stroke *(Box 16)*. Even modest blood pressure reduction in hypertensive people could prevent half of the stroke events worldwide. Other major risk factors mentioned above in the context of coronary heart disease are equally important for cerebrovascular disease, in particular smoking. Alcohol consumption also increases the risk.

Cancer

Cancer of the lung was the highest-ranking cancer in 1997, both for the total population and for the population aged 15 to 64. The most significant global trends in cancer mortality are listed below. Certain cancers are dealt with at greater length in the women's part of this section and its counterpart in the section on older people. *Fig. 10* shows the burden of cancer in 1997.

Long-term trends in survival are available only for the United States and some European countries, which are experiencing an overall improvement that is more marked in males. In 1990, the prognosis for cancer at a given stage was similar in all affluent countries. A study of survival in some developing countries has shown sig-

Fig. 10. The burden of cancer, 1997

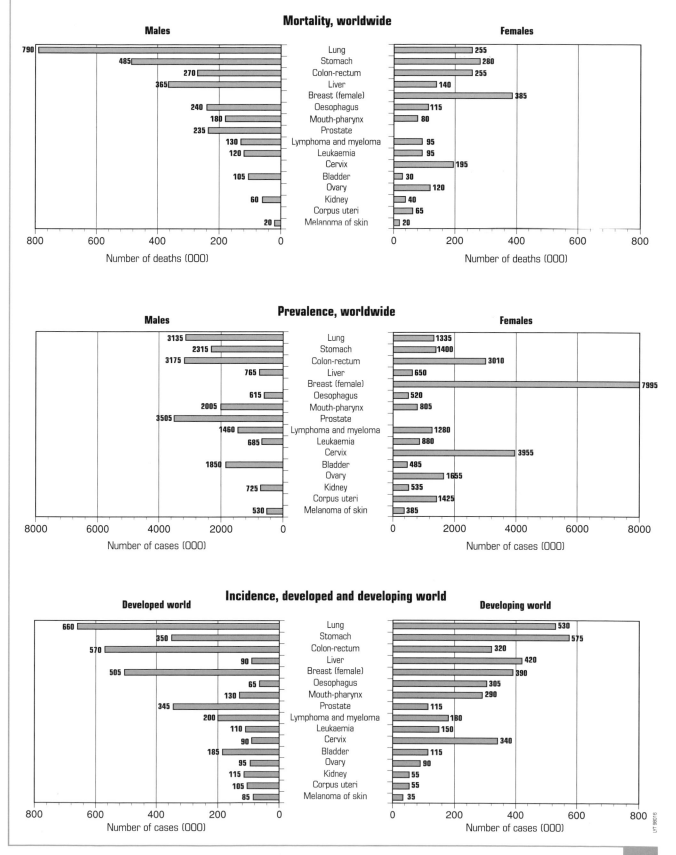

Mortality, worldwide

Males | **Females**

	Males	Females
Lung	790	255
Stomach	485	280
Colon-rectum	270	255
Liver	365	140
Breast (female)		385
Oesophagus	240	115
Mouth-pharynx	180	80
Prostate	235	
Lymphoma and myeloma	130	95
Leukaemia	120	95
Cervix		195
Bladder	105	30
Ovary		120
Kidney	60	40
Corpus uteri		65
Melanoma of skin	20	20

Number of deaths (000)

Prevalence, worldwide

Males | **Females**

	Males	Females
Lung	3135	1335
Stomach	2315	1400
Colon-rectum	3175	3010
Liver	765	650
Breast (female)		7995
Oesophagus	615	520
Mouth-pharynx	2005	805
Prostate	3505	
Lymphoma and myeloma	1460	1280
Leukaemia	685	880
Cervix		3955
Bladder	1850	485
Ovary		1655
Kidney	725	535
Corpus uteri		1425
Melanoma of skin	530	385

Number of cases (000)

Incidence, developed and developing world

Developed world | **Developing world**

	Developed world	Developing world
Lung	660	530
Stomach	350	575
Colon-rectum	570	320
Liver	90	420
Breast (female)	505	390
Oesophagus	65	305
Mouth-pharynx	130	290
Prostate	345	115
Lymphoma and myeloma	200	180
Leukaemia	110	150
Cervix	90	340
Bladder	185	115
Ovary	95	90
Kidney	115	55
Corpus uteri	105	55
Melanoma of skin	85	35

Number of cases (000)

nificantly lower survival for those tumours which are curable but require expensive drugs or technology coupled with specific expertise. Examples are lymphomas, leukaemias and cancer of the testes; also, breast cancer mortality is more elevated than would be predicted from incidence. Poor prognosis indicates lack of appropriate treatment.

In men, the effect of smoking still determines the high risk of dying from **lung cancer** in developed countries. However, incidence and mortality are declining among the young generations in rich countries, with very few exceptions (such as France, Japan and Spain). Mortality is falling in men in the United States, and began to fall in the European Union in 1985. On the other hand, a continuing rise is foreseen in Asia and Latin America. In women, mortality is on the rise in almost all developed countries, with the exception of Ireland and the United Kingdom.

Mortality from **stomach cancer** has declined and it no longer ranks first among world cancer deaths.

Incidence of **breast cancer** is increasing in the intermediate or low-risk populations (Asia, eastern and southern Europe and Latin America). In high-risk countries such as those in northern and north-western Europe, Australia, New Zealand and North America, there was a real increase until the late 1980s, after which the introduction of breast screening has modified the picture.

The incidence of **colorectal cancer** increases along with economic development. In rich countries, early diagnosis and improved survival keep mortality in control. However, screening will not be widely available in many countries currently at intermediate risk (in eastern Europe and Latin America) where the incidence is on the rise. It is possible, therefore, to predict a general parallel increase

of mortality rates in the near future.

Incidence of **prostate cancer** increased dramatically in developed countries after a cheap screening test (prostate-specific antigens) became available. However, mortality is increasing rather slowly, suggesting over-diagnosis and little improvement of prognosis. In the European Union, mortality is expected to increase by some 25% between 1990 and 2010.

Incidence of **lymphoma** is increasing in all developed countries. Due to improved survival, mortality is rising more slowly.

In spite of increasing incidence of **testicular cancer**, mortality is declining, due to substantial improvement in treatment and survival.

Respiratory diseases

Respiratory diseases are second only to cancers as causes of death and disability in adults, and rank among the three principal causes of lost workdays worldwide. Chronic obstructive pulmonary disease – a grouping of chronic bronchitis and emphysema, for which cigarette smoking is the most important risk factor – kills 2.9 million adults a year. At least 15% of middle-aged smokers in developed countries have abnormal lung function.

Asthma is a major chronic airway disorder affecting 155 million people of all ages worldwide. Asthma often appears very early in childhood and if it is inadequately treated, the lifelong consequences can be substantial and disabling. The major burden of asthma falls on the developing world. Increasing prevalence is associated with spreading urbanization, exposure to domestic mites, vehicle exhausts and passive smoking.

Respiratory diseases are second only to cancers as causes of death and disability in adults.

Diabetes

The rising prevalence of diabetes mellitus is closely associated in much of the developing world with industrialization and socioeconomic development. Twenty years ago, diabetes was considered an uncommon disease with an adult prevalence of 1-3% in European and North American populations, and much rarer in developing countries. The extent of its emergence worldwide has become apparent only relatively recently (*Map 7*). WHO estimates that over 143 million persons are now affected.

By 2025, the worldwide total is expected to rise to 300 million persons. This increase will be due mainly to population growth, ageing and urbanization. In 1997, 63% of persons with diabetes were resident in the developing countries. By 2025 this proportion will rise to 76%. In both 1997 and 2025, the three countries with the largest number of persons with diabetes are, and will be China, India, and the United States.

Whereas in developed countries, the greatest number of persons with diabetes are aged 65 years and above, in developing countries, most are aged between 45 and 64. This tendency is expected to accentuate by 2025. In the developing countries, increasingly, people will be affected by diabetes in the most productive period of their lives. Persons developing diabetes at an earlier age have longer in which to develop the long-term complications such as blindness, kidney failure and heart disease.

Although diabetes manifests itself most commonly in adult life, there is growing evidence that its origins lie much earlier and are related to inappropriate dietary patterns and exercise habits. Worldwide, substantial increases in the frequency of obesity are occurring, in many cases at a relatively early age. Obesity is closely related to diabetes.

Map 7. Diabetes mellitus

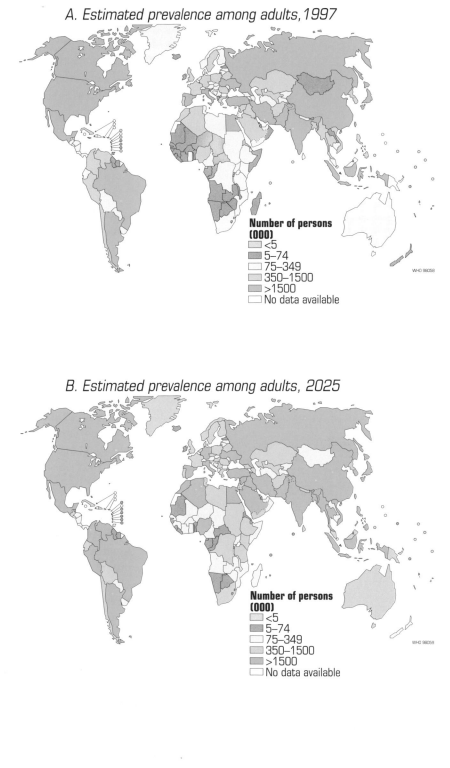

A. Estimated prevalence among adults, 1997

Number of persons (000)
- <5
- 5–74
- 75–349
- 350–1500
- >1500
- No data available

WHO 98058

B. Estimated prevalence among adults, 2025

Number of persons (000)
- <5
- 5–74
- 75–349
- 350–1500
- >1500
- No data available

WHO 98059

Fatal injuries

In 1990 there were almost 2 million violent deaths from homicide, suicide and acts of war: some 820 000 suicides, 560 000 homicides and 500 000 victims of war or civil conflict. In many developed and developing countries, 20-40% of deaths in men aged 15-34 are the result of homicide or suicide.

Chronic rheumatic diseases

Chronic rheumatic diseases (e.g. osteoarthritis, rheumatoid arthritis, low back pain, gout, osteoporosis and other diseases of the joints and soft tissues) are leading causes of disability. In the United States, they are among the most prevalent chronic conditions, affecting approximately 40 million persons in 1995 and a projected 60 million persons in 2020. A 1994 analysis of disability prevalence by age for Australia, Botswana, China and Mauritius showed that the frequency of disability increases roughly 3-5 times between 30-44 and 60-64.

Mental disorders

More working days are lost as a result of mental disorders than physical conditions. Identifying and treating mental disorders therefore not only reduces individual misery, it improves the functioning of the working population.

The diminishing prevalence of mental retardation is attributable to prevention of iodine deficiency in pregnancy and early childhood; to better prenatal diagnosis with tests such as amniocentesis; and to improved antenatal care and delivery practices. Screening of the newborn for the inherited metabolic disorder phenylketonuria, instituted in the 1950s, and for neonatal hypothyroidism, introduced more recently,

have also contributed to lower prevalence.

The most significant developments in mental health care in the past half-century are the more humane attitude to patients and the advent of a broad range of new pharmaceuticals affecting the brain, which have been used in the treatment of previously incurable mental disorders. The greatly diminished number of large mental hospitals is evidence of this trend, as well as the altered approach to psychiatric care.

Mental disorders contribute little to mortality but make a huge contribution to the global burden of disease. Moreover, people with depressive disorders have reduced levels of survival. The management of affective disorders, dementia, schizophrenia, post-traumatic stress, epilepsy, and alcohol and drug abuse consumes a great amount of health care resources.

Depressive disorders appear to be more common in younger age groups, suggesting that these disorders will increase disproportionately. On the other hand, the number of persons with schizophrenia (the frequency of which remains stable over time) will rise in proportion with population growth, particularly in early adulthood, when the disease tends to manifest itself.

The high prevalence of mental illness has resulted in the increased consumption not only of prescription drugs but also of alternative medicines. Abuse of psychoactive drugs and alcohol are rising problems in many countries. WHO has promoted measures to stem the rise, including treatment and rehabilitation policies for those dependent on psychoactive substances and alcohol.

Infectious diseases

In 1997, there were over 7 million new cases of *tuberculosis*, and

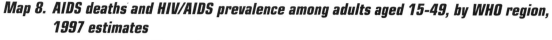

Map 8. AIDS deaths and HIV/AIDS prevalence among adults aged 15-49, by WHO region, 1997 estimates

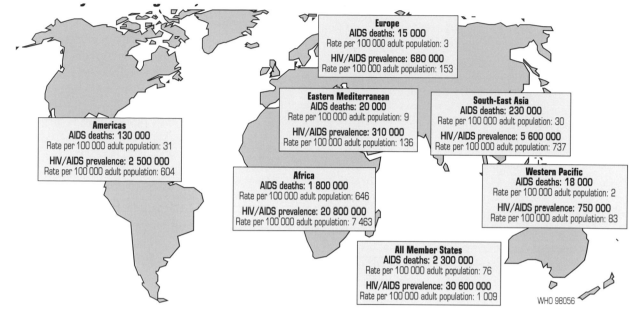

Europe
AIDS deaths: 15 000
Rate per 100 000 adult population: 3

HIV/AIDS prevalence: 680 000
Rate per 100 000 adult population: 153

Eastern Mediterranean
AIDS deaths: 20 000
Rate per 100 000 adult population: 9

HIV/AIDS prevalence: 310 000
Rate per 100 000 adult population: 136

South-East Asia
AIDS deaths: 230 000
Rate per 100 000 adult population: 30

HIV/AIDS prevalence: 5 600 000
Rate per 100 000 adult population: 737

Americas
AIDS deaths: 130 000
Rate per 100 000 adult population: 31

HIV/AIDS prevalence: 2 500 000
Rate per 100 000 adult population: 604

Africa
AIDS deaths: 1 800 000
Rate per 100 000 adult population: 646

HIV/AIDS prevalence: 20 800 000
Rate per 100 000 adult population: 7 463

Western Pacific
AIDS deaths: 18 000
Rate per 100 000 adult population: 2

HIV/AIDS prevalence: 750 000
Rate per 100 000 adult population: 83

All Member States
AIDS deaths: 2 300 000
Rate per 100 000 adult population: 76

HIV/AIDS prevalence: 30 600 000
Rate per 100 000 adult population: 1 009

WHO 98056

around 3 million died of it, making this disease the leading infectious killer of adults.

The disease is being controlled in many parts of the world, however. It has become clear that the DOTS strategy can achieve high cure rates in any country which is determined to succeed. The treatment success rate of cases in DOTS areas was 78%, compared with 45% in non-DOTS areas. The use of DOTS has expanded nearly tenfold in the past five years, cure rates have nearly doubled and drug-resistance is lower in places where DOTS has been used. But as impressive as this progress may seem, it is simply not enough when compared with the scale of the global epidemic.

AIDS deaths in 1997 totalled 2.3 million, of which 1.8 million were among adults aged 15 and above *(Map 8)*. Assuming that currently unbroken trends in many parts of the world will continue, it is estimated that more than 40 million people will be living with HIV/AIDS in the year 2000.

Although prediction of the long-term course of the epidemic is difficult because of the potential impact of prevention efforts, it is not unreasonable to assume that the number of people living with HIV/AIDS will continue to grow well into the 21st century *(Box 17)*. However, even if current increases in new infections seen in many parts of the world could be stopped or reversed, morbidity and mortality will continue to increase for another decade as a result of the long latency period between infection and the development of the disease.

Gains in survival achieved over the past few decades will, in some places, be cancelled out by the effects of HIV infection. Life expectancy in Botswana rose from under 44 years in 1955 to 58 years in 1990. Now, with 25-30% of the adult population infected with HIV, life expectancy is expected to drop back to levels last seen in the late 1960s. By the end of the decade, Zimbabwe will see a 10-year reduction in the life expectancy of a child born in 1990. Other sub-

Box 17. The evolution of AIDS

Recognized as an emerging disease only in the early 1980s, AIDS has rapidly established itself throughout the world, and is likely to endure and persist well into the 21st century and probably beyond.

AIDS has evolved from a mysterious illness to a global pandemic which has infected tens of millions in less than 20 years. It is now prevalent in virtually all parts of the world.

There are currently an estimated 30.6 million people living with HIV/AIDS, and 5.8 million new infections occurred in 1997. Since the beginning of the epidemic there have been an estimated 11.7 million deaths from AIDS, 2.3 million of them in 1997. The total number of AIDS orphans (HIV-negative children who lost their mother or parents to AIDS when they were under the age of 15) is near 8 million since the beginning of the epidemic.

The AIDS virus affects people who are particularly vulnerable. The main behavioural characteristics that facilitate the spread of HIV are unprotected sexual activity with different partners and sharing of equipment by injecting drug users. Women with HIV can also transmit it to their newborn children.

Adolescents and young adults who are becoming sexually active for the first time are particularly exposed, and are therefore an important target group for preventive action.

The AIDS virus is a virtually invisible passenger that uses the human body as a vehicle throughout a long incubation period before causing illness more than 10 years later in many cases. During part of that time HIV can be transmitted by an infected but symptomless individual to other people, who likewise will be its unwitting vehicle for further years and ensure its wider spread. In addition, the virus can mutate within an individual's body, so that by the time it is transmitted to someone else, it has changed some of its characteristics. This lack of "stability" is part of the complex make-up of HIV which will make the development of new drugs - and possibly a vaccine - very difficult.

From being first regarded as a "minority group" disease, AIDS has gradually been shown to be essentially a heterosexually transmitted infection. However, the evidence that transmission is most likely to occur with unsafe sexual behaviour has engendered complacency among populations which consider themselves outside that danger zone - either socially, behaviourally or geographically. This misperception or denial of risk is often a factor for further spread of the virus.

In some industrialized countries, AIDS is regarded as a disease restricted to the developing world. Such complacency is one more reason why AIDS will persist for a very long time. For the history of disease shows that when complacency occurs and vigilance weakens, infectious agents take full advantage of the situation.

The prospects for HIV/AIDS control depend largely on recognizing the scale of the threat and on political commitment to implementing policies to counter it. A key aspect of national AIDS programmes is early intervention addressing sex education, condom promotion and STD care; creating an enabling environment to facilitate behavioural change; and providing the necessary means to do so. Research is resulting in better understanding and treatment of HIV/AIDS. Combined drug therapy has lengthened life for many patients, but is inequitably distributed.

Saharan African countries show similar trends.

The potential for continued spread of HIV/AIDS in Asia and the Western Pacific is real and requires determined and sustained prevention efforts. Several countries have already experienced intense epidemics in certain population groups, or in some cases, in the population at large. In these countries, including Cambodia, India, Myanmar and Thailand, AIDS has imposed new demands on health care systems.

Drug injection is behind the dramatic surge in HIV infection in several eastern European countries, accounting for the majority of the 100 000 new infections estimated to have occurred in 1997. In Ukraine, where around 70% of infections have been in drug users over the past three years, some 25 000 cases of HIV infection have been reported so far, half of them in 1997. It is possible that a similar pattern will be seen elsewhere in the region.

In Latin America and the Caribbean, AIDS has already overtaken traffic injuries as a cause of death. However, a recent drop in AIDS mortality – similar to that seen in western Europe and North America – has been recorded in Sao Paulo, Brazil, and is attributed to the increasing use of antiretroviral therapy. In the United States in 1996, AIDS dropped into second place among leading causes of death in people aged 25-44 for the first time since 1992 (injury took over in first place). In western Europe also, the annual incidence of new cases of AIDS has begun to decline.

Unfortunately, access to antiretrovirals in the developing world is often difficult or impossible. It is encouraging, however, that in some developing countries such as Thailand and Uganda, the effects of preventive interventions are beginning to be seen. As a result of the increase in condom use and declines in other sexually transmitted diseases, the number of people expected to become HIV-positive in Thailand is now less than previously projected. Population growth is now expected to remain positive, whereas in 1994, population projections for Thailand indicated negative population growth by 2010. It appears likely, nevertheless, that many if not most of the 30 million people currently infected may well die – perhaps within the next decade.

Each year, there are 300-500 million clinical cases of *malaria* and 1.5-2.7 million people die of the disease. Of these deaths, 90% occur in sub-Saharan Africa, mainly in children under 5. The adult victims of malaria are those who were not previously exposed and thus have no immunity. Young men and women bear only 5-7% of the malaria burden. For many it is virtually an occupational disease because of their work in land development, mining, construction and seasonal migratory agriculture in malarious regions.

Apart from being a disabling and sometimes fatal disease in itself, malaria in non-immune pregnant women, or previously immune women in their first pregnancy, causes spontaneous abortion in up to 60% of cases and a maternal mortality rate of up to 10%. Malaria in adults also has a serious economic impact in terms of both lost productivity and treatment costs. Direct losses due to the disease in Africa in 1989 were calculated to be $ 800 million; by 1997 the figure had risen to $ 2.2 billion. This is largely due to the rising costs of treatment resulting from antimalarial drug resistance. Treatment costs for a normal bout of malaria can be as low as $ 0.15; to treat resistant strains can cost $ 7 per patient. In the malaria-endemic countries of South America, an episode of the disease causes the loss of between 1 and 14 days of work. Increasing numbers of cases are reported among international tourists and business travellers, of whom some 30 million from non-endemic countries visit malaria-endemic countries each year.

Resistance to the antimalarial chloroquine was reported on the Thai-Cambodia border and in Colombia in 1961, and spread in the late 1970s to Africa, where it has been reported from practically all endemic African countries. Chloroquine is still clinically effective in most primary health care settings, but its loss of efficacy in some areas has been accompanied by an increase in malaria morbidity and mortality.

Occupational diseases and injuries

WHO estimates that every year there are 217 million cases of occupational disease and 250 million cases of injuries at work, including 330 000 fatal cases. There are about 50 million new cases per year of occupational respiratory diseases. The 10 major work-related illnesses are respiratory diseases, musculoskeletal disorders, cancer, injuries, cardiovascular diseases, reproductive disorders, neurotoxic disorders, noise-induced hearing loss, dermatological disorders and psychological disorders.

Without preventive action, the burden of occupational diseases and injuries will escalate. By the year 2000, the global labour force will grow to some 3 billion people. Participation of women in the workforce will increase. Many workers will be exposed to occupational hazards such as toxic chemicals and dusts, allergenic agents and carcinogenic agents, and to serious injuries causing more than one month's absence from work.

Without preventive action, the burden of occupational diseases and injuries will escalate.

Box 18. Spotlight on gender

WHO, in applying a gender approach to health, moves beyond describing women and women's health in isolation, bringing into the analysis differences between women and men. It examines how these differences determine differential exposure to risk, access to the benefits of technology and health care, rights and responsibilities, and the control of people over their lives. In practice, a gender approach leads to:

- More consideration of all the factors that affect women's health, not only biological factors but social and economic status, cultural, environmental, familial, occupational and political factors.
- More attention to all of women's roles, not only their roles as wives and mothers.
- More attention to the roles and responsibilities of men, and the inequalities between men and women, with an examination of men's roles, perspectives and beliefs in relation to women's health concerns.
- More involvement of men in bringing about change.
- Listening to what women have to say about health and what they would like to know about it, rather than simply transferring information to women.
- Stronger measures to ensure that the voices of women are heard in identifying health issues and in research, planning, carrying out and monitoring the response to them.
- More attention to the entire duration of a woman's life, from birth to death - health for everyone is a cumulative matter.
- Greater recognition and support of women as active participants in the development of health care for themselves, their families and communities.

Most of these conditions lead to a reduction in working capacity or a permanent disability. The rising costs of occupational illness and injuries make health promotion and safety in the workplace a sound investment. In 1993, the cost of workers' compensation in the United States alone amounted to $ 57 billion. Data from 14 countries in Latin America and the Caribbean show that 38 million workdays were lost through occupational injuries each year during the 1980s. If this figure is extended to the population of the entire subregion, it can be assumed that approximately 95 million workdays are lost each year.

Special concerns of women

The United Nations Decade for Women (1976-1985) raised awareness of the link between women's status, fertility, and development. Societal policies can reduce gender inequalities (Box 18). Because of the strong preference for male children in many parts of the world, women receive inferior nutrition and health care from birth. Persisting discrimination will impede the improvement of women's health. Policies that aim to reduce gender inequalities focus on educating and empowering women and on encouraging both sexes to challenge gender stereotypes.

Coronary heart disease and stroke account for close to 60% of all adult female deaths in a typical developed country and are also the major cause of death among women aged 50 years and above in developing countries. A WHO study published in 1996 on the risk of haemorrhagic stroke associated with the use of oral contraceptive pills showed that the pill does not increase the risk in women below 35, who form the great majority of pill users worldwide. In current users over 35, however, the study found a small increase in risk. This was also found in relation to ischaemic stroke in current pill users, but was lower in women under 35, in non-smokers and in those who did not have high blood pressure. For both types of stroke, the study found no increased risk in women who had used the pill in the past. Women's risk of stroke can be reduced by avoiding using the pill if they have high blood pressure, and for users of the pill, by avoiding smoking.

Worldwide there are almost 700 000 cases of *breast cancer* each year, 57% of which occur in developed countries. Early detection is the main strategy for prevention, through physical examination of the breasts by trained health workers, breast self-examination, and mammography. Trials have shown that through screening – mammography followed by effective treatment – breast cancer mortality can be reduced by 30% in women aged 50 years and above. There is as yet no clear evidence of benefit from screening programmes for premenopausal women. The organization and implementation of mass screening programmes are far beyond the resources of developing countries, and breast self-examination remains the main option.

Cervical cancer is a preventable major cause of death, with 425 000 new cases are diagnosed each year, mostly in developing countries. The disease is one of the few cancers with a readily detectable and treatable precursor stage. In developing countries, screening is rarely accessible to women in rural areas, or to ageing women, who are at greatest risk. Screening once every five years and appropriate treatment can result in a reduction of 85% in mortality; screening once every 10 years could result in a 64% reduction. Screening older women, even once in their lifetime, will prevent more cases of cervical cancer than screening a small proportion of younger women every few years.

Around 585 000 women die each year of ***pregnancy-related causes***, 99% of them in developing countries. These are among the leading causes of death for women of reproductive age in many parts of the world. Where women have many pregnancies, the risk of related death over the course of a lifetime is compounded. In Africa, the risk is around 1 in 16, compared with 1 in 65 in Asia and 1 in 1400 in Europe. About 80% of maternal deaths are due to direct causes, that is, obstetric complications of pregnancy, labour and the puerperium, to interventions, omissions, in-

correct treatment, or to a chain of events resulting from any one of the above *(Fig. 11)*. The single most common cause – accounting for a quarter of all maternal deaths – is obstetric haemorrhage, generally occurring postpartum, which can lead to death very rapidly in the absence of prompt life-saving care, including drug treatment to control bleeding and, where needed, blood transfusions.

Puerperal infections, often the consequence of poor hygiene during delivery, or untreated reproductive

Fig. 11. Causes of maternal deaths, latest available year

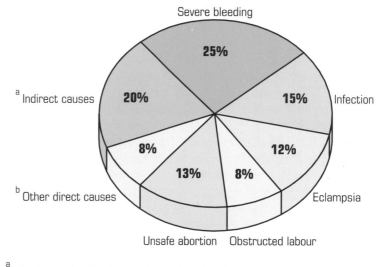

a Indirect causes including, for example: anaemia, malaria, heart disease.

b Other direct causes including, for example: ectopic pregnancy, embolism, anaesthesia-related.

tract infections (including those that are sexually transmitted) account for some 15% of maternal mortality. Such infections can be easily prevented. Hypertensive disorders of pregnancy, particularly eclampsia (convulsions), result in some 13% of all maternal deaths; they can be prevented through careful monitoring during pregnancy and treatment with relatively simple anticonvulsant drugs in cases of eclampsia. Around 7% of maternal deaths occur as a result of prolonged or obstructed labour. Other direct causes include ectopic

Box 19. Family planning

In the 1960s there was growing concern among countries about the negative impact of uncontrolled population growth on economic and social development, especially in developing countries. Human reproduction and especially contraception and family planning, previously taboo subjects at the World Health Assembly, were now openly discussed. In 1965, the Health Assembly adopted a resolution directing WHO to conduct research on medical aspects of sterility and fertility control methods and health aspects of population dynamics. A unit for this purpose was set up in mid-1965 at WHO headquarters. It subsequently became the Special Programme on Research, Development and Research Training in Human Reproduction.

Meanwhile, other organizations within the United Nations system and among the large foundations had become increasingly active in the area of population and family planning. Important new organizations were created during this period, such as the International Planned Parenthood Federation (1952), the Population Council (1952), and the Population Trust Fund – UN (now the United Nations Population Fund).

Three large intergovernmental conferences on population held in Bucharest (1974), Mexico City (1984) and Cairo (1994) brought together representatives of governments, specialized agencies, organizations of the United Nations system, intergovernmental organizations, nongovernmental organizations and the media to discuss issues of population and development and formulate plans of action. All these meetings endorsed population and family planning as integral to overall development. They established linkages with parallel concerns being discussed in other forums, such as health, the environment, children, women and human rights.

Population policies to provide the policy and legislative framework for the provision of family planning are essential. The successive population conferences and other important meetings have encouraged the development and adoption of such policies, and by 1991 (the latest dates for which figures are available) 96% of governments had policies directly supportive of the provision of family planning care, compared with 55% in 1974.

Fertility regulating methods that are safe, effective, reversible, easy to use and affordable are also essential. Research on technology development and assessment by WHO and others in collaboration with industry, government research councils and institutions throughout the developed and developing world have contributed substantially towards making such methods available.

pregnancies, embolisms and deaths related to interventions such as anaesthesia.

Around 20% of maternal deaths are due to indirect causes, that is, the result of pre-existing disease or disease that developed during pregnancy, which was not due to direct obstetric causes but was aggravated by the physiological effects of pregnancy. One of the most significant is anaemia, which can cause death through cardiac arrest and is also an underlying cause in a substantial proportion of deaths. Other important indirect causes of death include hepatitis, cardiovascular diseases, diseases of the endocrine or metabolic system, and diseases of the central nervous system.

The percentage of contraceptive users has increased from around 14% in 1960-1965 to an estimated 60% of women of reproductive age in 1994 (*Box 19*). Women are using family planning in increasing numbers in every region of the world. In developing countries, five times as many couples are now using contraception as in the 1960s. Worldwide, however, the full range of modern methods is unavailable to up to 350 million couples.

Present in most societies, but unrecognized, unreported or tacitly accepted, *violence* against women is a major health issue. Reliable information about its extent is unfortunately scant. Between 16% and 52% of women in some parts of the world suffer physical violence from their male partners. At least one in five women suffer rape or attempted rape in their lifetimes. Rape and sexual torture are systematically used as weapons of war. Psychological trauma, sexually transmitted diseases, unwanted pregnancies and reproductive health problems are among the consequences. Female genital mutilation is a traditional cultural practice, but also a form of violence against the girl child which affects her life as an adult woman. The number of girls and women who have been subjected to this practice is estimated at more than 130 million worldwide.

WHO's response

By the late 1980s and early 1990s it was clear that, with increasing co-infections with HIV and the spread of multidrug-resistant strains, the **tuberculosis** epidemic was worsening. In 1991, the World Healt Assembly called for the strengthening of district-centred tuberculosis programmes and the widespread implementation of directly observed, standardized, short-course chemotherapy (DOTS) and in 1993, WHO declared a global tuberculosis emergency.

The DOTS strategy incorporates components that were discovered, developed or expanded by a number of organizations and individuals over the past 45 years. These components are being used in one integrated strategy to document and manage the cure of tuberculosis cases, thus reducing the sources of infection in the community. Although there is no doubt about the effectiveness of DOTS in curing patients, it is still a strategy waiting to be used. Sustained political commitment is a major determinant of success. Governments must recognize the long-term benefits of providing the resources and staff necessary to ensure the proper implementation of DOTS. The benefits to individuals and society as a whole are overwhelming in comparison to the investment involved. Current research and surveillance initiatives are giving WHO a clearer picture of the threat of multidrug-resistant tuberculosis, as well as providing more accurate verification of data – both of which help the world respond more effectively to the epidemic. Because breakthroughs in diagnostic tools, drugs and vaccines may be years in the making, the world's future success in eliminating tuberculosis as a public health threat will rely on the parallel strategies of aggressive expansion of DOTS and a continued commitment to research.

In the 1980s, WHO alerted world authorities to national epidemics of **HIV/AIDS**. Since 1986, the Organization has helped Member States to establish or strengthen their national AIDS programmes; to carry out rapid assessment; to improve diagnostic, laboratory and blood screening capacity; and to plan national activities and long-term responses based on reliable projections. A report on the implications of the new antiretroviral treatments was published in 1997.

The development of a cheap, safe and effective vaccine is a priority, although this is not likely to be achieved for at least 10 years. Any major initiative in this area requires that the partners play three major roles: supporting and coordinating research; negotiating with industry to ensure that the products of research will be available to those most in need; and seeking mechanisms to encourage vaccine research, which is commercially far less attractive than research on new drugs. The development of a microbicide is equally urgent as the use of such a product is a method that is simple, can be controlled by women, and could be inexpensive. This highly promising area, likely to produce the quickest and widest benefits, needs an urgent injection of funds and effort. Drug therapy, on the other hand, is far from being a practical option (on grounds of cost, compliance, efficacy and resistance) or widely applicable as yet.

The majority of **occupational diseases** can be prevented through action in the work environment, improvement of working conditions and the reduction of harmful exposures. WHO's work on occupational health dates back to 1950, when it set up a joint committee with ILO. At the beginning of the 1990s, WHO instituted a new agenda for work, development and health, which led to the development of the Global Strategy for Occupational Health for All. Member States are urged to devise national programmes, with special attention to

The development of a cheap, safe and effective vaccine is a priority.

full occupational health services. WHO promotes health in the workplace in a wider sense through advocating the concept of the healthy company or healthy organization.

In 1997, WHO cosponsored and participated in the international symposium on maritime health in Norway and the international symposium on occupational asthma and allergy held in the Russian Federation, as well as the international conference on occupational health in the informal sector which took place in Indonesia. A joint ILO/WHO initiative to eliminate silicosis is planned in 1998. The disease is common in labourers in mines, quarries, construction, ceramics, the metal industries and other dust-generating activities.

Special concerns of women

Many WHO programmes are now addressing women's needs, but few have begun to examine systematically differences between the needs of men and women. Sex-disaggregated data are needed for any analysis of gender differences. WHO is developing a policy on gender and health which should facilitate this work. Several of the regional offices are collecting data in order to develop national and regional profiles of women's health.

WHO's norms and standards for post-abortion care represent best international practice and form the basis for the technical support that WHO provides to Member States and other partners. To date, systematic reviews have been undertaken and recommendations issued in relation to a range of issues, covering clinical management and complications, post-abortion family planning and managerial issues.

The Global Commission on Women's Health focuses on three key areas: education for the health of girls and women; violence against women; and maternal morbidity and mortality. Activities at the country and regional levels have focused on data collection and research in areas where gaps in knowledge about women's health exist, e.g. to examine the household factors affecting maternal morbidity and mortality.

WHO activities in reproductive health in 1997 included the expansion of the research initiative on the role of men in reproductive health; publication of data from the WHO collaborative study of cardiovascular disease and steroid hormone contraception; the completion of data collection – and initiation of final analysis – of a large post-marketing surveillance study of Norplant contraceptive implants; and the launching of several regional initiatives on female genital mutilation, acceptability of emergency contraception, increasing rate of Caesarean section and quality of antenatal care.

Older people

The challenges of ageing

For more people than ever before, the prospect of a healthy and extended old age is becoming a reality. People are not only living longer; research shows that in some cases they are also living in better health, with their rates of disability going down at the same time as their life expectancy goes up. For example, the National Long Term Care Surveys in the United States show significant declines in disability prevalence among older people between 1982 and 1994 (Box 20, Fig. 12). On this evidence, the world is learning how to grow old successfully.

The progressive ageing of populations in the 20th century is a triumph for the human species. Glo-

> The progressive ageing of populations in the 20th century is a triumph for the human species.

bal population ageing reflects the unprecedented gains in life expectancy described earlier in this report. It is due to a combination of factors, especially the dramatic declines in infant and child mortality, reductions in maternal deaths, and the benefits that come from overall socioeconomic development – improved nutrition, declining infections, better standards of living, progress in education, health care, and biomedical technology.

This ageing trend offers both great opportunities and formidable challenges for all societies. But for many, those opportunities may be denied and those challenges may become unmanageable in the coming century. It is essential that the potential social and economic impacts of improved life expectancy are fully appreciated and acted upon today. The well-being of society depends on the good health of its older members in their later years. For policy-makers and individuals alike, this means planning for the future.

The global challenge

Half a century ago, most people in the world died before the age of 50. Today, the great majority survive well beyond that age, particularly in many industrialized countries. The global population aged over 65 years is increasing by 750 000 a month. A child born in Japan today can expect to live to be 80 years old. By 2025 there will be more than 800 million older people in the world, two-thirds of them in developing countries, and a majority of them will be women.

Increases in the older population by up to 300% are expected in many developing countries, especially in Latin America and Asia, within the next 30 years. There will be 274 million people over the age of 60 years in China alone – more than the total present population of the United States.

Box 20. Living longer, feeling better

Biomedical research has had great positive effects on the health and physical functioning of the human population; by stimulating the growth of biotechnology, it has greatly affected the economies of developed nations. These effects on the health of the aged in the United States can be demonstrated using data from the National Long Term Care Surveys (NLTCS). Manton and his colleagues at Duke University found that the prevalence rate of chronic disability and institutionalization declined significantly, by almost 15% for the aged United States population from 1982 to 1994 (age 65 and older). This confirmed the decline in chronic disability prevalence of about 8% observed from 1982 to 1989 and suggested that the rate of decline in the prevalence of disability among aged Americans had actually increased (to 1.5% per annum) between 1989 and 1994.

Not only did the prevalence of, and institutionalization rates for, disability decline, but the prevalence of many chronic degenerative diseases measured by the NLTCS, and those thought to generate chronic disability, showed significant reductions. The declines in chronic morbidity suggest that chronic disability prevalence rates will continue to fall, at least over the period between the time of chronic disease onset and its eventual progression to a stage generating serious chronic disability. Longer-term declines are implied by lower disability prevalence rates, and higher survival rates at age 65-69 across three elderly cohorts from NLTCS sample populations in 1982 and followed to 1991.

Personal communication from Kenneth G. Manton, Larry S. Corder & Eric Stallard, Center for Demographic Studies, Duke University, Durham, NC, USA.

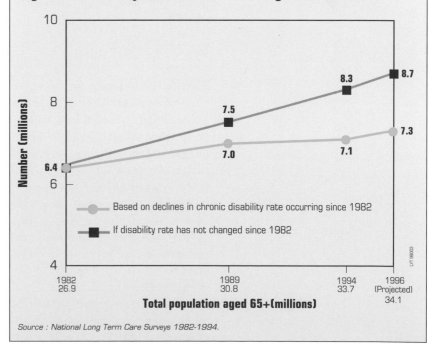

Fig. 12. Chronically disabled Americans aged 65 and above

Based on declines in chronic disability rate occurring since 1982

If disability rate has not changed since 1982

Source : National Long Term Care Surveys 1982-1994.

Population ageing

is having profound

effects on society.

It is a quiet,

almost unseen

social revolution.

At present, 13% of the population of the United States is aged 65 and above, compared to 4% at the beginning of the 20th century. The proportion is expected to reach approximately 20% by 2030. Although the population is ageing more slowly in industrialized countries, these countries will have relatively more people in the "oldest old" bracket. For example, there were only 200 people aged 100 years in France in 1950. By the year 2000, the number is expected to rise to 8500, and by 2050 it is projected to reach 150 000 – a 750-fold increase in 100 years.

The global challenge of ageing is made more complex by other demographic changes that are occurring simultaneously. In the next 25 years, the population aged 65 and above is likely to grow by 88% compared to an increase of 45% in the working-age population. This implies that a steadily declining number of people of productive age will have to provide for an expanding number of dependants, not merely in the form of direct support to older relatives but also through taxation, the provision of health and social services, and social security.

The social challenge

The adults of today are the older people of tomorrow. They are already asking: What kind of old age will we have? How will it differ from that of our parents and grandparents? What will be our quality of life? What will be our place in society? The answers largely depend on what people do now as individuals to ensure healthy ageing, and what governments and communities are prepared to do on their behalf.

Maintaining health and quality of life in an ageing population will be vitally important socially and economically. In the 21st century, post-poning the adverse effects of old age for as long as possible will be a major political and personal preoccupation. Health-related policies are needed to tackle the problems faced by those already in old age and those who will be the older people of the future.

Population ageing is having profound effects on society. It is a quiet, almost unseen social revolution that is gradually gaining pace and will accelerate and become ever more evident in the next 25 years. Its influence will be felt at every level, from family life and living arrangements, employment, the provision of health services and pension systems, to the state of the economy (Box 21).

In some of the more advanced nations, the day is not far off when older people will outnumber children, and the number of people reaching their hundredth year will be counted in tens of thousands.

While society is ageing, it is also changing in other, related ways. Traditionally, families have looked after their older members. Today's old tend to have fewer children to care for them, and in many cases those children have grown up and moved away to live at great distances from their parents.

Although daughters and sons are still the primary caregivers, their ability to care for their older relatives has been altered by changes in lifestyles. Women, the traditional caregivers, have increasingly become part of the workforce, and so unavailable for their customary role. To fill these gaps, the community is increasingly expected to intervene, by providing social services, home visits, hospitals, nursing homes, and sheltered accommodation for its older dependants, and to favour community care rather than institutionalized care.

Already, population ageing is beginning to revolutionize health care and social systems, with new public policies on health and social care – public and private sector pluralism, reduction in public spending – being widely adopted throughout the world. To many observers, these trends seem likely to exacerbate the disadvantaged position of many older people.

Even in wealthy countries, most old and frail people cannot personally meet more than a small fraction of the costs of the health care they need. At present, it seems clear that neither developed nor developing countries will be able to provide long-term, specialized care for the vast numbers of aged individuals in the population in the coming decades. But this scenario is not inevitable. Caring for the aged could be a great source of new employment.

Most of the increase in older populations will occur in developing countries, which will face the most serious challenges in providing a "welfare package" of services for their older people, given their economic difficulties, the lack of social service infrastructures, and the decline of traditional caring provided by family members.

Growing older is associated with increasing disability and greater dependence on others. Generally a person is regarded as dependent if he or she needs the help of another person in order to perform the basic activities of daily living, such as washing, getting dressed, moving about, eating and drinking. Most older people will eventually need help of this kind to some extent. It may be provided by any combination of relatives, neighbours, the community and health and social services, and it may be needed for periods of many years.

The cost of such help can seldom be borne entirely by the older individual or the family. The question therefore arises of who bears the cost,

Box 21. Disablement and functioning - Towards a common language: ICIDH-2

In line with its broad understanding of health, WHO is involved in a global initiative to revise the *International Classification of Impairments, Disabilities and Handicaps* (ICIDH) to capture an important paradigm shift towards a biopsychosocial understanding of human functioning and disablement. The revised version (ICIDH-2) is a classification of human functioning at the body, person and societal levels that takes into account the social and environmental context in which people live.

Medical diagnosis alone does not predict health care needs of individuals, nor does it predict the utilization, outcomes or costs of health services. Moreover, the presence of a medical condition is not a reliable guide for work performance, disability benefits or social integration of the individual.

With the increasing importance of chronic and noncommunicable illness, the ageing of the population and the increased emphasis on social policy solutions to health issues, a multidimensional classification is urgently needed. As a product of a worldwide consensus-building effort, the revised ICIDH (renamed *International Classification of Impairments, Activities and Participation*) will meet the need for an international common language for the consequences of diseases and other health conditions. ICIDH-2 will also provide users with operational tools for measurement and comparison.

The ICIDH-2 will provide a scientific basis for the study of functioning and disablement. It will serve as a common international language, across different users and sectors, for global data collection, research, health resource allocation and management, and social welfare programming. Because ICIDH-2 covers the human experience in all personal and societal domains, it can provide the basis for empirically-grounded policy and legislative change.

The ICIDH-2 favours a universal approach to functioning and disablement, in contrast to the minority model that sees disablement as a defining attribute of a minority of people. Disablement is a universal feature of humanity, manifested for everyone in different levels of functioning.

Similarly, since human functioning and disablement can only be understood against the background of existing social and physical factors, the ICIDH-2 includes a classification of contextual factors, i.e. environmental and personal factors that modulate the experience of disablement for individuals.

Arising out of a multisectoral partnership involving both providers and consumers, the ICIDH-2 points in the direction of an invigorated international partnership in health care management. As a framework for disablement, the ICIDH can further the commitment of the United Nations to an international disablement social policy founded on human rights and the universality of disablement.

and how that provision is to be funded. One obvious way of making adequate services available to the larger numbers needing them is to impose higher taxes on the working population. Increasing taxes, how-

> As people live longer, they must plan throughout life to take better care of themselves.

ever, is politically unpopular and many governments are under pressure to reduce taxes rather than raise them, which implies a reduction rather than an expansion of the services in question.

Most countries are now seeking alternative types of welfare package, such as combinations of public sector and private sector health insurance and pension schemes, funded by direct or indirect taxation and voluntary contributions, that will ensure long-term care for older people. Sweden has one of the most systematic strategies, with a wide range of services for older people. Commercial long-term care insurance plans are rapidly expanding in the United Kingdom. In Germany, funding for such insurance is predominantly public. A public long-term care insurance programme is likely to be introduced in Japan in the next few years. Half the costs will be paid by premiums levied on all those older than 40 years, and half will come from general taxation. In Australia, most long-term care is provided by the private sector through a mix of profit and non-profit organizations. New forms of partnerships between governments and private health insurers are being considered by some countries, based on schemes already in existence in some parts of the United States. This "mixed approach" to funding the dependency of older people at a level broadly capable of meeting needs for care, assistance and accommodation, appears to be gaining support.

The individual challenge

As people live longer, they must plan throughout life to take better care of themselves, on the assumption that a large proportion of their lives will extend beyond what has been traditionally regarded as their most productive years. Although "older people"

have long been recognized as a distinct social category, the starting-point of socially defined old age today is becoming less clear. In many countries, old age and the socially accepted roles associated with it are undergoing radical change. Old age is no longer accepted unquestioningly as beginning at a fixed chronological age, such as the point of retirement from work or the state pensionable age of 60 or 65 years.

In industrialized countries during much of the second half of the 20th century, most people were led to expect an abrupt transition from full-time work to full-time retirement at an age when many of them felt reasonably fit. They also assumed that retirement pensions and welfare services provided by the state would be adequate to cover their needs in old age. These expectations are now being fundamentally altered, by individuals, employers and governments. Individuals are being encouraged to prepare for old age financially by saving and investing more, and staying longer in work.

Many people do not want to retire at 60 or 65; about a third of respondents in a survey in the United States felt they had been forced by circumstances to retire earlier than they wanted to. In Canada it has been estimated that about 25% of retirees left the workforce involuntarily. The German government has introduced measures to make the transition to retirement more flexible, increase the effective pension age, reduce occupational health risks and stimulate the creation of new jobs adapted to the needs of older workers. People who want to work longer are being encouraged to do so; many of them feel obliged to do so, because of financial insecurity and uncertainties about future levels of state assistance.

Remaining productive, however, depends on remaining in good

enough health. Individuals therefore must take greater responsibility for their health at the earliest opportunity. This means adopting habits such as a healthy diet, adequate exercise, and avoidance of tobacco early in life, and maintaining them for the rest of their years.

Although hereditary factors play an important role in determining life expectancy and health, the individual's lifestyle is, along with the environment, one of the greatest modifiable influences. Health promotion, which is aimed at every other age group, does not exclude older people. Rather, it aims to stimulate habits and lifestyles conducive to a better old age, and can make a crucial difference in determining how different individuals reach old age. This notion has been encapsulated by the term "healthy ageing", and is a concept actively promoted by WHO and other agencies. Many countries now have health promotion programmes designed specially for older individuals, covering areas such as physical exercise, healthy nutrition, prevention of frailty and injury and chronic disease management.

The gender challenge

Women make up the majority of the older population in virtually all countries. In at least 67 developing countries, the projected increase in the number of women aged over 65 years between 1997 and 2025 exceeds 150%. During the same period, the number of older women in Asia (presently 107 million) is projected to soar to 248 million, and in Africa, from 13 million to 33 million.

Women have different circumstances, challenges and health concerns from men as they age. Older women are more likely to be widowed, to live alone and to live in poverty. Largely this is because globally

women live longer than men – an average of eight extra years in developed countries – and tend to marry men older than themselves. However, some of women's extra years are accounted for entirely by years of dependency. In the United States, this means that while only one in seven men who attain the age of 65 can expect to spend a year or more in a nursing home before death, one woman in three at 65 has the same prospect.

For women in developing countries who survive the early life span stages to reach middle age, life expectancy approaches that of women in developed countries. By far the major factor explaining this trend is reduced maternal mortality, due to declining fertility and improved maternal care. Life expectancies at age 65 show much greater similarity between developed and developing countries, at around 19 and 15 years respectively. The gap will narrow as mortality declines not only at younger ages but also at later ages. The main trend in ageing in developed countries is the increase in the oldest old, that is, those 85 years and older. The great majority of this age group are women, and this trend will continue in the foreseeable future.

As women live longer than men, the quality of their longer life becomes of central importance. Quality of life, measured in terms of older women's capacity to maintain physical, social and mental well-being notwithstanding varying levels of illness and disability, is of as much relevance as increased life expectancy and years of life free of disability. The major preventable causes of morbidity and mortality all take effect over extended time periods. Primary prevention strategies will be most effective when initiated as early as possible. Coronary heart disease, stroke and lung cancer are the conditions which primary prevention needs to address, while sec-

As women live longer than men, the quality of their longer life becomes of central importance.

ondary prevention strategies are applicable to other cancers.

Taking action to improve the health of ageing women is imperative if they are to achieve an acceptable quality of life in their extended old age and if all societies are to avoid the consequences that otherwise will ensue. The health of older women therefore receives special attention in the following section. However, the very fact that it is a special issue illustrates another reality: by this stage of women's lives, most of their male contemporaries have died. The reasons why men die sooner than women is also an issue which needs further investigation.

The health challenge

Ageing is a normal dynamic process. It is not a disease. While ageing is inevitable and irreversible, the chronic disabling conditions that often accompany it can be prevented or delayed, not only by medical interventions but more effectively by social, economic and environmental interventions.

The longer older people remain in good health, disability-free and productive, the better will be their quality of life and the greater their contribution to society, and – perhaps – the smaller will be the cost of providing health and social services for them. Equally, the longer the health of the working population can be sustained without disability, the more productive it will be and the more able to support older dependants. This will also benefit the working population as it ages.

Healthy life expectancy is influenced by a relatively small number of chronic disabling conditions that become more common with increasing age. They include circulatory diseases, such as cardiovascular disease and stroke; cancers; musculoskeletal conditions such as arthritis and oste-

oporosis; neurological or mental disorders such as dementia and depression; degenerative disorders such as loss of sight and hearing; and chronic obstructive pulmonary disease.

The paramount health challenge must be to prevent, postpone or treat these conditions. It is a challenge best met by a partnership of individuals and health care providers. The great variation in rates of chronic diseases around the world shows that many can in fact be prevented, or at least delayed. For example, age-specific rates for cardiovascular disease have halved in Japan and the United States in the past 30 years. Cancer and heart disease are more related to the 70-75 age group than any other, but beyond 75 years exists another population – the oldest old who have survived this hazardous phase of life. They have now become more prone to impairments of hearing, vision, mobility and mental function.

The following section refers to the major chronic conditions mentioned above, with special reference to their significance in women.

Circulatory diseases

The increasing number of older people in all societies and the high burden of cardiovascular disease (CVD) in older people make it urgent that appropriate health policy recommendations are made for this group. Over 80% of deaths from CVD occur in people over 65. Worldwide, CVD is the leading cause of death and disability in people over 65, but there is great potential for treating it.

The high prevalence of CVD risk factors in older people, particularly raised blood pressure and raised serum cholesterol, suggests the need for widespread treatment. Management of mild elevations of blood pressure can be achieved by non-pharmacological measures, including reduction

Ageing is a normal dynamic process. It is not a disease.

of salt and excess alcohol consumption, and physical activity. Moderate to severe hypertension can be treated with diuretics and beta-blockers.

Elevated serum cholesterol is common in older people and is a risk factor for coronary heart disease (CHD) in both men and women, and this relationship persists into very old age. As with younger people, drug therapy should be considered only after serious attempts at modifying diet have been made.

Intervention trials have shown that reduction of blood pressure by 6 mm Hg reduces the risk of stroke by 40% and of heart attack by 15%, and that a 10% reduction in blood cholesterol concentration will reduce the risk of coronary heart disease by 30%. Dietary changes seem to affect risk factor levels throughout life and may have even more impact in older people. Relatively modest reductions in saturated fat and salt intake, which would reduce blood pressure and cholesterol concentrations, could have a substantial effect on reducing the burden of cardiovascular disease. Increasing consumption of fruit and vegetables by one to two servings daily could cut cardiovascular risk by 30%.

Cigarette smoking is the most important modifiable risk factor for CVD in young and old alike. Fortunately it is usually less prevalent in older people than in younger people. The dramatic decline in cigarette smoking in some wealthy countries shows that smokers can be persuaded to give up.

For example, in the United States smoking declined in men aged 65 and above from 28% in the mid-1960s to 15% in 1990. However, in women in the same age group there was an increase from 10% to 12%. Reductions in stroke and CHD rates from smoking cessation increase as time since

quitting increases, but some benefits are realized immediately. For example, stroke risk decreases after two years' abstinence and becomes the same as that of never-smokers after five years.

In developed countries, there has been a consistent decline in stroke mortality over the last 40 years, with an acceleration in this decline in the mid-1970s. The fall in stroke deaths has been greater than that in deaths from CHD. For example, in Canada, Japan, Switzerland and the United States stroke mortality has declined by more than 50% in men and women aged 65-74 since the 1970s. Although the reasons are not fully understood, the limited evidence available suggests that a decline in case-fatality may be related to decreased severity of the disease, with the acute event becoming more mild, probably as a result of prevention efforts. Improved management in the acute phase may also have contributed.

As increasing age is considered to be the main risk factor for stroke and circulatory diseases more generally, the burden of these diseases will become heavier as greater proportions of the population in developing countries reach older ages.

Coronary heart disease and stroke are the major causes of death and disability in *ageing women*. The common view that they are men's health problems has tended to obscure their significance for ageing women's health and there is a need to bring their importance into sharper focus. They account for close to 60% of all adult female deaths in a typical developed country, and are also the major cause of death among women aged 50 years and above in developing countries. In the majority of developed countries for which trend data are available, declines in death rates from heart disease and stroke have been greater for women than

Management of mild elevations of blood pressure can be achieved by non-pharmacological measures, including reduction of salt and excess alcohol consumption, and physical activity.

Most cancers arise

at an advanced age,

and the risk

increases steeply

with age.

men, but cardiovascular disease will continue to be the major health issue for older women. Improvements in death rates have been much smaller in many developing countries.

Women are usually 10 years older than men when symptoms of heart disease first appear, and may be up to 20 years older before a heart attack occurs. In the United States, 55% of women over 75 years with coronary heart disease are disabled by their illness. The disease will probably become epidemic in older women unless they take preventive action throughout their lives, yet studies show that women do not usually count heart disease among the health problems they consider most important.

The impact of increased smoking rates among women is now becoming more evident. Death rates from smoking-related diseases have plateaued in men whereas they are increasing in older women. Cigarette smoking by women has not yet become widespread in developing countries, and there is still time to take global action to protect older women from diseases due to smoking.

Cancer

The gradual elimination of other fatal diseases, combined with rising life expectancy, means that the risks of an individual developing cancer during his or her lifetime are steadily increasing. Most cancers arise at an advanced age, and the risk increases steeply with age. The cancer burden is therefore much more important in populations having long life expectancy, relative to other groups of diseases.

As shown in *The World Health Report 1997*, the average age at death from six of the most common forms of cancer ranged from 61 to 69 for a sample of six countries. In France and the United States, breast cancer on average deprives women of 10 years of life expectancy, while prostate cancer reduces male average life expectancy by only one year.

As a result of medical advances, one-third of all cancers are preventable, and a further one-third, if diagnosed sufficiently early, are curable. For the remaining one-third, appropriate palliative care can bring about substantial improvements in the quality of patients' lives.

The five leading cancer killers worldwide are also the five most common in terms of incidence. Together they account for about 50% of all cancer cases and deaths. Among men, the leading eight killer sites for cancer are the lung, stomach, liver, colon-rectum, oesophagus, mouth-pharynx, prostate, and lymphoma. In women they are cancers of the breast, stomach, colon-rectum, cervix, lung, ovary, oesophagus and liver. The major killer cancer in women in developing countries is breast cancer, followed by stomach cancer. In developed countries, breast cancer also ranks first, followed by colorectal cancer.

An analysis of the risk factors involved in the development of the major cancers shows that a few major factors dominate – tobacco, diet, alcohol, infections and hormones – all of which lend themselves to preventive actions. The long latent period for most cancers dictates the importance of early detection.

In terms of prevention, screening for cervical cancer has contributed to steep declines in this disease in many countries. To combat breast cancer, mammography is now generally proposed for women over 50 in those countries where the disease has a high incidence. Prostate cancer, most common in men over 70 years, also lends itself to early detection, although the value of screening is debated.

Lung cancer is the most preventable of all cancers as over 90% is attributable to smoking. Levels of morbidity and mortality among older women due to lung cancer are now similar in developed and developing countries, and likely to grow worldwide, given the increasing numbers of women who smoke. Lung cancer in women has increased fourfold over the last 30 years in many developed countries, and has overtaken breast cancer as the leading cause of cancer death in women in the United States, where women first took up smoking in large numbers. This pattern is being repeated elsewhere in developed countries, where between one-quarter and one-third of women have started smoking. In many Latin American countries, up to two-thirds of young women smoke; levels are considerably lower in most African and Asian countries.

Chronic obstructive pulmonary disease (COPD)

This category includes chronic bronchitis and emphysema, which are especially prevalent in older age groups. Although these conditions are more common in men, their prevalence in women will undoubtedly increase, because cigarette smoking is the main risk factor, and smoking among women is globally on the rise. The direct cost of managing COPD, which frequently requires hospitalization, is high. Most deaths due to COPD occur after the age of 65.

Musculoskeletal conditions

These conditions reduce mobility and agility, and so have a major impact on self-care. For ageing men and women, exercise is an important preventive activity against all major musculoskeletal conditions. Yet few older women exercise on a regular basis in developed countries. Lack of exercise and inappropriate nutrition have led to an increase in the proportion of women who are overweight or obese. By contrast, in developing countries it is the excessive physical demands on women throughout their life that most adversely affect physical strength and mobility. Dealing with heavy loads leads to damage of the joints. In addition, nutritional deficiencies reduce the physical strength of women as they age. In developed countries, undernutrition is a problem among the oldest of old women.

Osteoporosis and associated fractures are a major cause of death, illness and disability, and a cause of huge medical expense worldwide. Bone fractures are the main complication, and given that they are most common in older people, the influence of increasing life expectancy on the number and regional distribution of hip fractures will be dramatic. Worldwide, it is estimated that the number of hip fractures could rise from 1.7 million in 1990 to around 6.3 million by 2050. Women represent 80% of those who have a hip fracture; their lifetime risks for osteoporotic fractures are at least 30% and probably closer to 40%. In men, the risk is 13%.

Women are more prone because their bone loss accelerates after the menopause. Prevention is possible with hormone therapy at the menopause. Lifestyle factors are also associated with osteoporosis (diet, physical activity, smoking), opening a perspective for primary prevention. The primary aim is to prevent fractures: this may be achieved by increasing bone mass at maturity, by preventing subsequent bone loss or by restoring the bone mineral. Lifestyle modifications, particularly increased calcium intake and physical activity, could be of great importance.

For ageing

men and women,

exercise is

an important

preventive activity.

The risk of

developing dementia

rises steeply with age

in people over

60 years.

Dementia

The ageing of the global population will inevitably result in significant increases in the number of cases of dementia, of which the incurable Alzheimer disease is the most common form. The risk of developing dementia rises steeply with age in people over 60 years. Alzheimer disease is a brain disorder characterized by gradual onset and progressive decline in cognition. The average course of the disease is approximately a decade, with a range of 3 to 20 years from diagnosis to death. As the disease advances, memory is increasingly lost, and changes in mood and behaviour follow.

The possibilities for prevention are extremely limited because the major determinants – age, genes and family history – cannot be modified, and an effective treatment is yet to be found. However, recent progress in understanding the diagnosis and pathogenesis of Alzheimer disease and related disorders has benefited many patients. Early and accurate diagnosis avoids the use of costly medical resources and allows patients and family members time to prepare for future medical, financial and other challenges. While no current therapy can reverse the progressive cognitive decline, several pharmacological agents and psychosocial techniques have been shown to provide relief for the depression, psychosis and agitation often associated with dementia.

Generally, the management of dementia is based on long-term care, preferably at home, with support from a community-based health team. Living with and caring for a person with dementia can be very burdensome and caregivers are at high risk of becoming exhausted. The needs of these carers should be kept in mind when planning services for people with dementia. Women are more likely to suffer than men because of their greater longevity. Most of those caring for people with dementia are ageing women, either spouses or adult daughters.

Blindness and visual impairment

These are major causes of disability in older people, especially in developing countries where there are fewer resources for prevention and treatment. At present, about 25 million older people are blind; the number is expected to double by 2020.

WHO's response

In 1979 the World Health Assembly adopted its first resolution specifically targeted to health care of older people, which led to the establishment of a global programme. Its goals were to promote health and well-being throughout the entire life span and to assist Member States in developing strategies to ensure the availability and provision of comprehensive and holistic health care to older populations.

A policy paper prepared by WHO for the 1982 World Assembly on Ageing convened by the United Nations provided a basis for the Vienna International Plan of Action on Ageing which became the framework for WHO activities between 1982 and 1987. The Plan encouraged Member States to develop demographic and health profiles; to formulate programmes for community-based health care for ageing individuals, with special focus on health promotion and self-help care; and to advocate issues related to the health of older people with scientific and professional organizations.

WHO organized scientific meetings on ageing-related issues such as nutritional status, cardiovascular diseases, mental health, prevention of respiratory infections, family life and support, prevention of accidents, and health promotion. Published in 1984, *The uses of epidemiology in the study of the elderly* stimulated new approaches to research on ageing. Activities from the late 1980s to the mid-1990s were focused on determinants of healthy ageing, osteoporosis and age-associated dementias. In 1994, the programme was reoriented towards "ageing and health".

Today, the WHO programme deals with both old age and ageing. It sees older people as not compartmentalized but part of the life cycle. It emphasises health promotion, with a focus on healthy ageing, or ageing well. It takes account of gender differences evident in both health and ways of living, and the cultural settings in which individuals' age determine their health in older age. It is concerned also with strategies to maintain cohesion between generations and the many ethical issues of population ageing.

An expert committee on determinants of healthy ageing is scheduled to meet in 1998 to discuss these perspectives in depth. This committee's guidance will be sought on how WHO and its Member States can best play a major role in presenting the health component of the International Year of Older Persons (1999).

Other WHO activities are directed towards specific aspects of the health of older people. For example, the main strategies for preventing blindness and deafness have focused on the development of national programmes based on primary health care

More than 100 countries have set up blindness prevention programmes, and many of these have been highly successful in reducing certain causes of blindness, such as trachoma. The main constraints are insufficient resources for large-scale provision of care, such as cataract surgery. Recent developments in new, low-cost technology are very promising (e.g. intraocular lenses), but need to be made available on a large scale in developing countries.

During 1997, a WHO Alliance for the Global Elimination of Trachoma was established, to intensify action against that disease together with interested nongovernmental organizations and other partners, making use of new methods for rapid assessment and more effective treatment of the disease. Other collaborative activities have included support to cataract surgery in Africa, planning for eye care in China and in Haiti, and an economic analysis of blindness prevention. WHO has also undertaken applied research, in collaboration with the United States National Eye Institute on cataract surgery in India, and specific evaluations of national programme results in China and Nepal.

In the Americas, 26 countries are developing ocular health services to address the major problems of cataracts, diabetic retinopathy, glaucoma, and the need for inexpensive eyeglasses.

Work for the prevention of hearing impairment has included field-testing of uniform assessment procedures in selected countries, and development of strategies against noise-induced hearing loss.

More than 100 countries have set up blindness prevention programmes.

Chapter 4
The changing world

E conomic and social gains during the past 50 years have been dramatic and unprecedented, particularly for developing countries. Though the global population doubled during the period, per capita gross domestic product (GDP) increased by at least 2.5 times, GDP more than five times and exports more than 10 times *(Table 7)*. Considerable progress has been made in reducing the incidence of absolute poverty (with a more modest reduction in the number of poor) and in achieving somewhat better living standards for those who have remained in poverty.

Social gains have also been significant during the past 50 years. Life expectancy at birth increased from 46 years in the early 1950s to 64 in the early 1990s, and infant mortality rates declined from 156 per 1000 live births to 62 per 1000 during the same period. Food supply has more than doubled in the past 40 years, much faster than population growth, and the proportion of people chronically undernourished fell from about one in three to one in five. Adult literacy rates rose

from less than 50% in 1970 to more than 75% in the early 1990s; and the proportion of children attending school rose from less than half to more than three-quarters. During the last two decades, coverage of infants with immunization against the six major vaccine-preventable diseases reached more than 80%. However, the pace of such postwar progress has been neither steady nor uniform, as the following analysis will show.

Economic trends

Growth of the economy

During the period *1950-1973*, the world experienced a golden age of unparalleled prosperity with unusually favourable performance of the economy and dynamism observable in all regions. World per capita GDP grew by about 3% a year – more than three times as fast as during the earlier half of the 20th century – from about $ 2140 in 1950 to $ 4120 in 1973. However, the overall long-run pattern of income spreads between 1950 and 1973 was strikingly divergent. The intercountry spread in per capita GDP grew steadily larger from 35 to 1 in 1950, to 40 to 1 in 1973 (but then there was also a "catch-up" phenomenon). Economic growth was interrupted around 1975 by a sharp reduction, possibly resulting from strong inflationary pressure, the breakdown of the fixed exchange rate system and the sudden rise in oil prices. The momentum of the earlier period has never been regained since, except in East Asia.

This chapter is largely based on the latest available publications of other international agencies with respect to areas under their responsibilty. Detailed references can be found in the statistical annex.

Table 7. Growth of GDP and GDP per capita[a]

	Growth of GDP (annual percentage change)		GDP per capita (US $)		
	1981-1990	1991-1996	1980	1996	1997
World	3.1	3.3	4 883	5 966	6 123
Developed market economies	2.8	1.7	16 547	21 995	22 497
Economies in transition[b]	2.0	-6.4	5 464	4 012	4 062
Developing countries	3.8	5.8	2 102	3 147	3 282
of which LDCs	2.4	3.5	1 097	1 132	1 159

[a] On the basis of purchasing power parity.
[b] Including the former German Democratic Republic until 1990.

Fig. 13. Population by age and sex, 1995 and 2025

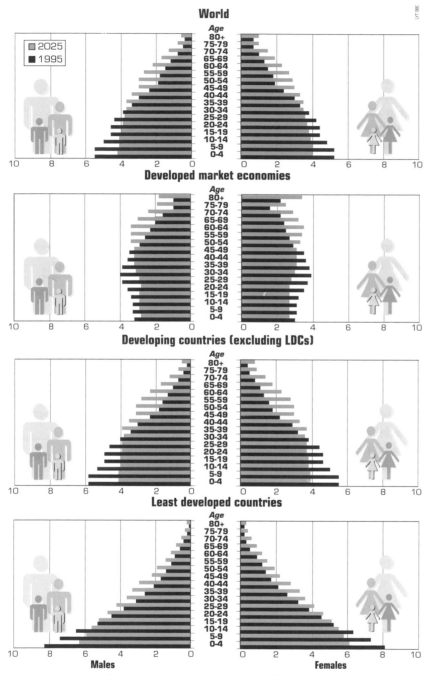

Percentage of total population by level of development

The rate rose from 1.2% during 1965-1975 to 2.2% during 1975-1985 and reached 2.6% during 1985-1990. Despite this accelerating growth, by 1990 international migrants accounted for only 2.3% of the world's total population. However, their distribution by region was far from uniform.

In Australia and New Zealand, international migrants made up 18% of the total population in 1990; in western Asia, nearly 11%; in North America, less than 9%; in the traditional market economy countries of Europe, over 6%; and in Asia (excluding western Asia), Africa and Latin America, less than 2.5%.

Net international migration contributed 45% of the overall population growth in the developed world for 1990-1995, but it lowered slightly the overall growth rate of the population in the developing world by 3%. Whereas the annual growth rate of international migrant stock in the developed world increased only moderately from 2.3% per year during 1965-1975 to 2.4% during 1985-1990, the annual growth rate of the total number of migrants in the developing world increased ninefold, from 0.3% during 1965-1975 to 2.7% during 1985-1990. Despite the rapid growth of the number of international migrants in the developing world, by 1990 the proportion of international migrants among the total population of the developing world remained low at 1.6%, as against 4.5% of the population in the developed world. However, in Europe almost 88% of the population growth during the period 1990-1995 was attributable to international migration, with unemployment of the educated in the developing countries being a contributing factor.

Refugees are an important component of the number of international migrants in the world. The total number of refugees worldwide is estimated to have increased markedly during 1985-1990, going from 10.5 million to 14.9 million and accounting for 12.4% of the world's migrant stock in 1990. In fact, the refugee stock reached a maximum early in 1993, when it stood at 18.2 million. Since then, the number of refugees has been decreasing so that by early 1996 it stood at 13.2 million. This decline has resulted from major repatriations made possible by the solution of several long-standing conflicts and from the growing reluctance of countries of asylum to grant refugee status.

Age composition and dependency ratios

In 1997, there were about 2.3 billion young persons aged less than 20 years in the world (40% of the total population). Children under 5 constituted 10% of the world population, and older persons 7% (389 million). The rest were aged 20-64 years.

Population growth not only varies by level of development, there are also differential rates of growth of various components of the global population (Fig 13). For example, the global population of children grew at 1.57% per year between 1955 and 1975, 0.6% between 1975 and 1995 and is expected to grow by 0.25% between 1995 and 2025. The older population aged 65 and above, however, increased by 2.3%, 2.4% and 2.6% respectively during these periods. Of the 140 million increase between 1975 and 1995 in the population aged 65 and above, 46 million (33%) is attributable to the developed countries and 7 million (5%) to the LDCs. Increases for the period 1995-2025 are estimated to be 91 million (21%) for the developed countries and 28 million (6%) for LDCs.

Though the child population decreased by 8 million in the developed

countries during 1975-1995, there was an overall increase of 74 million in the developing world, more than 40% of which concerned the LDCs. During 1995-2025, however, it is expected that the child population will decrease by 6 million in the developed countries but increase by 54 million in the developing world, more than 90% of which will concern the LDCs.

Overall there is also a shift in the composition of the dependency ratios (Fig 14). For every 100 young dependants aged less than 20 years in 1955, there were 12 older dependants aged 65 and above. In 1975 the ratio was 100 to 12, in 1995 it was 100 to 16 and by 2025 there are expected to be 31 older dependants for every 100 young dependants.

The number of women of childbearing age (15-49 years) increased annually by 1.8% during 1955-1975 and by 2.1% during 1975-1995, and is expected to increase by 1% per year during 1995-2025, an increase of 522 million. Adolescent women aged 15-19 account for about 20% of all women of reproductive age now in the developing world, but are expected to represent 16% by 2025. Worldwide the number of these women will increase by at least 56 million during 1995-2025, rising to 307 million by 2025, most of them in the developing countries..

Fertility

The total fertility rate (TFR) – the number of births per woman of childbearing age – has been declining from 5 in 1955 to 4.2 in 1975 and to 2.9 in 1995. It is expected to reach 2.3 by 2025. The world average, however, conceals large differences among countries and regions. TFRs in 1995 ranged from 1.2 in Italy to 7.6 in Yemen. In 1995 the TFR for the developed world was only 1.7 compared

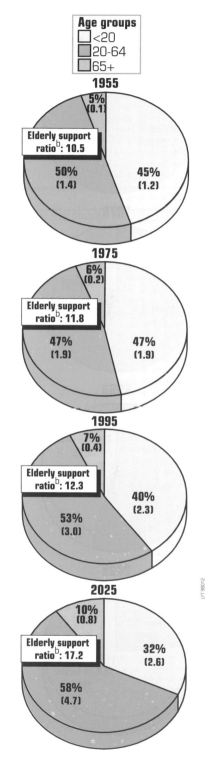

Fig.14. Age structure of the global population, 1955-2025[a]

Age groups
- <20
- 20-64
- 65+

1955
- 5% (0.1)
- Elderly support ratio[b]: 10.5
- 50% (1.4)
- 45% (1.2)

1975
- 6% (0.2)
- Elderly support ratio[b]: 11.8
- 47% (1.9)
- 47% (1.9)

1995
- 7% (0.4)
- Elderly support ratio[b]: 12.3
- 53% (3.0)
- 40% (2.3)

2025
- 10% (0.8)
- Elderly support ratio[b]: 17.2
- 58% (4.7)
- 32% (2.6)

[a] Percentages of total global population; figures in brackets refer to the number of persons in billions.
[b] Elderly support ratio: population aged 65 and above as a percentage of the population aged 20-64.

Box 22. Alcohol and socioeconomic stress

The period of transition to democracy in the countries of the former USSR has been associated with a catastrophic increase in mortality. Between 1987 and 1994 male life expectancy at birth in the Russian Federation fell by over seven years, to 57.6 years. In some parts of the country, the drop was even greater and life expectancy fell to 49 years, a figure comparable with many parts of sub-Saharan Africa. Life expectancy at birth for women also fell, although to a much smaller extent, resulting in 1994 in a 13-year difference between men and women – the largest sex difference ever documented.

These changes are unprecedented in an industrialized country in peace-time. Theories about their cause have included inaccurate data, collapse of the health care system, environmental damage, alcohol and psychosocial stress. A team of Russian, British and French researchers, using a recon-structed series of previously unpublished mortality data, has recently shown that the trends are real and has accumulated compelling evidence for the important role of alcohol.

Alcohol consumption has always been a feature of Russian life. In 1985, decisive action was taken to address the social consequences of high levels of alcohol consumption, with a major anti-alcohol campaign, leading to a dramatic reduction in supply. Within a few years, however, the amount of alcohol available began to rise again, largely due to illegal production.

The fall in age-specific death rates from a variety of causes after the anti-alcohol campaign was almost an exact mirror image of the rise after 1989, strongly suggesting that the same factors are involved in both. Many of the causes of death affected, such as accidents and violence, alcoholic poisoning and pneumonia, have recognized links with alcohol. The one surprise was cardiovascular disease, where the prevailing consensus is that moderate alcohol consumption is protective. Evidence is emerging, however, that binge drinking has specific effects on the heart, with a recent Finnish study report-ing a seven-fold increased risk of sudden cardiac death among those drinking three or more litres of beer at a time. This is consistent with a key finding from the Russian data of a significant increase in sudden cardiovascular deaths at weekends, especially among young and early middle-aged men. Other work has shown that a high proportion of Russian men dying suddenly have specific evidence of alcoholic damage to their heart muscle.

These findings have implications for other countries undergoing social and economic transition. They also highlight the importance of considering alcohol as a major cause of premature death in other countries. Alcohol consumption has been shown to be a major cause of the failure by Hungary to match the gains in life expectancy of neighbouring countries such as Po-land and the Czech Republic. A better understanding of the linkage between excessive alcohol consumption, social and economic stresses, and health is likely to be of relevance to some other regions and countries in the world undergoing periods of rapid transition.

Personal communication from Martin McKee & David Leon, European Centre on Health of Societies in Transition, London School of Hygiene and Tropical Medicine, United Kingdom.

an unequalled future and the grave threat of unparalleled disaster. Recent years have witnessed a re-emergence of a positive view of urbanization. As the world approaches the 21st cen-tury with close to 6 billion inhabitants and with nearly half this number liv-ing in urban centres, it is now ac-cepted that a predominantly urban population is not only an inevitable part of a wealthy economy, but also one that brings many advantages. The challenge is how to manage cities and other human settlements and ensure healthy living conditions in an increas-ingly urbanizing world.

About 45% of the world's popula-tion now live in urban areas and in a few years, for the first time in history, urban dwellers will outnumber those in the traditionally rural areas as the global urban population increases from 2.6 billion in 1995 to about 4 bil-lion in 2015. The United Nations Centre for Human Settlements (UNCHS-Habitat) estimates that by the end of the 21st century, more peo-ple will be in urban areas of the de-veloping world than are alive on the planet today. The number of persons living in urban areas increased glo-bally from 872 million (32% of the world population) in 1955 to 1.5 bil-lion (38%) in 1975, and to 2.6 billion (45%) in 1995. It is expected to reach 4 billion (54%) by 2015 *(Fig. 16)*. Al-though there is a growing number of what are termed "megacities" (with a population exceeding 10 million) they represented only 3% of the world population in 1995. New kinds of ur-ban systems are also developing in many parts of the world, often around the largest cities where a denser net-work of smaller cities develop and become more dynamic than the large city itself. While the growth of the urban population is faster than over-all population growth in the develop-ing world, the annual growth rate de-clined from 4% during 1955-1975 to

3.8% during 1975-1995, and is expected to decline further and reach 2.9% per year between 1995 and 2015. However, the composition and distribution of urban agglomerations have been changing dramatically during the past few decades. While the number of megacities increased from one in 1955 to five in 1975, and to 14 in 1995, the number of urban agglomerations with a population exceeding 1 million increased from 90 in 1955 to 178 in 1975, and to 324 in 1995. There are expected to be 408 in 2015. The proportion of the urban population living in these agglomerations has also increased from 26% in 1955 to 36% in 1995, and may be 37% in 2015. This means that a significant proportion of the world's urban population live in small market towns and administrative centres, strengthening urban-rural linkages in economic and social support systems. It also reflects the steadily declining proportion of the world's population making a living from agriculture and related areas. The "city summit" in Istanbul in 1996 outlined new directions for human settlements and an enabling approach that could also ensure satisfaction of the social, economic and environmental goals of sustainable development.

The occurrence of the major vector-borne diseases is closely related to naturally existing *environmental conditions*. In addition, the incidence, severity and distribution of vector-borne diseases are affected substantially by human activities such as water and agricultural development, and by urbanization. As nearly all malaria is associated with environmental conditions, it is estimated that 90% of the global burden of this disease (e.g. an estimated 1.5-2.7 million deaths and 300-500 million cases globally) is attributable to environmental factors. Schistosomiasis is another tropical disease which is strongly re-

lated to environmental conditions. Spread via a parasite in freshwater snails, it infects more than 200 million people. Other major vector-borne diseases influenced by environmental conditions include lymphatic filariasis, dengue fever, leishmaniasis and Chagas disease. Diarrhoeal diseases which are closely associated with lack of access to clean water and food, and personal hygiene, cause 3 million deaths annually.

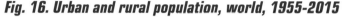

Fig. 16. Urban and rural population, world, 1955-2015

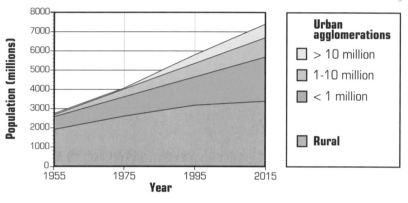

Table 8 summarizes the multiple linkages between exposure situations and the major diseases/conditions they can cause. Most of these are potentially related to several environmental exposure situations. Poor environmental quality is estimated to be directly responsible for around 25% of all preventable ill-health in the world today, with diarrhoeal diseases and acute respiratory infections heading the list. Up to two-thirds of preventable ill-health due to environmental conditions occurs among children.

Driving forces create the conditions in which environmental health threats can either develop or be averted. Government policies and programmes – which will vary according to the prevailing value system – change the direction and/or magnitude of driving forces and can there-

Table 8. Potential relationships between exposure situations and diseases/conditions

Health conditions of concern	Exposure situations					
	Polluted air	Excreta and household wastes	Polluted water or deficiencies in water management	Polluted food	Unhealthy housing	Global environmental change
Acute respiratory infections	•				•	
Diarrhoeal diseases		•	•	•		
Malaria and other vector-borne diseases		•	•	•		•
Other infections		•	•	•	•	
Cancer	•			•		•
Cardiovascular diseases	•					•
Mental disorders					•	
Chronic respiratory diseases	•					•
Injuries and poisonings	•		•	•	•	•

fore alleviate or exacerbate a broad array of environmental health threats. The main driving forces are: population dynamics; urbanization; poverty and inequity; technical and scientific developments; consumption and production patterns; and economic development. Environmental threats to human health can be divided into "traditional hazards" associated with lack of development and "modern hazards" associated with unsustainable development.

Traditional hazards related to poverty and insufficient development include: lack of access to safe drinking-water; inadequate basic sanitation in the household and the community; indoor air pollution from cooking and heating, using coal or biomass fuel; and inadequate solid waste disposal.

Modern hazards are related to development that lacks health-and-environment safeguards, and to unsustainable consumption of natural resources. They include: water pollution from populated areas, industry and intensive agriculture; urban air pollution from motor vehicles, coal power stations and industry; climate change; stratospheric ozone de-

pletion and transboundary pollution.

Water, food and air are the principal exposure routes of environmental health hazards. Also heavily implicated are the manner in which household wastes and sewage are handled, and the conditions in which people live and work.

More than 1 billion people do not have ready access to an adequate and safe water supply, and a variety of physical, chemical and biological agents render many water sources unhealthy. Today, more than 800 million of those unserved live in rural areas *(Fig.17)*. Water supply also varies widely in terms of region and country. For instance, urban areas generally have higher coverage than rural areas. In cities, water is often provided to districts whose populations can pay for services. Water supply and sanitation coverage has changed considerably over the years. In the mid-1970s, of the approximately 2.5 billion people in the developing world, only 38% had safe drinking-water, and 32% adequate sanitation. At the beginning of the 1980s, water supply coverage was 75% in urban areas and 46% in rural areas, while sanitation reached 60% in urban centres and 31% in rural environments. In developing countries, 75% of the population had access to water supply and only 35% had access to sanitation in 1994.

Food is essential to a healthy life, but it can also be a major route of exposure for many pathogens and toxic chemicals. These contaminants may be introduced into food during cultivation, harvesting, processing, storage, transportation and final preparation. Biological and chemical agents in food represent the two major types of foodborne hazard. Biological agents tend to pose acute hazards with incubation periods of a few hours to several weeks before the onset of disease, whereas chemical hazards usually involve long-term, low-level exposures.

Air pollution, both indoor and outdoor, leads to an estimated 3 million premature deaths globally. For example, the acute and long-term consequences for health of the recent forest fires in South-East Asia are a case in point of the serious threats to health from air pollution on a regional scale. When inhaled, air pollutants affect the lungs and respiratory tract; they are also taken up by the blood and transported throughout the body. And since air pollutants are deposited on soil and plants and in water, they can contribute to further human exposure if contaminated food and water are ingested. Indoor air pollution can be particularly hazardous to health because it is released in close proximity to people. The most prominent source of indoor air pollution in developing countries is household use of biomass and coal for heating and cooking, usually involving open fires or stoves without proper chimneys.

Ozone layer depletion due to use of chlorofluorocarbons has increased rapidly in recent years and the "ozone

Fig. 17. Water and sanitation coverage, rural and urban population, developing world, 1994[a]

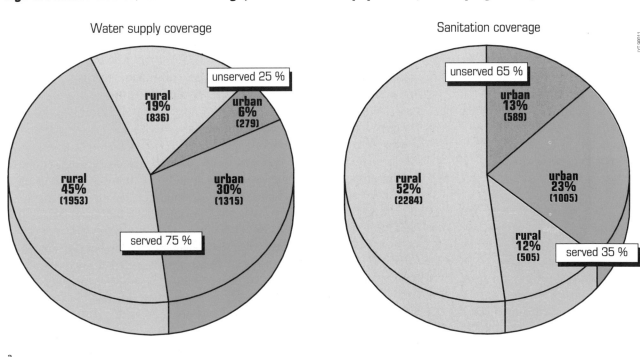

a Percentages relate to population in rural and urban areas concerned; figures in brackets refer to population in millions.

Box 23. Climate change – Health risks for the 21st century

Unprecedented changes taking place in the global climate because of greenhouse gas emissions could lead to wide-ranging impacts on human health, according to some leading scientists. Such climate changes are gradual and complex, and their environmental consequences are difficult to predict, but they could result in marked increases in death and illness from both infectious and noninfectious diseases. Various recent scientific studies based on mathematical models indicate that a global mean temperature increase of 1-2 degrees C would enable mosquitos to extend their range to new geographical areas, leading to increases in cases of malaria and several other infectious diseases - especially in populations living just outside the areas where these diseases currently occur.

The proportion of the world's population at risk of malaria, presently estimated at 2.4 billion people, could increase from around 45% to 60% by the year 2050. The estimated number of annual deaths from malaria would rise from between the present 2-3 million to 3.5-5 million. There is already some evidence that malaria incidence is increasing in a number of highland regions, for example in Kenya, in a manner that is compatible with recent regional warming - although other ecological factors may also be involved.

Dengue, another mosquito-borne disease, currently threatens 1.8 billion people. An estimated 50 million people are infected annually, and the disease causes about 25 000 deaths. A temperature rise of 1-2 degrees C could result in an increase of the at-risk population by several hundred million, with 20 000-30 000 more dengue deaths a year in 2050. A recent study by the World Resources Institute, in conjunction with WHO experts, predicted that by 2020 - if the current trends in greenhouse gas emission continue - there would be 700 000 avoidable deaths occurring annually because of additional exposure to atmospheric particulate matter (PM) produced by the burning of fossil fuels, with 80% of these deaths occurring in developing countries. The health effects of PM include cardiovascular and respiratory illness. The researchers have calculated that up to 8 million PM-related deaths worldwide in the first 20 years of the next century could be prevented by the implementation of a climate policy designed to reduce carbon emissions significantly. They have concluded that regardless of how or when greenhouse gases alter climate, reducing them now will save lives worldwide by lessening particulate air pollution, and that the beneficial effects of reduced particulate pollution appear to be far greater in rapidly developing countries than in developed countries, although they are substantial in both regions. The study was presented at a United Nations climate change conference in Kyoto, Japan, in 1997.

Some effects of global climate change and stratospheric ozone layer depletion (a separate but coexistent problem) could be beneficial. For example, in areas with relatively colder climates, an increase in ambient temperature could result in a decrease in cardiovascular mortality. But most effects are expected to be adverse. For example, stratospheric ozone depletion would increase skin cancer incidence, but scientists calculate that the excess mortality involved from increases in skin cancer would be much less than that due to the expected rise in malaria deaths from climate change.

hole" over the South Pole now reaches populated areas. A similar trend is seen around the North Pole and the associated increase of solar UV-radiation exposure may in the next decades cause an increase of cataracts, skin cancer and immune system damage. The Intergovernmental Panel on Climate Change has concluded that a warming of the Earth's surface due to human activities producing greenhouse gases is occurring (Box 23).

The number and quantities of chemicals used, both in developed and developing countries, are constantly increasing. The total number of chemicals on the market is now close to 100 000, while the value of the total global annual production of chemicals is about $1.5 trillion. The population groups most affected by chemicals are poor, illiterate people with little or no access to appropriate training or basic information on the risks posed by chemicals to which they are exposed directly or indirectly every day. Although both men and women are exposed to the health risks related to the use of chemicals in the rural environment and to chemicals used in cottage industries and in the home, women's health can be particularly affected. Infants and children are more susceptible to a variety of chemicals, such as heavy metals and several persistent organic pollutants.

In favourable circumstances, work contributes to good health and economic achievement. With economic development, many countries have experienced a shift from the hazards that characterized work in agriculture, mining and other primary industries, to those that characterize manufacturing industries or service industries. Many workers, however, are exposed to health hazards that contribute to respiratory diseases, cancer, reproductive disorders, allergies, cardiovascular disease, psychological stress, eye damage and hearing loss, as well as some communicable diseases. New occupational disease problems have emerged, and the incidence of reported occupational disease has accordingly increased in certain developed countries.

Housing is of central importance to quality of life. Ideally, it minimizes disease and injury, and contributes much to physical, mental and social well-being. The home environment should afford protection against the hazards to health arising from the physical and social environment. Yet numerous factors in the home environment may influence health negatively *(Box 24)*. At least 600 million urban dwellers in Africa, Asia and Latin America live in life- and health-threatening homes and neighbourhoods. Most live in cramped, overcrowded dwellings with four or more persons to a room in tenements, cheap boarding houses or shelters built on illegally occupied or subdivided land. Tens of millions are homeless and sleep in public or semi-public spaces – for instance pavement dwellers and those sleeping in bus shelters, train stations or parks. Perhaps as many as 600 million also have inadequate or no access to effective health care, which means that the economic impact of disease or injury is magnified.

The combustion of raw biomass products produces hundreds of chemical compounds including suspended particulate matter, such as carbon monoxide, oxides of nitrogen and sulfur. The principal adverse effects of these compounds on health are respiratory, but in poorly ventilated dwellings, especially when fuels such as charcoal and coal are used to heat rooms in which people sleep, carbon monoxide poisoning is a serious hazard.

Estimating levels of poverty based on poor-quality housing – ***housing***

Box 24. The health burden of poor housing

Any study of the health burden of poor housing has to consider the health burden arising not only within the home but also in the area around the home. Here are nine features of the housing environment that WHO has singled out as having important direct or indirect effects on the health of their occupants:

- The structure of the shelter (which includes consideration of the extent to which the shelter protects the occupants from extremes of heat or cold, insulation against noise and invasion by dust, rain, insects and rodents).
- The extent to which the provision for water supplies is adequate – both from a qualitative and a quantitative point of view.
- The effectiveness of provision for the disposal (and subsequent management) of excreta and liquid and solid wastes.
- The quality of the housing site, including the extent to which it is structurally safe for housing and provision is made to protect it from contamination (of which provision for drainage is among the most important aspects).
- Overcrowding which can lead to household accidents and increased transmission of airborne infections such as acute respiratory infectious diseases, pneumonia and tuberculosis.
- The presence of indoor air pollution associated with fuels used for cooking and/or heating.
- Food safety standards – including the extent to which the shelter has adequate provision for storing food to protect it against spoilage and contamination.
- Vectors and hosts of disease associated with the domestic and peri-domestic environment.
- The home as a workplace – where the use and storage of toxic or hazardous chemicals and unsafe equipment may present health hazards.

---

poverty – and on absence of basic infrastructure and services gives a more realistic picture of urban poverty, particularly in the developing world (as elaborated in *The World Health Report 1997*). For a significant proportion of more than 600 million people living in life- and health-threatening homes and neighbourhoods, improvements in levels of infrastructure and service provision and support can be achieved at low cost. UNCHS-Habitat points out that such improvements are often with

Investing in people's

health and their

environment is a

prerequisite for

sustainable

development.

good possibility of cost recovery. The reason for the very poor housing and living conditions in which a sizeable proportion of people live is not that they are unable to pay for housing with basic services, but that such housing is unnecessarily expensive or simply not available.

The eradication of poverty, particularly housing poverty, is essential for sustainable human settlements and thus for sustainable development. Science and technology have a crucial role in shaping housing conditions and living and working environments, and in sustaining ecosystems. Quality of life depends on the indoor and outdoor conditions and spatial characteristics of villages, towns and cities. However, it is imperative that governments recognize their role as active agents in building an enabling environment for applying knowledge and experience in these areas for sustainable human settlement development. The challenge is for society to be willing to meet these needs and for governments to formulate innovative policies and programmes for action to make our human settlements safe and liveable. A plan to this end was elaborated at the United Nations Conference on Human Settlements (Habitat V), held in Istanbul in 1996.

WHO's response

From 1950 to 1970, WHO emphasized environmental sanitation. In 1971, the Fifth general programme of work noted that a dark side of industrialization and urbanization was the emergence of factors detrimental to health, e.g. pollution, road accidents and stressful city life, and that the previous concept of environmental sanitation had evolved into that of environmental health. During the 1980s, considerable impetus was given to the improvement of commu-

nity water supply and sanitation by the International Drinking Water Supply and Sanitation Decade (1981-1990). Recently however, sanitation has been given very low priority in comparison to other general development needs, including water supply. Rapid population growth in developing countries, particularly in urban areas, has contributed significantly to the dramatic proportions of the sanitation deficit. For this reason, the World Health Assembly will consider a new strategy on sanitation for high-risk communities in 1998.

The Earth Summit held in Rio de Janeiro, Brazil, in 1992 heralded a new approach to national and international development and environment planning. World leaders recognized the importance of investing in improvements to people's health and their environment as a prerequisite for sustainable development. Continuing commitment to securing human health and a healthy environment is now widespread, as evidenced by a number of declarations and statements that have emanated from recent international conferences. WHO's Commission on health and environment provided a substantive input into the preparation of Agenda 21, the blueprint for action towards human-centred sustainable development, and WHO's global strategy on health and environment was developed as a response. As part of the follow-up process, a worldwide effort is under way to prepare national plans for sustainable development. Conferences of health and environment ministries convened by WHO in the Americas, Eastern Mediterranean and Europe have been instrumental in accelerating the process, and agreements have been reached on deadlines for completing such plans. For example, in Europe, by the end of 1997 more than 50% of all countries had prepared national environmental health action plans.

In 1997, WHO published *Health and environment in sustainable development: five years after the Earth Summit,* which brings together quantitative data on health-and-environment issues with examples from regions and countries. Other publications include *Linkage methods for environment and health analysis – technical guidelines,* which, together with its companion volume, the *General guidelines,* was used in teaching workshops on epidemiology for decision-making. Other activities have contributed to further strengthening the international and national systems for radiation emergency medical preparedness and response, the medical and epidemiological monitoring of populations affected by the Chernobyl accident, and the understanding of biological and health effects of low-dose radiation.

In response to growing public health concerns in Member States, WHO is coordinating and encouraging research into possible associations between low-frequency electromagnetic fields and a number of diseases such as childhood leukaemia, breast cancer, and diseases of the central nervous system. In 1997, the representatives of 31 agencies from 17 countries identified the most important gaps in the existing scientific knowledge. This has enabled WHO to make recommendations to the international scientific community concerning research priorities in this field over the next four years.

A sanitation promotion kit was developed in 1997 as the foundation of a new WHO strategy on sanitation. Country workshops and hygiene education seminars were held in all regions to promote sanitation as a major instrument to reduce diarrhoeal mortality in infants. A comprehensive guidebook was issued on the management of health care wastes.

Following international concern about the dangers posed by chemicals to humanity and the environment expressed by the United Nations Conference on the Human Environment in 1972, the International Programme on Chemical Safety (IPCS) was established in 1980 as a collaborative programme of WHO, ILO and UNEP. During the past two decades, IPCS has made full evaluations of some 200 chemicals. Guidance has been provided on safe levels of some 100 chemicals in drinking-water, 35 chemicals in air, 655 pesticides and 30 veterinary drug residues in food, and of 1205 food additives. Guidance has also been provided on diagnosis and treatment of toxic exposures to some 250 chemicals, and on the safe use of 1300 chemicals in the workplace. In 1993, IPCS initiated a project to globally harmonize approaches used by different countries for the assessment of risk. IPCS issues, on a biannual basis, a CD-ROM containing the various published outputs of the chemical programmes of WHO and its partners. International organizations are also cooperating with IPCS to develop a global information network on chemicals, and to provide information electronically, with access through the Internet.

Twelve environmental health criteria monographs were published in 1997. These are comprehensive documents which provide internationally peer-reviewed assessments of risk to human health and the environment from exposure to chemicals. The IPCS chemical incidents project provides guidance to the health sector on preparedness for and response to direct or indirect exposure of populations. A harmonized format for international exchange of data on chemical incidents is currently being field-tested with the assistance of a WHO collaborating centre (University of Wales Institute, Cardiff).

WHO is coordinating research into possible associations between electromagnetic fields and a number of diseases.

Major investment in international work will have to be made if the goal of evaluating a further 500 chemicals by the year 2000, as requested by the UN Conference on Environment and Development, is to be met. Research is also needed to better elucidate the etiology of diseases caused by chemicals, including those which may be caused by endocrine-disrupting chemicals, as well as other impacts of chemicals on the health of vulnerable population groups, particularly women, children and the elderly.

Food and nutrition

Food security, defined as the access for all people at all times to enough food for an active and healthy life, underpins the "food for all" initiative launched at the World Food Summit in 1996. Much of the work in this area was concerned mainly with food security and until recently focused on the adequacy (or inadequacy) of food availability to meet the nutritional needs of the population.

In almost all countries there are people who suffer from hunger and malnutrition – a pathological state resulting from too little consumption of essential nutrients – but the extent and the pattern differ substantially from country to country. One way to examine the nutrition situation and monitor developments in world food security is to look at the food supply available for consumption. Average dietary energy supply in calories derived from national food balance sheets and population data show that, although enough food is supplied globally, at least 840 million people in the developing world had inadequate access to food in the early 1990s (i.e. below the nutrition threshold that represents a minimum level of energy requirements). This figure, though high, reflects a substantial degree of

progress since the beginning of the 1970s, when the number of persons with inadequate access to food was about 920 million. In relative terms it declined from 35% of the population in the developing world to 21%, primarily as a result of progress in East Asia (including China) and parts of South Asia, such as India and Pakistan. Worldwide average daily per capita dietary energy supply increased from less than 2300 calories in 1961-1963 to 2440 in 1969-1971, to 2720 in 1990-1992 and is expected to reach a value of 2900 calories by 2010. The population with an average dietary energy supply per capita per day of more than 2700 calories increased from 145 million in 1969-1971 to more than 1.8 billion in 1990-1992 and is expected to be 2.7 billion by 2010.

For several developing countries, the 1970s was a decade of improvement, faster than that of the 1960s, with rapid progress continuing up to about the mid-1980s but at a slower pace thereafter. However, several countries and even whole regions failed to make progress and even experienced outright reversals. The situation is most serious in Africa, where the number of classically undernourished people in sub-Saharan countries more than doubled during this period. Even though the global average may increase to 2800 calories per day by 2010, there may not be significant nutrition progress. The population with inadequate access to food may decline only from 840 million to 680 million, although this would represent a reduction from the present 21% of the population of the developing countries to 12% in 2010.

The green revolution which began in the 1960s has been seen as a global technological achievement, the effects of which are still being felt today. Innovative approaches focusing on economic, social and environ-

In almost all countries

there are people

who suffer from

hunger and

malnutrition.

mental factors that affect the food production process should also be addressed, however. To this end FAO proposes **urban agriculture** as a possible solution to the concerns related to food insecurity in the next 25 years.. Urban agriculture is defined as food production that occurs within the confines of cities, for example in backyards, community vegetable gardens or unused spaces, and is mostly small-scale and scattered. City farming has a long tradition in many societies, especially in Asia and Europe. The contribution of urban agriculture to food security (defined as the holding of a certain supply of food to be available and accessible at all times) appears to be substantial in many developing cities. 200 million urban farmers worldwide supply food to 700 million people, or about 12% of the world population. Surveys have shown for example that urban farming provides 50% of vegetable consumption in Karachi and 85% in Shanghai. Women form the bulk of producers in both Africa and Latin America.

Nutritional status of the population depends on food consumption and not solely on production and availability of food. Dietary energy

supply measurements assume that available food is distributed and consumed in relation to requirements, which is rarely the case. Several measurements of the human body directly related to intake have therefore been developed. Children's body measurements, for example, are particularly sensitive to changes in the intake of protein and calories as well as to the onset of disease. Protein-energy malnutrition (PEM), generally referred to simply as malnutrition, is an imbalance between the supply of protein and energy and the body's demand for them to ensure optimal growth and function. Such an imbalance leads to wasting, stunting and underweight when energy intake is inadequate, and to overweight and obesity when it is excessive (Fig. 18).

The most commonly used indicator of PEM is the percentage of children whose weight-for-age falls below a reference value (international growth curves) usually set by WHO and the United States National Center for Health Statistics. Underweight prevalence in children under 5 has declined in developing countries, from 46% in 1975 to 31% in 1995, but progress has not been uniform. Recent WHO estimates suggest

Fig. 18. Percentage of population underweight and overweight, selected countries, around 1993

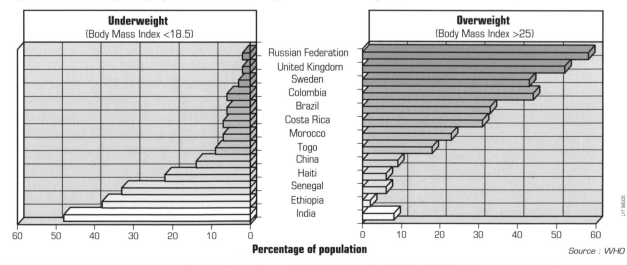

Growth in the number

of severely

overweight adults

is expected

to be double that of

underweight adults.

that worldwide in 1995, 168 million children under 5 were classified as underweight (31% of the total). In developing countries, about 206 million (38%) were stunted, and about 49 million (9%) wasted. The risk of being malnourished as measured by underweight is 1.2 times higher in Asia than in Africa, and 3 times higher in Africa than in Latin America. The number of under-5s living in each geographical area – 54 million in Latin America, 121 million in Africa, and 363 million in Asia – renders the distribution among regions even more unequal. South-central Asia has by far the highest malnutrition levels, both in terms of prevalence rates and absolute numbers. In this subregion alone, about 50% of under-5s (86 million) are malnourished, accounting for half the total number of malnourished children in developing countries.

Mortality rates in children under 5 are 2.5 times higher in those that are moderately underweight, and 5 times higher in the severely underweight. About 50% of deaths among these children were associated with malnutrition, while for about 300 000 under-5 deaths in developing countries, malnutrition was the direct cause. It is also estimated that about 22 million children under 5 years are overweight. WHO estimates that in developing countries about 245 million adults are moderately underweight and 93 million severely underweight. At the same time, there are over 200 million adults who are moderately or severely overweight, of whom 58 million are in developing countries. Overall it appears that in any country – developed or developing – prevalence of malnutrition (underweight and overweight) is about 50%.

WHO estimates that underweight prevalence in developing countries should decline to about 28% (165 million) among children under 5 years by 2025. For adults, even the most optimistic trend gives a global value for 2025 of 82 million for severely underweight and 131 million for moderately underweight; severe overweight prevalence in 2025 is estimated at 300 million adults. Growth in the number of severely overweight adults is expected to be double that of underweight adults during 1995-2025. In order to assess the implications of these trends for the future health of mankind, the following figures should be considered: excess adult mortality in 1995 attributable to undernutrition is estimated at about 0.5 million deaths and to overnutrition at about 1 million; mortality rates increase by about 25% and 100% respectively in underweight and overweight persons.

Prevalence of micronutrient malnutrition in respect of iron, iodine and vitamin A is more widespread than PEM (*Table 9*). An estimated 2 billion people are anaemic, with nearly 3.6 billion iron-deficient. Anaemia prevalence is highest (around 50%) in pregnant women and preschool-age children in developing countries. Iodine deficiency disorders affect about 15% of the world's population, 834 million having goitre, 16.5 million cretinism. Vitamin A deficiency (subclinical) affects about 285 million (42%) of under-5 children globally; about 0.5% are severely affected (xerophthalmia). Iodine deficiency disorders are declining rapidly however, thanks to near-universal salt iodization. Sustainable elimination by 2000 or 2010 is possible. Clinical vitamin A deficiency could with sustained effort be eliminated by 2025. The main problem is in dealing with iron deficiency, but with widespread iron fortification programmes, slow reduction would be possible.

WHO's response

A safe food supply that will not endanger consumer health through chemical, biological or other forms of contamination is essential for proper nutrition. WHO has provided leadership in the field of food safety assurance over the past 50 years by giving guidance on food safety and quality control systems, promoting good manufacturing practices and educating food retailers and consumers about appropriate food handling. Activities have included providing Member States with expert scientific opinion, and advising them on the development and enforcement of food legislation, jointly with FAO as the Secretariat of the Codex Alimentarius Commission. WHO has also provided leadership at the international level, with the development of guidelines for the implementation of the hazards analysis and critical control point system as a management tool for food safety assurance, and in the assessment of food technologies (e.g. food irradiation and fermentation) that prevent foodborne infections and intoxications and reduce post-harvest losses. More recently WHO has dealt with the safety evaluation of foods produced using modern biotechnology, through collaboration with other international agencies, national governments and NGOs.

In 1997, WHO prepared a document on *Food safety and globalization of trade in food* in cooperation with WTO, which draws the attention of public health authorities to the implications of the WTO Agreement on the Application of Sanitary and Phytosanitary Measures for national food legislation (see also *Box 5*). Other consultations (convened jointly with FAO) concerned risk management and food safety, and food consumption and exposure assessment to chemicals in food. A study group con-

Table 9. Micronutrient malnutrition, developing countries, 1995 and 2025

Prevalence	Number of persons (millions)	
	1995	2025
Goitre	834	350
Iron deficiencies	3 580	2 750
Vitamin A deficiencies	2.85	0.17

vened with FAO and IAEA concluded that food irradiated to any dose appropriate to achieve the intended technological objective is both safe to consume and nutritionally adequate, and no upper dose limit need be imposed.

To strengthen and support surveillance of foodborne diseases, WHO has issued a document entitled *Surveillance of foodborne diseases: what are the options?* A databank on foodborne disease outbreaks was established to collect epidemiological data on foodborne disease outbreaks, and a consultation was held on prevention and control of enterohaemorrhagic *E. coli* O157:H7 infections.

Education

In the 21st century, the world will be shaped by new and powerful forces that include the globalization of economic activity and the growing importance of knowledge as a prerequisite for participation in fundamental human activity. During the 1990s, the global development community renewed its search for ways to broaden the scope and improve the quality and accessibility of basic education. Worldwide primary and secondary school enrolments rose from about 250 million children in 1960 to more than 1 billion in 1995. Enrolments in higher education have more than doubled since 1975, and the number of literate adults tripled from 1 billion in 1960, to more than 3 billion in 1995.

The worldwide adult literacy rate increased from 70% of the population aged 15 years and over in 1980 to 78% in 1995, and it is expected to reach about 83% in 2010 *(Fig. 19)*. While progress is narrowing the gender gap, striking disparities between males and females and among countries still persist. While increased enrolments of children in formal schooling are crucial, masses of illiterate and poorly-educated adults are still inadequately prepared as parents, workers and citizens in the emerging global society. Improvements in literacy rates have been more pronounced among the younger age group. Both developed and developing countries are therefore paying more attention to the basic education of adults. Nonformal or out-of-school education is increasingly seen as a necessary component of a comprehensive strategy to provide education for all.

Unemployment

The International Labour Organization (ILO) estimated the world labour force at about 2.7 billion in 1995, with 78% in developing countries. As a result of both demographic factors and behavioural changes, developing countries' share in the total world labour force is expected to continue to increase, reaching 81% by 2010 (2.8 billion), but the average annual rate of growth is expected to slow from 2.2% (over the period 1950-1995) to 1.9% over the next 15 years, with variations among countries.

While the world economy continues to absorb the bulk of a rapidly rising global workforce, which is better educated, possesses greater skills and is more mobile than at any time in the past, unemployment has emerged as a problem and the effectiveness of labour markets has become a policy issue. Approaches to solving the problem of unemployment are being formulated in the context of rapid changes in economic conditions and in the quantity and quality of labour.

Since the 1970s, changes in the technology and organization of production in the developed economies and a slower rate of productivity and real output growth have made the achievement of low unemployment in a non-inflationary environment much more difficult than had been anticipated, and certainly much more difficult than it appeared to be 50 years ago. At that time, the Universal Declaration of Human Rights provided for the right of individuals to productive employment, and many developed economies adopted policies aimed at achieving full employment, or at least high levels of employment.

Over 120 million people worldwide are officially unemployed and many more underemployed, causing massive personal suffering, increased poverty, marginalization, exclusion, inequalities, reduced well-being, loss of dignity, widespread social disintegration and huge economic waste. The ILO considers an individual to be unemployed if he or she is currently without employment, is actively seeking employment and is available for employment within some time period mutually acceptable to both the prospective employee and a prospective employer. In many developing countries, unemployment remains a major unresolved problem and there has been a rise in underemployment, with a majority of the labour force remaining in low-productivity work that offers no escape from poverty. In a majority of industrialized countries, unemployment has persisted for over two decades while most transition economies have experienced a rapid rise in unemployment since 1990.

Youth unemployment is a serious problem in several developing countries, where at least 20% of male

> Over 120 million people worldwide are officially unemployed.

Fig. 19. Adult literacy, 1980-2010[a]

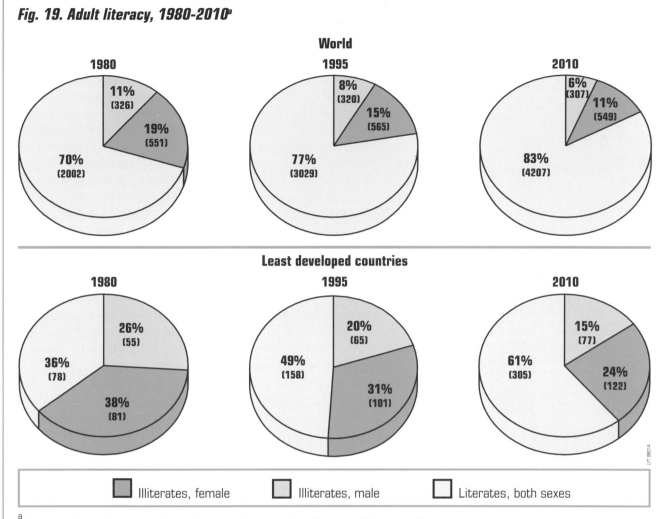

World

1980 — 11% (326) · 19% (551) · 70% (2002)

1995 — 8% (320) · 15% (565) · 77% (3029)

2010 — 6% (307) · 11% (549) · 83% (4207)

Least developed countries

1980 — 26% (55) · 36% (78) · 38% (81)

1995 — 20% (65) · 49% (158) · 31% (101)

2010 — 15% (77) · 61% (305) · 24% (122)

☐ Illiterates, female   ☐ Illiterates, male   ☐ Literates, both sexes

a
Percentage of total adult population; figures in brackets refer to the number of literates and illiterates in millions.
Source: UNESCO.

youth aged 20-24 years are unemployed. The relative share of people seeking their first job, the majority of whom are young workers and women, within the total unemployed population has been increasing over the past decade. Economies in many regions, particularly in Africa, have not been able to absorb new labour market entrants.

Economic restructuring in many countries has contributed to reducing demand for ***educated labour***, particularly where the public sector used to represent the main source of demand for such skills. Growth alone is no guarantee that employment will rise – the pattern of growth must be labour-absorptive, and this in turn is determined in part by the quality and quantity of labour. Lack of employment opportunities among the highest skilled labour and educated professionals are pushing them to leave their country in search of work abroad – a phenomenon known as the "brain drain".

The problems of unemployment, underemployment and poverty are severe in the developing world. The majority of the labour force remains trapped in low-productivity employment in the rural and informal sectors which offer little relief from poverty. On average, unemployment in the industrialized countries is also much higher now than it was in1950-1970. It is 50% higher in the United States and about seven times higher in Germany than in the 1960s. With the increasing integration of the world economy, issues of employment and labour standards have assumed a global dimension, since trade and investment flows have become an increasingly important influence on domestic employment prospects and policy options. The scope for national policy autonomy is restricted and the effectiveness of traditional policy instruments reduced, particularly in labour and social policy.

Poverty

Although there have been setbacks and difficulties, the global economic expansion of recent decades has brought great economic and social progress to many areas of the world. Mass poverty has been eliminated in the economically more advanced countries and significantly reduced in many developing countries. Measured in constant terms, incomes per capita in 1995 were about 90% higher in the developing countries than they were in 1970. The figure for the developed countries was about 60%. Infant mortality rates have fallen and life expectancy has risen. There have been advances in education, health care, living conditions and technology.

However, this prosperity has not been universal. Economic growth has been slow or non-existent in many poorer countries. Recent estimates by the World Bank of the number of people living below a common global poverty line indicates that in West Asia and sub-Saharan Africa per capita incomes had fallen to 80-90% of their 1970 level, in North Africa and Latin America incomes had risen by 25-50% of the 1970 levels, in South

Asia incomes had risen by more than 60% of the 1970 level, while in East Asia (including China) 1995 per capita incomes were more than twice the 1970 levels. The countries that saw a decline in their per capita incomes over the period constituted about 12.5% of the total population of developing countries in 1990, most of these being low-income countries. About a quarter of the world population lives in dire poverty and in many regions it is increasing. There is also a widening gap between the living standards of this quarter and those of the more privileged who enjoy rising standards of living. There is, however, an increasing international commitment to ensure that the poor share the benefits of economic expansion and social development, and in many countries special attention is now being paid to those living in absolute poverty and those who are disadvantaged as a result of discrimination, age, disability or infirmity (Box 25).

Both the absolute poor and the non-poor are trapped in a situation where economic growth and social development are interdependent. Low incomes mean limited capacity to save and invest, limited means for obtaining health services, high risk of personal illness, limitations on mobility, and limited access to education, information and training. Poor parents cannot provide their children with the opportunities for better health and education to improve their lot. Lack of motivation, hope and incentives creates a barrier to growth, and poverty is passed from one generation to the next. To rise out of poverty, the poor need the enhanced opportunities provided by faster economic growth as well as improved ability to respond to the opportunities available.

The central goal of development is increasingly recognized as the strengthening of human resources so

With the increasing

integration of the

world economy,

issues of employment

and labour standards

have assumed

a global dimension.

Box 25. Vulnerability reduction – A new approach

The World Health Report 1995 – Bridging the gaps drew attention to the widening gap between the health of privileged and underprivileged groups and concluded that poverty is the world's "deadliest disease". Noting that health and socioeconomic development are inextricably linked, the report also presented compelling arguments for focusing on the needs of vulnerable groups as a strategy for achieving sustainable human development.

The practical relevance of this strategy was demonstrated in late 1997, when WHO inaugurated the Mediterranean Centre for Vulnerability Reduction and thus formally launched a new approach to the prevention and management of major risks in vulnerable groups. The approach recognizes that certain communities are at "chronic" risk of emergencies due to factors that range from geographical location and climate, through the proximity of dams, industry, and other technological hazards, to poverty and the social exclusion it imposes.

While some of these factors cannot be altered, communities can nonetheless be helped to protect themselves, to cope and recover, and thus to prevent risks from turning into emergencies, and emergencies into disasters. The approach aims, in short, to stop the downward spiral of adverse event, emergency relief, dependance, withdrawal of short-term aid, deterioration of conditions, increased vulnerability, emergencies, and recurrence of disaster, with even worse results.

Although comparatively new, vulnerability reduction is firmly rooted in what WHO, the United Nations Development Programme, and other development agencies have learned about the dangers of fragmented sectoral assistance and the advantages of seeking long-term results.

The approach draws on strategies that are known to work. Efforts to reduce vulnerability and to manage risks are fully compatible with the principles of sustainable human development. Both rely on participatory techniques applied to local communities at risk. Both are closely linked to environmental concerns and adopt people-centred strategies. Both acknowledge that the best help is self-help, and both aim to achieve community self-reliance through decentralized and integrated multisectoral approaches.

The Mediterranean Centre for Vulnerability Reduction was created to serve as a regionwide technical institution and centre of reference and excellence for the Mediterranean basin. The Centre's primary concern is to develop the technical approaches and programmes needed to help communities at risk to strengthen their own capacity for vulnerability reduction and risk management.

The scope of activity includes the following types of risks:
- epidemics caused by infectious diseases;
- technological risks, including chemical and radiological hazards;
- natural risks, such as floods, earthquakes, cyclones, and landslides;
- societal risks, such as those caused by social exclusion and extreme poverty.

Tunisia, which provides the Centre's premises and infrastructure, has close links to the concept of vulnerability reduction and nationwide experience in its practical application. In recent years, the entire Tunisian population has mobilized support for a wide-ranging initiative aimed at fighting poverty and eradicating social exclusion by the year 2000. In the view of the government, such a programme, accompanied by broad popular support, represents the surest strategy for preventing social instability, which so often has its roots in inequalities, social exclusion, and extreme poverty.

as to improve education, health and productivity. The economic and social benefits of literacy are obvious. The cost to society of preventable illness and premature death is both economic and personal. Moreover, when all groups do not share equally in opportunities, the cost is borne not only by those discriminated against but by society as a whole. For this reason, policies directed at strengthening human resources, improving health and enhancing interaction on the basis of equity are the key to economic growth and poverty reduction.

Poverty reduction for those of working age has focused on increasing productivity through investment in human and physical capital, leading to higher levels of output and in-

The connection

between education,

health and earning

capacity is better

understood.

come. The connection between education, health and earning capacity is better understood. Policies are being formulated to prepare the unskilled for better jobs, augment the supply of scarce skills, upgrade the training of the poor, improve the functioning of the labour markets and improve the health status of the population of working age. For the full benefits of such policies to be reaped by the poor, a major effort may be needed to upgrade schools, clinics, sanitation and other public services.

Recent evidence suggests that raising literacy levels and reducing mortality and ill-health rates is more difficult for countries with a lower level of GNP per capita. Even so, policy interventions have been launched to increase literacy and survival prospects, even at low levels of per capita income. Raising incomes through faster economic growth, combined with appropriate social development policies, has contributed to a decline in poverty in the world and even in some regions, to an elimination of the manifestations of poverty.

National strategies for combating absolute poverty should include a modernization process that could accelerate and sustain long-term growth of labour productivity and enhance individuals' health and knowledge potential to contribute to society. To ensure that workers' output and earnings increase, the labour force must be better educated and more adaptable and be supported by improved technology and management, all of which require investment in human and physical capital.

Above all, good governance – the rule of law, equity, participation by all in society and the provision of efficient basic services – is essential if growth is to take place rapidly and provide maximum benefit for the poor. At the community level, implementation of poverty programmes should be in support of the activities carried out by local and self-governing institutions and should facilitate local involvement to raise productivity and the material conditions of the poor.

Chapter 5
Achieving health for all

Overall survival

prospects of the

population worldwide

have improved,

but disparities in

health levels have

in many cases

increased.

In 1997, 158 Member States (representing 91% of the global population) reported to WHO the findings of an evaluation of progress in the implementation of the strategy for health for all in their countries. Based on data and information provided by these reports, supplemented from international sources, WHO estimates that:

- In 1995, 102 Member States, with a total population of 3.4 billion (60% of the global population) had reached at least the minimum life expectancy at birth of above 60 years; infant mortality rate of below 50 per 1000 live births; and under-5 mortality rate of below 70 per 1000 live births.
- Immunization coverage of infants in 1996 was nearly 90% for BCG and about 80% for DPT3, measles and poliomyelitis. For tetanus toxoid, however, coverage of pregnant women was below 50% of live births in developing countries.
- In the developing world in 1996, coverage for antenatal care was 65% of live births; for deliveries in health facilities, 40%; and for skilled attendance at delivery, 53%. About 90% of newborns weighed at least 2500 g at birth, and the available limited data show an increase in infant care coverage since 1986.
- In 1994, at least 75% of the population in the developing world had access to safe water, and 34% to sanitation services, compared with 61% and 36% respectively in 1990.
- Over one-third of the world population still lack access to essential drugs. On average, only 50% of patients take their medicines correctly, and up to 75% of antibiotics are prescribed inappropriately, even in teaching hospitals.

Findings show that substantial, though only partial, progress has been made in achieving the goals of the global strategy for health for all. Overall *survival* prospects of the population worldwide have improved, but *disparities* in health levels between and within countries have persisted and in many cases increased. In spite of political commitment by Member States and the development of health systems based on primary health care, issues of inequalities in health status and health care access seem not to have been adequately or effectively addressed during the past two decades. The stage has been set however for developing and sustaining health systems that are dynamic, effective and able to meet changing health care needs.

More details are given in this chapter, which can be supplemented by reports prepared in each WHO region for the third evaluation of the implementation of the global strategy for health for all, and reviewed by the respective regional committees in 1997.

Health for all and primary health care

Since 1952, the World Health Organization, in its capacity as the directing and coordinating authority on international health work, has periodically

> There was a realistic
>
> expectation that
>
> by the year 2000
>
> no country, or
>
> no individual citizen,
>
> should have a level
>
> of health below an
>
> acceptable minimum.

assessed the global health situation. Reports on the world health situation were used to convey salient findings and main problems and achievements to the World Health Assembly. *Table 10* gives selected extracts from the first eight reports on the world health situation spanning from 1954 to 1989. The Fifth report, covering the period 1969-1972, underlined in particular the slow progress in improving the health status of developing countries, and the widening gap in health status and access to health care between and within countries. The report alerted the global community through the World Health Assembly to the continuing inability of health services to reach out to those in dire need and to provide, on a permanent basis, access to health care for the entire population at a price that they could afford. Over 5 million children were dying annually of diarrhoea, and more than half of all child deaths could be traced to malnutrition, and diarrhoeal and respiratory diseases. Failure to control such diseases of poverty prevented further reductions in mortality rates, and in incidence rates of major diseases such as malaria, schistosomiasis, filariasis, cholera and leprosy – which had even increased.

The imperative for change

Too few resources were being invested in the health sector, and these were usually spent on meeting the needs of 10-15% of the population. Richer countries had been attracting doctors from the poorer ones – over three-quarters of the world's migrant physicians were to be found in only five countries: Australia, Canada, Germany, the United Kingdom and the United States. Although the training of a physician was eight times more expensive than that of a medical auxiliary, many developing countries were still stressing the training

of physicians. Moreover, ordinary people had little control over their own health care, as health professionals were rarely willing to trust them to make decisions about their own health.

In 1977, the World Health Assembly reaffirmed that health is a basic human right and a worldwide social goal, that it is essential to the satisfaction of basic human needs and quality of life, and that it is to be attained by all people. The Assembly called for the vigorous transformation of existing health care strategies to facilitate the attainment of health for all as defined in the Constitution of WHO, and decided that the main social target of governments and of WHO should be the attainment by all the people of the world by the year 2000 of a level of health that would permit them to lead a socially and economically productive life. In other words, as a minimum, all people in all countries should have at least such a level of health that they are capable of working productively and of participating actively in the social life of the community in which they live.

There was a realistic expectation that by the year 2000 no country, or no individual citizen, should have a level of health below an acceptable minimum, and that the world community would later adopt a new strategy to take people further towards the goal of health for all in the future. The target date of 2000 was intended as a challenge to all Member States. If this initiative was successful, the next intermediate target would be to achieve further improvements in health beyond the year 2000, with a better quality of life for all people, taking into account changes in the demographic, socioeconomic, environmental and epidemiological situation.

The strategy for health for all

Achieving even this minimum level of health for all people in all countries implied transforming health care delivery and health services support and management so that health services were made accessible to each and every member of the community.

As stated in the Declaration of Alma-Ata adopted in 1978, the key to attaining the goal of health for all by the year 2000 is primary health care. Primary health care is essential health care based on practical, scientifically sound and socially acceptable methods, and made universally accessible to individuals and families, at a cost they can afford. It should address their main health problems, providing promotive, preventive, curative and rehabilitative services accordingly. Since these services reflect and evolve from the local economic conditions and social values, they vary in different countries and communities, but should include at least education concerning prevailing health problems and the methods of preventing and controlling them; promotion of proper nutrition; an adequate supply of safe water and basic sanitation; maternal and child health care, including family planning; immunization against the major infectious diseases; prevention and control of locally endemic diseases; appropriate treatment for common diseases and injuries; and provision of essential drugs.

The three prerequisites for successful primary health care are a multisectoral approach, community involvement and appropriate technology. All health programmes and the health infrastructure should be built on primary health care. The individual, the family and the community are the basis of the health system, and the primary health worker, as the first agent of the health system that the community deals with, is the central health force. A thorough reorientation of the existing health systems is required to be made as soon as feasible in each country – developed or developing, rich or poor – through an evidence-based managerial process and through health systems research. In order to achieve this, the prime driving force is political commitment.

Political basis

Public health is the art of applying science in the context of politics so as to reduce inequalities in health while ensuring the best health for the greatest number. Health outcomes are related to political democracy, social and cultural development, and economic efficiency. Countries with a culture of democratic values and egalitarian aspirations tend to be less hierarchical, and participation of people in the design of their own future is more acceptable, and even desired. In countries that exhibit a rigid social and political structure, the participation of people in shaping their own future has been perceived by some as a loss of their own power and a risk. The style of socio-economic development of a nation, its political orientation and the priority assigned to social sectors, including investment in health promotion and disease prevention, illustrate the level of commitment to the global goal of health for all.

Due to the political nature of health care, it is not surprising to note that in all WHO regions intersectoral coordination and the formulation and implementation of a healthy public policy have been the most difficult achievements. The third evaluation of the global strategy for health for all brings out the following issues:

> Public health is the art of applying science in the context of politics so as to reduce inequalities in health while ensuring the best health for the greatest number.

		Socioeconomic development	Health system
Report 1 1954-56	Main problems		● Degree of incompleteness varied considerably between different diseases, countries and parts of the same countries and from one period to another (notification of communicable diseases). ● Two parallel and more or less disconnected systems of «medical» and «health» services – greater attention to medical side.
	Main achievements		● Modern concept of health as a state of physical, mental and social well-being and not merely the absence of disease and infirmity offered new horizons to health workers. ● Importance of public health recognized by nations/governments as a factor in social and economic development. ● People's awareness for their own participation to build up the health of the nation. ● Effort to improve the quality of human life – adding life to years. ● Realization that health cannot be imposed: its promotion requires teamwork within the community
Report 2 1957-60	Main problems		
	Main achievements	● There had been scientific, economic and political changes, from 1959 to 1960 which positively influenced health development. ● Political changes, independence, enough freedom of thought and action and of association in the councils of the world. ● The great boom of education in some developing countries.	● Understanding that the problem of health must be based on precise information and precision implies measurement. ● Work on establishment of indicators which would mark definitely the signs of improvement and achievements in health matters.
Report 3 1961-64	Main problems		
	Main achievements		● Substantial increase in general government health expenditure. ● Express desire to organize health planning as a part of total planning for socioeconomic development. ● Establishment of central bodies for health research in the countries.
Report 4 1965-68	Main problems	● Large-scale migration from rural to urban areas.	
	Main achievements	● More attention being given to social and economic factors influencing health.	
Report 5 1969-72	Main problems		● General morbidity statistics very incomplete or non-existent in most countries.
	Main achievements		● % of GNP on health – general trend increasing. ● Public health research becoming more attractive. ● Concept of national health planning in general accepted by developing countries.
Report 6 1973-77	Main problems	● Urbanization (all over the world) and migration (in Europe). ● 80% of adult population illiterate in low-income countries.	● % of GNP spent on health in developing countries, 2-3% (a few US$ per capita expenditure).
	Main achievements		● 30th World Health Assembly in 1977: Health-for-all strategy – primary health care. ● % of GNP spent on health – slow increase. ● Global expenditure on health research – increase.
Report 7 1978-84	Main problems	● Number of illiterate persons increased from 1970-1980. ● 1000 million people living in absolute poverty, 90% of whom in rural areas. ● GDP per capita had fallen – especially in Latin America and Caribbean. ● Increase in unemployment from 1970-1980.	● Some factors affected the evaluation process: not yet suitable methods, no definite baseline for measuring, lack of information support to managerial process.
	Main achievements	● Illiteracy of adults from 48% in 1970 to 40% in 1980.	● Impressive analytical contribution from 177 Member countries for first evaluation. ● Endorsement of health-for-all strategy from almost all countries. ● Positive trends in mobilizing communities for health and allocation of resources.
Report 8 1985-89	Main problems	● Disparities between the least developed and other developing countries had increased. ● Degradation of living conditions in developing countries, especially in urban areas.	● Slow progress due to slow reorientation of disease control programme towards people's needs, difficulties in involving all those concerned with health, weak management of health care delivery system etc. ● National health expenditure devoted to local health services had decreased in least developed countries. ● In 1/4 African countries per capita expenditure on health was under US$ 5.
	Main achievements	● Per capita GNP – some increase in developed countries. ● Adult literacy rate increased from 62% in 1985 to 66% in 1991.	● Slight increase in % of GNP spent by national governments for health in developing countries. ● Increasing number of countries adopted policy of decentralization and delegation of responsibility to district level. ● People increasingly involved in improving their own health.

Health status	Health services
• Very high infant mortality rate and maternal mortality rate in developing countries. • Half of the children died before they reached the age of five years. • Disease problems: malaria, 1.5 million deaths, smallpox still a menace. • Prevalence (millions): trachoma 400, malaria 150, yaws 50, onchocerciasis 20, leprosy 12.	• Very low vaccination coverage (no exact data). • Water supply and waste disposal systems quite inefficient. • Great shortage of water supply and sanitation in larger cities: 10-30% of dwellings without these facilities.
• General trends towards the improvement of health status (decline in increase in height and weight and improvement in nutritional status).	• Application of some simple technology (chlorination, fluoridation, long-acting penicillin, etc.). • Dental health services had been expanding rapidly in many countries.
• Still very high infant mortality rate and maternal mortality rate in developing countries. • Half of the children died before reaching the age of five years. • Rate of poplation growth of 3% and more per annum in some countries. • Increase in number of venereal diseases, mental disorders and anxiety states and accidents.	• Proventive and curative medicine are not easily «integrated» (antithesis between preventive and curative medicine). • Antisocial concentration of medicine and nursing skills in the larger cities.
	• Reawakening of the interest in the environment influenced development of «sanitary policy» which helped in the control of communicable diseases.
• Recurrence of certain diseases: venereal, rabies, viral hepatitis, trypanosomiasis, plague. • «Population pressure» – dramatic projection of the population growth. • Malnutrition: anaemia, goitre. • Substantial reduction in infant mortality rate (in Africa by 20-30 %). • Decrease of some communicable diseases (cholera, smallpox, leprosy, yaws, trachoma, etc.). • Further development and enlargement of health services (hospitals, health centres, manpower). • Recorded progress in general education (proportion of children attending schools has risen from 2.3% to 9%, especially in Africa).	• Great disparity in wealth, health and educated manpower.
• High prevalence of parasitic diseases. • No sign of decreasing plague, venereal diseases, etc. • Increase of some diseases: cardiovascular, cancer, mental, accidents. • Big economic burden of some diseases: tuberculosis, syphilis, etc. (in USA). • Some efforts in control of communicable diseases influenced decline of some of them: smallpox (40% less than in previous years), polio in developed countries, leprosy, cholera. • Savings from some eradication programmes, for example measles in USA (1963-68), had averted 10 million acute cases, saved 1000 lives and prevented more than 3000 cases of mental retardation. • Proportion of the population over 65 expanded.	• Considerable attention had been paid to the education and training of manpower (more doctors, new schools, more nurses, etc.). • Some progress had been made in the provision of community water supply – especially in Latin America. • Main progress in structural development of health services, rather than in performance. • The period 1965-68 was notable for the growing appreciation of the dangers of environmental pollution.
• Malnutrition (protein-calorie malnutrition) a big problem – more than 100 million cases in children under 5. • Increase of population growth rate from 1.82% in 1950-55 to 2.08% in 1965-70.	
• Increase in life expectancy at birth, highest values in Europe and the Americas. • Some diseases show «withdrawal» – rapid decrease in number (smallpox in the Americas – since April 1971 – last case in Brazil, cholera fewer notified cases, etc.). • Treatment of some diseases effective: plague, tuberculosis, yaws, etc.	
• No improvement in some diseases/conditions: diabetes, acute respiratory infection, malaria, malnutrition, accidents, maternal mortality (developing countries), etc. • Food and nutrition, 1000 million globally without enough food. • Annual increase of global population: 80 million. • Infant mortality rate decreasing in developed (8.3-40.3/1000 live births) and in developing (130-200/1000) countries. • Life expectancy at birth increasing (male: 53.9 years, female: 56.6). • Population over 65 increased. • Smallpox – no new areas. • Endemic treponematoses – low prevalence. • Mortality from cardiovascular and ischaemic heart disease – decrease in some developed countries.	• Low % of children immunized – less than 10%. • Inadequate distribution of manpower: urban/rural. • % of population with access to safe drinking-water not satisfactory in rural areas in developing countries. • Contraceptive methods – slow increase. • Number of medical schools – increase. • Drinking-water supply improved in urban areas. • Drug control laboratories established in some countries.
• Infant mortality rate – still high: over 50/1000 live births in 79 countries. • Mortality from ischaemic heart disease increased in under 65s in most countries.	• Immunization coverage (DTP-3rd dose low – 15%) • Some improvements in water supply and sanitation – nullified by population growth and drought.
• Eradication of smallpox declared 1980 by 33rd World Health Assembly. • Infant mortality rate less than 50/1000 live births in 80 countries. • Life expectancy at birth over 60 years in 98 countries. • Diarrhoeal diseases – decline in mortality, morbidity. • Mortality from cardiovascular disease in developed countries – decline.	• Coverage with primary health care from 80 to 100%. • Immunization coverage by DTP– 15%.
• Maternal mortality rate still high in some developing countries (up to 737/1000 live births). • More than 3 million people dually infected by tuberculosis and HIV. • Increased number of HIV infections. • Nutrition of children in developing countries not yet satisfactory.	• Local health services still not reaching 10-20% of population. • 2 million children still dying because of not being immunized. • Maldistribution of health personnel (among countries, within countries, urban/rural, etc.). • Shortage of nurses – especially in Asia.
• Life expectancy at birth increase of 1 year from 1985 to 1990. • Infant mortality rate decrease from 76 per 1000 live births in 1985 to 68 in 1991. • Birth weight over 2500 g improved from 79% in 1985 to 88% in 1991. • Disparities in health status between developed and developing countries reduced, but problem remains.	• Immunization coverage increased globally – to 80%. • Safe water coverage increased from 68% in 1985 to 75% in 1991. • Adequate excreta disposal increased from 46% in 1985 to 71% in 1991. • Availability of essential health care increased globally.

- The political nature of health, illness and health care.
- The value of representative democracies in all countries where human, political and socioeconomic rights are truly respected.
- The inextricable play of economics, religion and culture with politics in decision-making and priority-setting in health.
- The value of peace and conflict resolution as essential conditions for physical, mental and spiritual health.
- The value of institutional designs that ensure government capacity to manage political struggles where the results affect people's well-being negatively.
- The essential importance of governance in managing transitions, crises and new paradigms.
- The implications of politics and policy-making for WHO's technical cooperation in the future: political contexts should be monitored in a systematic way so as to be able to foresee some possible impacts on health development; and to support ministries of health and other partners in the formulation of better health policies.

Experience of the past 20 years shows that governance is one of the decisive factors in securing the implementation of primary health care goals. It is also essential to strengthen the social, political and psychological capacity of people to facilitate the shifts in values and behaviours required to participate and be active in decision-making. Trust in the systems of justice, protection and security must be secured. Transparent assignment of resources, financial execution and social participation in the process of decision-making are also part of good governance.

Experience of the past 20 years shows that governance is one of the decisive factors in securing the implementation of primary health care goals.

Managing progress in implementation

To ensure that governments and WHO know whether they are making progress with the implementation of their strategies and whether these strategies are effective in addressing the health concerns and improving the health status of the people, the Organization's Member States agreed at the World Health Assembly in 1981 to monitor progress and evaluate the effectiveness of their strategies at regular intervals, and to report their findings to the WHO governing bodies. Implementation was monitored in 1983, 1988 and 1994, and evaluated in 1985, 1991 and 1997. The findings were then reviewed by the regional committees and by the World Health Assembly.

The process and progress in health systems development and the trends in health care coverage during the last two decades are highlighted below.

Health systems development

Up to 1978, the biomedical model of health systems predominated, and the health sector was confused with the medical sector. To develop a health system, doctors and nurses were trained, hospitals established, infrastructures created and medicines distributed, especially in towns and for populations that could afford them. Access to modern health care was extremely limited in many developing countries, particularly for rural populations. The limitations of the biomedical model were evident. Fortunately, following the Declaration of Alma-Ata in 1978, new channels and alternative experiments opened up increasingly credible options worldwide.

The three main elements of the strategy (which went far beyond the prevailing biomedical model) were: the development of peripheral services, an intersectoral approach and community participation. The strategy was adopted, more or less explicitly, by the vast majority of countries.

Changes in the economic and political situation in the 1980s proved to be a major obstacle to the implementation of the health-for-all strategy. It was adopted several years too late for the political and social movements that could have provided support and served as a springboard for development. So, before long, it was criticized, distorted, taken over and interpreted more and more restrictively. In general, however, the results of the health-for-all strategy have been encouraging as regards the development of peripheral health services, but little has been done to promote an intersectoral approach and community participation.

WHO continued to support the principles of health for all, but organized itself in such a way as to deal with prevalent *diseases* in developing countries. It pushed the medical approach as far as it could go, even in prevention, by giving greater emphasis to vaccinations and vertical programmes.

Appropriate preventive, curative and community care has a central role in the pursuit of the health-for-all targets. Using adequate policy instruments and cost-effective management of resources, appropriate care focuses on accessible primary care, supported by strong secondary and tertiary care, including services for people with special needs, in order to ensure a high quality of care, and maximum health gains.

Resources for health

Countries can be divided into three groups according to the predominant method of *financing* their health system: mainly based on taxation; chiefly based on social insurance; characterized by centrally-planned normative distribution of government budget funds. With a significant increase in most countries in the role of the private sector in the delivery of services, both equity and allocation issues are receiving more attention. Concerns have also been raised about the quality of care.

In all countries, the reform process is bedeviled by the growing costs of health services. The ageing of the population, associated with an increased need for health care, the availability of new treatments and technologies and rising public expectations, all exert financial pressures. Most countries are responding with a series of measures to control rising costs. In western Europe, for example, successful macroeconomic measures have given way to additional efforts to restrain escalating costs at the institutional level. In the countries in transition, this approach has been less successful, although there is some evidence of improving efficiency. The quest for cost-containment and more efficiency, and the imperative to identify more resources, frequently take precedence over the health-for-all principles and values. Consequently, from the patient's point of view, often what is referred to as "reform" does not contain any elements of improvement. Patients are asked to pay more and receive less.

A core concern in countries engaged in reforming their funding system is to balance the principle of solidarity with pressures to establish competition among insurers and providers. Private health insurance schemes are often operated in a manner that

With a significant increase in the role of the private sector in the delivery of services, both equity and allocation issues are receiving more attention.

The proportion

of the GNP allocated

to health has failed

to increase, or has

even diminished.

corrodes social solidarity. On the whole, the western European countries decided to retain their general health care policy orientation as before, but they have made major changes. More choice, competition and pluralism have been introduced in tax-based systems. Insurance-based countries are paying more attention to cost containment, primary health care and preventive services. In other regions, countries where the tax-based systems are deemed to be insufficient are reviewing the option of health insurance; for example, the Philippines has adopted an expanded comprehensive national insurance system, although the need to subsidize the poorer segments of society is limiting its success. In the Eastern Mediterranean, growth of health expenditure since 1990 has been rather slow, partly because of the difficult economic environment prevailing since the mid-1980s and the consequences of the structural adjustment programmes in several developing economies of the Region. Several countries have tried to mobilize the necessary funds through alternative financing schemes based on cost-sharing and the development of health insurance schemes.

A central issue for many countries, such as China, is improved coordination and management of multiple funding sources. Many health systems struggle to keep up with rising costs or are affected by national decisions to reduce expenditure on health. Various cost recovery mechanisms are therefore being explored. Malaysia and Mongolia are investigating user charges to finance certain health services, although possibly not critical care services.

In Africa, investment in health has virtually ceased. The social sectors, including the health sector, have been hardest hit by the worsening budget deficits. The proportion of the GNP allocated to health has failed to increase, or has even diminished. There is still a gross imbalance between expenditure on tertiary care and expenditure for local care, to the detriment of the latter. Progress in this area has been marginal.

In general, reliable and valid data on health care financing are sparse in most developing countries. In addition, data on expenditures in the private sector are often difficult to obtain. Yet in most countries of South-East Asia, for example, 60-75% of the total health expenditure occurs in the private sector. Direct out-of-pocket spending by households appears to account for a major portion of private spending in most countries in the Eastern Mediterranean, while private insurance premiums account for a limited fraction of private spending. This means that households bear a substantial proportion of health care costs while having little or no financial protection (i.e. insurance) in the event of major illness or injury.

In many developing countries, additional resources for the health sector are provided by nongovernmental organizations and bilateral and international donors. The role played by nongovernmental organizations in both the provision and financing of health services is growing in many countries as a consequence of diminishing resources in public sectors. As the prospects of financial assistance from many donor countries are not optimistic, owing to economic recession and cuts in developing assistance programmes, financial institutions are being approached for loans aimed at supporting health development programmes. In many less developed states, external sources of funding support disease control activities and critical health promotion services, such as campaigns related to maternal and child health and immunization. In these countries aid coordination remains a concern.

Few countries, even the most prosperous, are satisfied with the distribution of financial resources between promotive and curative services.

In Europe, redistribution of financial resources towards primary health care could not be confirmed by the few existing data. Some evidence about the outcome of such reform policies comes from other indicators, such as immunization rates and infant and perinatal mortality, which mostly improved, although this was not consistent. Disparities in access between social groups also persist, and in some cases have even worsened.

In the Western Pacific most countries devote sufficient resources to the health sector and thus express their priority concerns in terms of issues of equity, appropriate allocation of the resources and efficiency. This has become an important issue for China, where central funds are used to balance regional and rural funds. Malaysia, for example, recognizes that the public system should ensure that appropriate social safety nets are in place for those who, for economic reasons, have difficulty accessing appropriate care. In most countries of the Region, basic care of children, older citizens and those with other special needs is met by governments. In Cambodia and the Lao People's Democratic Republic, however, the allocation to the health sector is 2% or less of the gross national product, and is not sufficient to meet basic needs.

Data from some countries in the Eastern Mediterranean show that public resources are not equally distributed between geographical regions and between social classes. They tend to favour urban and well-off populations and to generate polarization with regard to accessibility to health care. This aspect is further worsened by privatization policies. An important share of recurrent budgets of ministries of health is allocated for tertiary care, thus limiting resources for primary health care services, and preventive and promotive programmes. On average, 43% of national health expenditure is devoted to local health care, down from 50% in the early 1980s.

Experience in some countries has shown, however, that decentralization may also have negative effects such as fragmented services, or inequity. Successful decentralization requires sufficient local administrative and managerial capacity and appropriate mechanisms for accountability and citizens' participation. In addition, there is evidence that certain areas such as the basic framework for health policy, or regulations concerning public safety, are better managed centrally. Decentralization of responsibility for primary health care to local authorities is not always accompanied by a shift of financial resources. In Europe, for example, the reluctance of hospital-based medical specialists to accept policies that strengthen primary health care and/or restrict direct access to secondary care are a continuing feature. Services are still often characterized by the existence of parallel vertical programmes. Integrated horizontal services are nevertheless being developed in some European countries, providing a full range of outpatient services supplemented by home care, in cooperation with the social welfare services.

Problems associated with *human resources* vary in different regions. In the Americas, the expansion of human resources has in particular been limited by recent cutbacks in spending by the public sector, precipitated by the downturn in the economy. Another factor has been high management turnover because

> Successful decentralization requires local administrative and managerial capacity and mechanisms for accountability and citizens' participation.

Most countries

are examining their

personnel policies;

strengthening

the capacities of

training institutions;

and reorienting the

curricula to meet the

changing needs of

the health services.

of changes in government and direction and the lack of a personnel policy and of appropriate incentives to motivate personnel.

In South-East Asia, on the other hand, the absolute and relative numbers of most categories of health personnel have risen. Most countries are examining their personnel policies and formulating plans; expanding and strengthening the capacities of education and training institutions; and updating and reorienting the curricula to meet the changing needs of the health services. Countries continue to make use of other training resources in the Region to supplement their own training opportunities.

Investment in human resources for health has been such that in most countries in the Eastern Mediterranean Region, the resources allocated for personnel consume 60-70% of the total budget of ministries of health. Recent demographic and epidemiological changes have resulted in an increase in the overall ratios of human resources for health, especially nursing and midwifery personnel. This can be attributed to the increased number of nursing institutes and increased demand, and is the outcome of health policies launched several years ago. Measures adopted include incentives to work in remote and rural areas (e.g. in Iraq), and the involvement of nongovernmental organizations in training health personnel (e.g. in the Islamic Republic of Iran).

In many African countries, the low output of health institutions and poor performance of health personnel remain major concerns. The brain drain continues, undermining the public sector's capacity to respond to health needs. The phenomenon of unemployment among school leavers is particularly affecting the health sector. Although some initiatives have been taken, they are of limited scope

and will need to be encouraged and expanded since they have proved their effectiveness in some cases.

In the Eastern Mediterranean, although human resources have been produced and deployed in larger numbers, their distribution is not balanced among the different levels of care, nor is it always equitable within countries, or balanced between various categories. Some countries (e.g. Lebanon and Pakistan) have more physicians than nursing/midwifery personnel because of cultural or employment factors, or shortages in education and training facilities. There are problems of absorbing graduates (e.g. in the Islamic Republic of Iran), and of low intake of nationals in nursing institutes, for cultural reasons. The recruitment and deployment of health personnel may be carried out by a central government body irrespective of real needs, and rapid progress in technology and increased public awareness of needs may also be causing pressure. Health personnel are concentrated in the capital or other cities, where university hospitals and other secondary and tertiary care institutions exist. This disparity – fewer physicians assigned to primary health care despite more physicians joining the services – raises several issues. In addition to the factors mentioned above, primary health care may not be attractive for physicians when it is remote and without incentives.

Examples in other regions include the Philippines, where the output of educational institutions does not match what the service needs. Among its many health initiatives, New Zealand is attempting to address this issue with specific purchasing agreements for educational institutions. Singapore has recognized the need to support the training of nurses in order to address similar concerns. China is exploring market mechanisms to meet health service needs – encouraging practitioners to run their own clinics or consultations, and encouraging healthy competition between medical institutions to improve efficiency and reduce costs, thus matching demand for care at different levels.

In the Americas, the most important constraint is the failure to develop a model of human resource needs in health in coordination with training institutions, and the trend towards professional medical specialization persists, with a steady rise in the number of physicians. The health workforce continues to be largely female and concentrated in nursing. Reduced employment in health and the changes in financing resulting from state reform have influenced policies related to the development of new human resources for health in most countries. At the same time there are no signs that the geographical and social distribution of health workers has improved; they remain highly concentrated in the cities, to the detriment of rural areas and urban peripheries. Virtually all countries are aware of the urgent need to rectify this situation. The appearance of new factors in the health sector job market (banks, NGOs, other agencies) has meant significant changes in the mechanisms and processes involved in the regulation of health care and the health professions. Meanwhile, however, structural action needed for solving the problem is often postponed or considered unviable.

In the Western Pacific, the main strategy is continually to upgrade the skills of the workforce through education and training, with particular emphasis on continuing education. Upgrading is seen as a particularly important issue in China. Cambodia is revitalizing its health system through a national continuing education programme. Continuing education is an explicit priority in Kiribati and the Philippines.

In Europe, the implementation of policies to develop primary health care is accompanied by the introduction of schemes for training general practitioners/family physicians, or for the retraining of physicians already in practice. Some countries are developing family physician services with a parallel community nursing service, where one did not already exist. Also there is a tendency to create academic departments of general practice/family medicine and to introduce the subject into the undergraduate curriculum of medical students.

Most countries in South-East Asia have also taken steps to increase production of certain categories of health personnel, including voluntary workers, in order to improve and expand coverage, especially at the community level. A few have established new categories of personnel and new training programmes in an effort to meet increasing and changing health service needs. For example, Maldives is now conducting a diploma course in primary health care to train middle-level managers and Myanmar has established a new institute which offers a degree in community health to prepare public health officers in charge of basic health services in peripheral areas. There is, however, a tendency of educational institutions to seek "quality" in the abstract, with insufficient attention to the real needs of the communities and their limited resources. Deficiencies in training facilities, teaching capability and resources are also constraints.

In the Americas, on the other hand, countries usually have a variety of institutions that, working in isolation, make decisions about training and education needs. The institutions responsible for training human resources have tended to neglect education in public health, health policy, and health management.

There is a tendency to create academic departments of general practice/family medicine and to introduce the subject into the undergraduate curriculum of medical students.

> Hospitals continue
>
> to consume the
>
> largest share of
>
> the health budget,
>
> sometimes at
>
> the expense of
>
> health centres.

In Africa, many countries made the development of *infrastructure* the focus of their health policy, but the results obtained were uneven in view of limited investment capacity. Hospitals continue to consume the largest share of the health budget, sometimes at the expense of health centres. Maintenance of facilities and equipment is inadequate, not only because of financial constraints but also for cultural reasons. Quite often, achievements could not be sustained without international cooperation.

In the Americas, in contrast to the 1970s, infrastructure development policy in the past 15 years has stagnated and is currently one of the components with the greatest need for support. Generally, health policy does not provide for the development of physical infrastructure such as facilities and equipment. This means that equipment is not procured on the basis of an evaluation of the health needs of the population. In the majority of countries, technical services are not an integral part of the health care system, nor are maintenance plans for hospital equipment. Equipment is not utilized because it is inappropriate, because of lack of personnel who know how to use it, or because of minor faults and a lack of spare parts. In addition, ministries of health generally do not have a sufficient budget for repairing and maintaining infrastructure and equipment, so that international assistance is often the only recourse.

The physical infrastructure in many South-East Asian countries has continued to expand, particularly at the primary and first referral levels. Health care facilities in the private sector have expanded, as reflected by the increasing number of private hospital beds. However, maintenance of infrastructure appears to be a problem in many countries, and communities are becoming involved in estab-

lishing, equipping and maintaining the health infrastructure in some countries. Most countries have given priority to upgrading the health infrastructure, particularly in rural areas. Remote health facilities are often linked by telecommunications. Improving the infrastructure is often hampered by staffing difficulties and shortage of spare parts. Moreover, improvements may not systematically benefit poorer populations. Nepal, Sri Lanka and Thailand have comprehensive networks of health facilities extending to the village level. Access to primary health care has been considerably improved, and work is now being undertaken to ensure planned development and maintenance. Assistance from international funding agencies has also been very useful in that respect.

In the Eastern Mediterranean, initiatives have recently been taken to ensure equitable distribution of the infrastructure. Many countries have opted to specify catchment areas as the unit for planning health services, and in general physical infrastructure has received considerable attention and investment, often benefiting from bilateral and multilateral assistance projects. Construction and renovation of secondary and tertiary hospitals has also developed, but at a slower rate. Accessibility to health services reached 82% in 1990 and has been sustained. Further expansion of coverage has been hampered by civil strife in some countries and by the high cost in remote areas. Outreach and mobile teams are used as alternatives to static units to serve scattered and remote populations. Linked to accessibility are two other parameters, coverage and utilization. The reported pattern of utilization varies among and within countries. Underutilization is sometimes due to a lack of availability of budgetary resources for drugs, physicians, health staff and equipment or to the availability of alternative acceptable services, whether provided by traditional, private or nongovernmental organizations. Facilities constructed thanks to donations from nongovernmental organizations or communities or through loans are often not included in proposals for recurrent budgets due to poor coordination between planning and financial departments.

Public facilities – buildings, equipment and supplies – are not usually well maintained, because of lack of financial resources and qualified personnel. Few countries have adequate repair and maintenance workshops, whether centralized or decentralized. Some countries contract out for maintenance and repair of biomedical equipment. Underuse of equipment may result from poor maintenance or from shortage of necessary supplies such as chemicals. Ministries of health cannot compete with private firms in attracting scarce qualified repair and maintenance technicians. There is a need for resources to be provided through bilateral and multilateral cooperation in this area.

Since hospitals are the main consumers of health care resources, they have been at the centre of health care reform in every European country. There have been many changes aimed at increasing patient satisfaction, rationalizing resources and achieving better outcomes. Most countries claim moderate to good development in this area, although the pace of change has been slower than desired. The number of hospital admissions has varied widely, even between countries with similar levels of economic and health development. Hospitalization all over Europe has shifted further from chronic and simple surgical procedures to acute, day hospitals and shorter length of stay, and complicated pathologies and treatments. On average, the number of hospital beds per 1000 population has decreased in all parts of the Region, most notably in some countries of eastern Europe. On the whole, however, the costs of hospital treatment have probably increased, both in absolute terms and as a proportion of total health expenditure. Progress has been made regarding alternatives to hospitalization such as day surgery, day care and home care.

Increasingly, countries in all regions are endeavouring to ensure *quality of care*, through the identification and constructive use of best practices and the optimal use of existing resources. In 1993, the European Forum for Medical Associations stated that ensuring quality of care is an ethical, educational and professional responsibility inherent in the medical professions. Good progress is being made in European countries following the achievement of consensus on quality indicators, e.g. for diabetes management and obstetrical and perinatal care. Outcomes in central European countries have been identical to those in western Europe, while at the same time quality of care has been achieved with less frequent use of technology-intensive interventions.

In the Americas, although some countries have set up a classification system to define the levels of potential risk to the health of the population, based on quality and safety criteria, greater organization is still needed for its use in practice. In one country for example, only 0.8% of the facilities evaluated had some method for treating hazardous solid waste.

In the Eastern Mediterranean, countries have undertaken assessment of health services to identify new entry points to improve performance. Some countries (e.g. Bahrain, Egypt, Jordan, Morocco) have initiated quality control programmes at selected levels of care. Capacity-

> Countries in all regions are endeavouring to ensure quality of care, through constructive use of best practices and the optimal use of existing resources.

Low-income countries with a food deficit continue to face declining food production and complex emergencies that have displaced massive numbers of people, (see *Chapter 4*). The prevalence of protein-energy malnutrition in children under 5 in developing countries declined from at least 42% in 1975 to over 31% in 1996, indicating that in general dietary protein had become widely available. Anaemia, mostly due to iron deficiency, was the most common nutritional deficiency worldwide in the 1970s and remains so. Over the past 20 years there has been some decrease in the prevalence of iodine deficiency disorders, particularly in recent years following near-universal salt iodization by 1995 in most countries affected. Vitamin A deficiency is decreasing worldwide, but severe forms are still common in parts of sub-Saharan Africa. Foodborne illnesses continue to be a major public health concern in both developed and developing countries.

Water supply and sanitation

In 1972, the United Nations Conference on the Human Environment brought environmental concerns to global attention for the first time. In the mid-1970s there were approximately 3 billion people in the developing world, only 38% of whom had safe drinking-water and 32% adequate sanitation. In 1978 the International Drinking-Water Supply and Sanitation Decade was launched with the stated goal of clean water and adequate sanitation for all by the year 1990.

In 1980, safe water supply was available to about 50% of the world population, while adequate sanitation was available to about 35%. In 1985, an average of 55% of the populations in developing countries had safe water. By 1990 the figure had risen to 66%. The figures for excreta disposal were 31% in 1985 and 53% in 1990. There are great differences between and within countries, particularly between urban and rural areas. From 1990 to 1994 the number of people without sanitation increased by nearly 300 million, totalling almost 3 billion for developing countries in 1994 (see *Fig. 17*). This figure is projected to increase to over 3 billion by the year 2000. From 1990 to 1994 nearly 800 million people gained access to safe water supplies but, due to population growth, the number of unserved decreased only from 1.6 billion in 1990 to 1.1 billion in 1994. The rural population remains at a disadvantage: in 1994, sanitation coverage in rural areas was a mere 18% whereas it was 63% in urban areas; access to water amounted to 70% in rural areas and 82% in urban areas.

There are positive developments however. The focus is shifting from drinking-water quality alone towards overall improvement of the environment. Public policies aimed at creating a healthy environment are becoming more generally accepted.

Maternal and child health

The range of health care needs that can arise during and just after pregnancy make the challenge of ensuring the access of all women to relevant services complex. Current global estimates show that in the developing world approximately 65% of pregnant women receive at least one antenatal visit during pregnancy; 40% of deliveries take place in health facilities; and slightly more than half of all deliveries are assisted by skilled personnel. This contrasts sharply with developed countries, where practically every woman receives regular care during pregnancy, delivery and the postpartum period.

Postpartum care has been a relatively neglected aspect of maternity

> Public policies aimed at creating a healthy environment are becoming more generally accepted.

care. It does not feature in the goals set at major international conferences and the lack of reporting is an indication of low priority. Less than one-third of developing countries report national data, and levels of coverage can be as low as 5%. Estimates based on the limited data available indicate a coverage of 35% at the global level. This low level of care is disturbing, since timely interventions during the postpartum period can prevent deaths of both mothers and newborn infants, and can reduce the incidence of long-term pregnancy-related illnesses.

In developed market economies and economies in transition, well over 90% of pregnant women received antenatal care in 1996. Deliveries took place in health facilities and were attended by skilled personnel. In the least developed countries, while nearly 50% receive antenatal care, only 30% deliver in health facilities or have skilled attendants. In other developing countries the numbers are around 70% and 60% respectively. Worldwide, only every third woman receives care from a skilled health professional in the postpartum period. Estimates of anaemia in pregnancy are less than 20% in developed market economies and economies in transition, but are above 50% elsewhere.

In 1965, only about 9% of all married women of reproductive age in developing countries, or their partners, were using a method of contraception. Today this figure is approaching 60% worldwide. However, the fertility-regulating needs of large segments of the world population remain unmet by the currently available methods and services.

These indicators of maternal health care utilization have a number of limitations. They do not, for example, reflect the content or quality of the care provided.

Just as maternal health is dependent on many factors, newborn and

---

Box 26. WHO's Expanded Programme on Immunization (EPI)

One of the most dramatic current goals for EPI is the *eradication of poliomyelitis* by the year 2000. While there are still difficulties in raising the resources needed to ensure that the job is finished on time, all the indications are that progress towards the goal is on target. Reported BCG and DTP3 coverages have remained steady since 1990 at about 90% and 80%, respectively. Countries in greatest need have reported a slow, but steady improvement for DTP3 coverage, increasing from 26% in 1988 to 44% in 1996. At least 86 countries have now introduced hepatitis B vaccine into their routine immunization programme, and at least 25 have introduced *Haemophilus influenzae* type B (Hib) vaccine.

The *managerial process* of immunization programmes has particular features which differ from those of other programmes. EPI has strongly recommended that annual operational plans be developed looking at all managerial aspects of health. Such activities have provided a good basis for measuring programme effectiveness.

EPI has been instrumental in establishing *links between partners* in immunization, enhancing the use of funds in ways which support other parts of the health sector as well as immunization.

EPI has focused attention on *countries in greatest need* – those requiring technical and financial support. Such countries have low national programme implementation capacity and have received little support compared to other countries which are financially and technically stronger. Support for immunization in the area of, for instance, training has resulted in improvements in other areas of health care.

For a long time, *surveillance* has been regarded as an unwelcome necessity for immunization programmes, and not carried out well. Through the polio eradication initiative, the entire surveillance system has been revitalized to the extent that many countries now report polio data weekly. In addition, an effort has been made to include other infectious diseases in the same reporting system, e.g. yellow fever, dengue and meningitis.

A basic requirement for all national immunization programmes is an intact and functional *cold chain*. This facility is useful for many other primary health care products not used by EPI. Stock control training for management of vaccines also facilitates the management of other commodities used in health centres.

EPI promotes *safe injections* for immunization and for all other purposes. EPI has developed auto-destruct syringes which can be used only once before they block and have to be disposed of. The method of disposal of any autodestruct or disposable syringe and needle is important, and EPI has developed and promoted the use of "safe boxes" which successfully dispose of them and prevent these sharp items from contaminating the environment.

While *vitamin A* is not a vaccine, the target group of infants and mothers is the same, at least in countries where the vitamin deficiency exists. By giving the inexpensive vitamin orally at the same time as immunizations, the cost for both commodities is reduced.

The most devastating illnesses (including measles) of children living in developing countries is dealt with by the strategy of *integrated management of childhood illnesses*. By supporting this initiative, EPI has helped to produce a comprehensive teaching programme for training health care workers.

Map 9. Polio

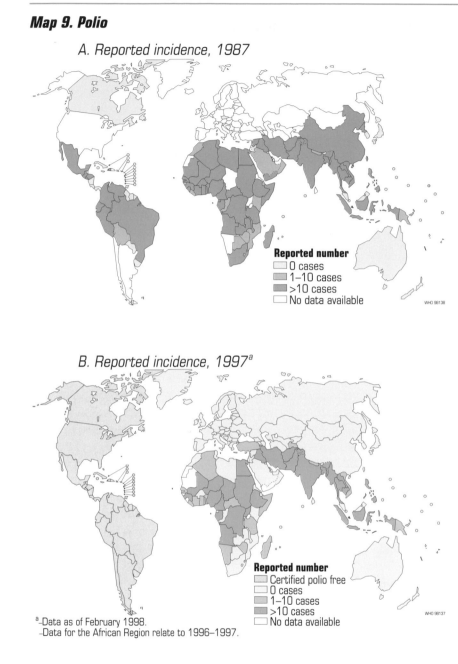

A. Reported incidence, 1987

Reported number
- 0 cases
- 1–10 cases
- >10 cases
- No data available

WHO 98138

B. Reported incidence, 1997[a]

Reported number
- Certified polio free
- 0 cases
- 1–10 cases
- >10 cases
- No data available

WHO 98137

[a]–Data as of February 1998.
–Data for the African Region relate to 1996–1997.

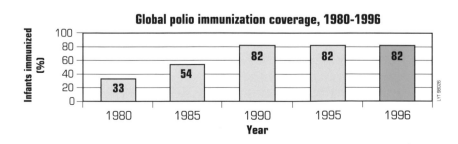

Global polio immunization coverage, 1980-1996

Infants immunized (%)

Year	1980	1985	1990	1995	1996
%	33	54	82	82	82

LYT 98026

child health are also strongly related to the social, economic and health status of the mother. Most infant morbidity and mortality could be prevented through the provision of adequate water supplies and sanitation facilities at community level, good nutrition of mother and child, and access to first-level care including good immunization coverage. Available – often limited – information shows that coverage of infant care by trained personnel has increased since 1985, but more importantly indicates the large differences that continue to exist between countries.

Immunization

In the early 1980s there were three concerns with regard to immunization: immunization levels were low; supplies of vaccines and infrastructure for their dissemination were inadequate; and the immunizable diseases were limited primarily to diphtheria, pertussis, tetanus, polio, measles and tuberculosis.

The Expanded Programme on Immunization was established in 1974 and immunization service delivery was rapidly improved by staff training; the development of secure cold chains; and the availability of routine immunization. Success was measured by vaccine coverage levels, and successful reduction in the incidence of some diseases through widespread immunization made it possible to consider the elimination of diseases such as measles and neonatal tetanus, or even the eradication of some diseases such as poliomyelitis (*Box 26*). Since 1991, polio has been eradicated from the Americas and many other parts of the globe. The target is its eradication by the year 2000. *Map 9* shows reported incidence in 1987 and 1997.

Global policies and strategies for immunization have been adopted by virtually all countries of the world. Overall immunization rates against the six vaccine-preventable childhood diseases have increased from less than 50% in 1980 to over 80% worldwide in 1995.

Neonatal tetanus is now a target for elimination with a possibility of success by 2000. A time-frame for the global elimination of measles will be set by the year 2000. The vaccine for hepatitis B has been added to the standard list, as has the vaccine for yellow fever in endemic areas. Meanwhile, some 20% of the world's children, most of whom are among the poorest and least privileged, continue to be unreached by immunization (*Fig. 20*). Some countries, even some with adequate infrastructure and financial capacity, report consistently low coverage.

In developing countries and economies in transition, constraints to the maintenance of even 80% immunization coverage include inadequate financing, poor facilities and the need to upgrade the entire system. In many least developed countries, especially in Africa, sustaining high coverage remains problematic owing to the almost universal constraints of insufficient funding, equipment, supplies, cold-chain and transport; lack of trained personnel; inadequate access to facilities; and poor receptivity on the part of the population.

In the developed market economies, immunization rates have been increasing since the early 1990s. In the economies in transition they declined in the early 1980s but have been increasing in recent years. In the developing countries, immunization rates have increased dramatically, while in the least developed countries, immunization rates increased from less than 20% in the early 1980s to more than 60% in the mid-1990s. In the developing countries, where neonatal tetanus remains a major

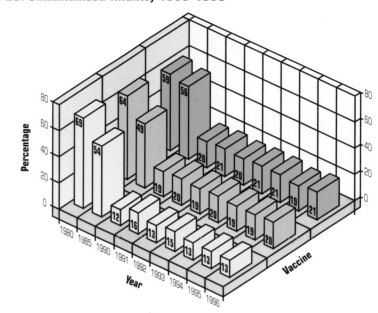

Fig. 20. Unimmunized infants, 1980-1996 [a]

☐ BCG   ☐ DTP3   ☐ Measles vaccine [b]

[a] These data include only those countries that have reported data as of 22 October 1997.

[b] Measles vaccine coverage is among children up to 2 years.

problem, immunization rates with tetanus toxoid have grown but still remain quite low at below 50% coverage.

Locally endemic diseases

Approaches and progress in the eradication, elimination and control of infectious diseases have been dealt with elsewhere in this report, especially in *Chapter 2*. In the context of primary health care, the approach to disease control is the following:

- Selected diseases are targeted for eradication, elimination and control where cost-effective interventions are available and their wider application operationally feasible, e.g. poliomyelitis, leprosy and filariasis.
- Integrated packages of cost-effective interventions are developed and promoted for disease clusters to ensure optimal impact on health status and make better use of re-

sources. Examples of this approach are the Expanded Programme on Immunization which aims to control six major childhood diseases through immunization; the Integrated Management of Childhood Illness that focuses on five major childhood killers; and the recent move towards integrating activities for the control of clusters of tropical diseases *(Box 27)*.

- Capacity at national and global levels is reinforced to recognize and respond rapidly and effectively to outbreaks of emerging and re-emerging diseases. For example, mechanisms are being established by WHO for a global surveillance system supported by a team of experts who can be at the location of an outbreak anywhere in the world within 24 hours of being officially notified.

Provision of essential drugs

In 1978, the lack of drugs for the public sector, especially for primary health care, was identified as a significant problem. Although countries were spending 20-40% of their scanty health budgets on importing drugs, most of the people in rural areas and urban slums had no access to these drugs. At all levels of the health system – from the national level to the hospital to the patient – many countries lacked drugs in sufficient quantities. At the same time, many drugs were available in private pharmacies but were out of reach of the majority of the population. Today although some problems (unequal access, irrational use, lack of resources) remain unchanged, new challenges have emerged. Securing rational use of drugs by health care providers and the public is not easy in an environment where resistance to antibiotics is increasing rapidly and where new diseases are emerging. Also difficult is the implementation of existing rules, regulations and standards to ensure that drugs on the market are safe, effective and of acceptable quality in the absence or the scarcity of human and financial resources, political commitment and physical infrastructure.

There have nevertheless been improvements in a number of countries in the Eastern Mediterranean and South-East Asia Regions. In

---

Box 27. *Integrated disease control*

An integrated approach to disease control requires the establishment of clear priorities on the basis of epidemiological analysis and existing resources and opportunities, as well as careful assessment of the potential effectiveness and sustainability of proposed interventions. Such an approach should be initiated as a development process, which could be progressively extended to other priority areas, and eventually become a sustainable health care service.

Action has been taken since 1996 to integrate activities between groups of diseases where appropriate, starting in five countries, the Islamic Republic of Iran, Mauritania, Saudi Arabia, the United Republic of Tanzania (Zanzibar) and Yemen. The geographical distribution of intestinal parasitic infections, schistosomiasis, filariasis, malaria, leprosy, vaccine-preventable diseases and other diseases and the approaches to their control are quite different in these countries. As a consequence these Member States, working closely with the programme on control of tropical diseases in WHO, have developed national plans of action for integrated disease control, which include surveillance activities, and which are now being implemented. This work was carried out by the ministries of health in collaboration with other ministries as well as with the WHO regional offices and the relevant programmes at WHO headquarters. Particular attention is being paid to the most common requirements for disease control and to the most pressing needs of the population.

With the tools and strategies now available, the integrated approach can become a reality in many areas where there are various communicable diseases and where the epidemiological circumstances and the resources are such as to provide a good opportunity for success. However, as much more experience is needed in this area, it will be necessary to continue the initiative for several more years.

Better coordination and the combining of resources would appreciably enhance the health impact of control efforts against communicable diseases in tropical areas, an approach that is attractive to both ministries of health and development agencies because it is more cost-effective. However, very careful joint planning is essential if the expected benefits are to be realized. The activities in the five countries should yield valuable information that will enable this approach to be progressively extended to other areas.

Africa, access to drugs is still inequitable even though it has been improved by introducing cost recovery as part of the Bamako Initiative and other similar initiatives (*Map 10*).

In the Americas, drug legislation and regulation have constituted a priority component of health sector reform in many countries – the objective being to create and/or update the legal framework to improve the supply and rational use of drugs. Three major problems have been identified with respect to public policies on essential drugs: the annual budget is low in terms of the need for coverage; the supply is ineffective; and while a distribution system exists, it does not function properly. There have been budget cutbacks in the social sector, and many countries have adopted different sources of financing, with patients paying more of the costs. The private sector constitutes 78% of the total pharmaceutical market in Latin America.

Drug consumption accounts for about one-third of total health spending in the Eastern Mediterranean, and in many countries a relatively high percentage of private spending goes towards the purchase of drugs. This pattern is especially pronounced in Egypt, Morocco and Yemen, where up to 70% of total health spending is for pharmaceuticals, most of it through private financing. Drug selection, procurement and distribution present the most problems, especially for countries in greatest need. Limited budgets for drugs have stimulated the search for alternative financing methods, such as cost-sharing or revolving funds to ensure accessibility of drugs for those in real need. Local drug production in Egypt, Islamic Republic of Iran, Jordan, Morocco and Pakistan covers more than 80% of the total drug consumption, and is rapidly growing in other countries of the Region,

Map 10. Populations with regular access to essential drugs
A. 1987 estimates

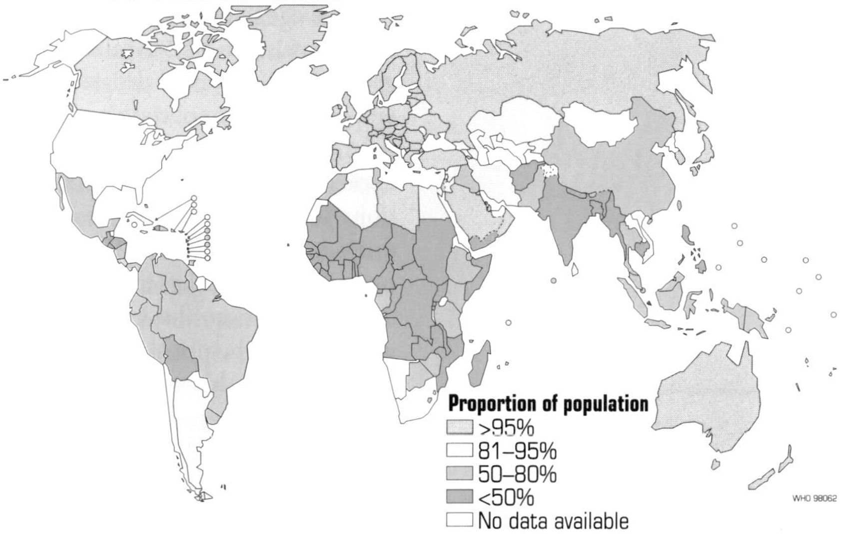

Proportion of population
>95%
81–95%
50–80%
<50%
No data available

B. 1997 estimates

Proportion of population
>95%
81–95%
50–80%
<50%
No data available

strongly supported by governments. However, most countries have no clear policy regulating drug production to ensure the availability of essential drugs and vaccines.

A common constraint in countries in South-East Asia is the limited government budget for drugs. Distribution systems are inefficient, are not well planned, and do not take into account seasonal variations in drug requirements related to epidemio-

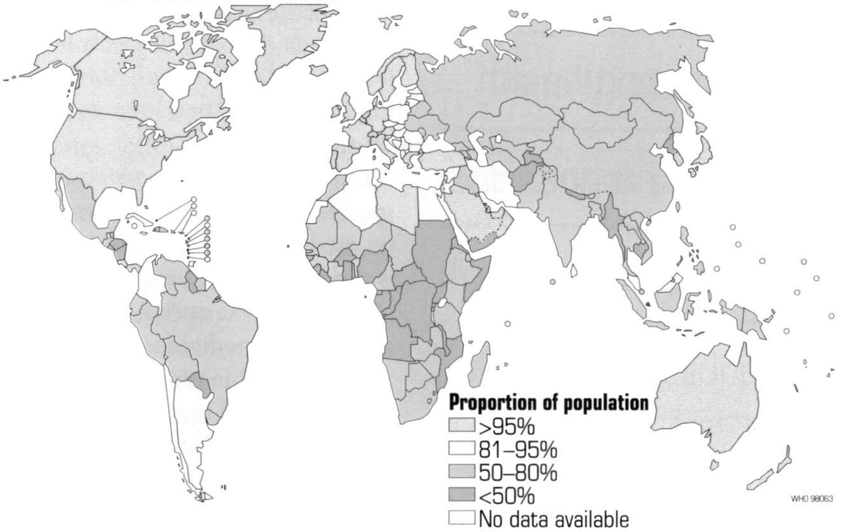

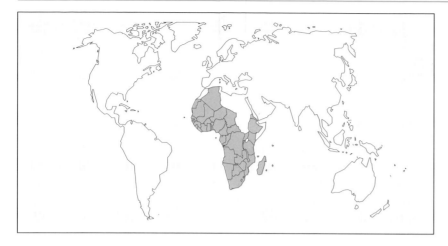

46 Member States
Population (1997): 612 million

GNP per capita

- Regional average (1995) $ 564
  min.: Mozambique $ 80
  max.: Seychelles $ 6 620

- Annual average growth rate
  (1985-1995)
  min.: Gabon   -8.2 %
  max.: Botswana   6.1 %

Algeria	Lesotho
Angola	Liberia
Benin	Madagascar
Botswana	Malawi
Burkina Faso	Mali
Burundi	Mauritania
Cameroon	Mauritius
Cape Verde	Mozambique
Central African	Namibia
Republic	Niger
Chad	Nigeria
Comoros	Rwanda
Congo	Sao Tome and
Côte d'Ivoire	Principe
Democratic	Senegal
Republic of	Seychelles
the Congo	Sierra Leone
Equatorial Guinea	South Africa
Eritrea	Swaziland
Ethiopia	Togo
Gabon	Uganda
Gambia	United Republic
Ghana	of Tanzania
Guinea	Zambia
Guinea-Bissau	Zimbabwe
Kenya	

Tables concerning demography, health indicators and GNP are based on United Nations and World Bank estimates. All other information is from regional sources.

Africa

Almost all the countries of the Region were under colonial rule up to the end of the 1950s. The 1960s witnessed a "bumper harvest" of independent African countries. Over 30 countries became independent between 1960 and 1969. The 1970s added six countries. Zimbabwe gained independence in the 1980s, and Eritrea, Namibia and South Africa joined in the 1990s.

Another important determinant during this period was political instability. In some countries this culminated in civil strife and wars: eight countries were affected, at one time or another. In most of such affected countries, hundreds of thousands of people were displaced and the refugee problems compounded the health problems of the day. In some other countries, political instability and the attendant absence of peace destabilized health sector development.

At independence, socioeconomic development was a challenge, and the opportunity of securing favourable trade terms was not missed by some countries. More school and health facilities were built, not only in the urban areas but also in the rural areas. By the end of the 1970s, access to health and education had im-

proved. Literacy rates increased but were still below 20%. The population growth rate was still relatively low at about 2.5%, and there was limited growth in urbanization. Of the 25 countries that were recognized as least developed countries at that time, 13 were in the Region.

The 1980s were the decade of economic reform, following the 1979 oil crisis. The objectives of the reforms, for most countries, were to respond to both internal and external disequilibria created by the worldwide economic crisis. They usually involved the implementation of the IMF/World Bank "packaged" structural adjustment programmes. The 1980s generally witnessed an increase in economic uncertainty, little or no investment, a decrease in food self-reliance and an increase in external debt. The population growth rate increased to 2.8%, and unchecked growth in urbanization created a new class of poor people in the urban areas.

By the 1990s, the negative effects of economic reforms became more vivid. Twenty-one countries had a lower real, as well as nominal, average growth rate in 1991-1995 than they had in 1980-1985.

Health trends

During the immediate post-independence period, health development in the Region called for re-

Selected health-for-all (HFA) indicators	1975			1997			2025			HFA targets	No. of Member States which have *not* met the HFA targets in 1997
	Average	Max.	Min.	Average	Max.	Min.	Average	Max.	Min.		
Life expectancy at birth (years)	46	64	35	53	72	38	65	77	51	> 60	39
Infant mortality rate (per 1000 live births)	125	197	47	89	169	16	47	99	7	< 50	40
Under-5 mortality rate (per 1000 live births)	200	294	51	139	251	16	66	139	6	< 70	40

sponses in four strategic areas: development of human resources for health; promotion of environmental hygiene; epidemiological surveillance and control of communicable diseases; and strengthening of health services.

Many countries made the development of infrastructure the focus of their health policy, to help improve the coverage and management of the health problems of their populations. But the results obtained were uneven because of limited investment capacity. Quite often, achievements could not be maintained except through international cooperation and community initiatives. Infrastructure expansion was noted in some cases but did not measure up to needs.

The deterioration of the economic and financial situation in recent years has been felt particularly in the health sector. Health investment has virtually ceased. The social sectors, including the health sector, have been the hardest hit by the worsening trend of budget deficits. There is still imbalance between expenditure on tertiary care and expenditure for local care, to the detriment of the latter.

The development of **human resources for health** has been a top priority and substantial efforts have been made to provide a generation of trained personnel of all categories, such as physicians, nurses, midwives, laboratory technicians, sanitary engineers, etc. However, in most coun-tries, the targets in terms of ratio to the population have not been achieved. Qualified specialists were produced but did not always remain in the countries or the public sector because of the brain-drain phenomenon, or because they were lured away by non-national institutions. In some cases, the training provided was not entirely adequate or appropriate.

The reform of medical education has received special attention. Efforts are being made to define the profile and the skills of the 21st century medical practitioner, to improve the functions of nurses and midwives and to redirect them towards primary health care services. Unfortunately, the impact of these reforms has not yet been felt. The low output of health institutions and poor performance of health personnel are still major concerns in a large number of countries. The impoverishment of health personnel is undermining the public sector's capacity to respond.

An increasing number of countries are worried about the general degradation of the **environment** and the inability of their health structures to address the problem. The substantial increase in the volume of industrial and domestic wastes poses a threat, given the inadequacies of waste disposal systems in a large number of countries. The risk of water contamination and soil degradation by chemical pollutants is also a real problem, yet to be solved in many cases.

Death rates: age- and sex-standardized, and age-specific, 1955-2025 estimates (per 100 000 population)

Age group	1955	1975	1995	2025
Age- and sex-standardized	1 173	873	636	462
0-4	2 709	1 690	722	374
5-19	287	160	86	52
20-64	730	544	409	340
65+	6 105	5 650	5 289	4 348

strategies in order to face poverty. These can be most readily seen in the massive incorporation of women into precarious working conditions and in the early insertion of adolescents and minors into the workforce.

Health trends

Mortality indicators have shown improvement in all the countries of the Americas over the last 35 years and, with rare exceptions, in all age groups. However, the favourable evolution in mortality and in the health conditions of the population hides enormous disparities between and within countries. For children under 1 year, the gaps in mortality were stable or decreasing for the countries in the moderate income group, but they were high and tended to increase in countries belonging to the lower income groups.

However, when age-adjusted mortality rates are compared between countries of similar income, reducible gaps in avoidable deaths are significant. The variation of mortality in the Region is notable. However, it is possible to state that in the country with the highest per capita income, 4.7% of mortality in the age group 45-64 could have been avoided, whereas in the country with the lowest income, preventable causes accounted for 62% of mortality in the under-65 age group.

Violence in the Region is responsible for 7-25% of mortality. If current trends persist, the problem is likely to increase, reaching epidemic proportions in some countries. In Latin America and the Caribbean, the average mortality and disability attributable to occupational accidents, is calculated to be four times greater than that notified by developed countries, at an estimated 300 daily deaths of workers.

Because one of the major functions of the Organization is to monitor the human condition in order to detect where inequities exist and whether the interventions designed to correct them are effective, methodological advances that allow the analysis of differences among and within countries have been developed. The distribution and spatial dynamics of inequalities in health status and living conditions are being analysed by coupling cartographic information with basic data on health indicators.

Much has been accomplished in the *struggle against disease* in the Americas. The Region remains free of circulating wild poliovirus, and there has been enormous progress towards the elimination of measles and neonatal tetanus. The number of episodes of acute diarrhoeal disease have been markedly reduced, and there have been significant reductions in mortality due to intestinal and acute respiratory infections. Despite these advances, diarrhoeal diseases, acute respiratory infections, and malnutrition continue to be the leading causes of death in the population under 5 in most of the medium- and low-income countries of the Region. Chronic undernutrition has replaced acute malnutrition in infancy, which, together with micronutrient deficiencies, makes up the nutritional deficiency of the lower-income countries.

The AIDS and HIV epidemic continues, while malaria has expanded its borders and the population at high risk has increased, and dengue continues to be a serious threat. In the case of malaria, morbidity (as measured by the annual parasite infection rate) began a steady increase in the mid-1970s. There was a decrease in 1993 which reversed in 1994 and 1995, reaching rates that are more than twice those registered two decades ago. A similar trend can be observed with the resurgence of dengue. Cholera has become endemic in several areas and countries of the Region, although case-fatality rates have continued to be low.

In order to provide a broader response to the threat posed by *new and emerging diseases*, the Organization will be dealing with foodborne illness and outbreaks through the newly redefined Pan American Institute for Food Protection and Zoonoses in Argentina and with new and emerging zoonoses such as hantavirus, plague and equine encephalitis through the Pan American Foot-and-Mouth Disease Center.

Despite the progress in expanding coverage, there are serious problems related to *water quality and water supply*, as well as to solid waste disposal. As a result of the cholera epidemic, countries have increased investment in water supply and sanitation. The 1995 coverage for the total population with access to water supply through house connections and other acceptable means was 73%. In the field of sanitation, by 1995 the total coverage of wastewater and ex-

Leading clusters of diseases/conditions, Region of the Americas, selected years (indicative list)

Disease category	1960	1980	1997	2025
Infectious and parasitic	1	1	2	4
Perinatal and maternal	2	3	5	5
Malignant neoplasms	5	5	4	3
Endocrine and nutritional				
Mental and behavioural				
Circulatory system	4	4	3	1
Respiratory system				
All external causes	3	2	1	2

creta disposal facilities had increased to 69%. Urban services remained constant at 80%; however, rural services were extended to approximately 40% of the population. One of the most critical sanitary problems in Latin America remains the lack of sewage treatment. A 1995 survey indicated that the percentage of sewage collected that receives treatment is just above 10%.

In response to increasing awareness among Member States that *noncommunicable diseases* account for nearly two-thirds of deaths in the Americas, that these diseases mainly result from risk factors that can be modified, and that increasing the emphasis on prevention could improve health status, the CARMEN programme was developed. It takes an integrated approach that combines clinical prevention for individuals with health promotion directed at the general population. CARMEN projects reach their audience through community, workplace and school settings, as well as through local health services.

The financial constraints in the social sectors over the past decade have increasingly revealed the serious limitations of institutions in terms of resource management, a situation that has worsened due to rising costs in the services. In 1994 the countries of Latin America and the Caribbean spent over $1 billion on health, or about $240 per capita.

Future prospects

In contrast to the 1970s, infrastructure development policy in the past 15 years has stagnated and is currently one of the components with the greatest need for state policy support. Infrastructure development is one component that requires strengthening within the health sector reform processes. Another is improving mechanisms to ensure the supply and availability of essential drugs and other supplies.

There have been significant changes in the formulation and implementation of national and health sector policy. Decentralization, social participation, and inter- and intra-sectoral coordination are part of the strategies that have been promoted and that in some places have yielded positive results.

The countries have accorded high priority to the care of children under 5 and women. Action has been geared towards improving coverage. However, the population's need for access persists owing to a variety of constraints. The Organization is responding by promoting the trend towards the delivery of integrated health services to priority population groups.

The need for financing and other resources has been considered a constraint to expanding and maintaining health programmes. In many countries decentralization to the local level and greater community involvement could contribute to the sustainability of activities.

Emphasis will also be given to the crucial importance of actions directed towards safeguarding the planet, particularly in light of events that are affecting natural resources and producing ecological changes. The emergence of new diseases which threaten human existence is linked to these changes. Natural disasters and their effects on drinking-water safety and the availability of food and shelter could have been given more attention, particularly in light of the Region's vulnerability to hurricanes, volcanic activity, earthquakes, and other natural disasters.

The vision of health for all represents a desired future state that is being approached by renewing commitment to the goal and by implementing suitable strategies and concrete actions. This vision may be summarized as a shared understanding of health in which the energies of the Hemisphere respond to the challenges that arise for the achievement of sustainable human development with dignity and equity.

With the new millennium approaching, Member States should renew their commitment to the goal of health for all and its health strategies within the context of the social, economic, political, environmental, and technological trends that are affecting the health of the populations, the environment, and the health services, giving priority to the adoption of policies to resolve their health problems in a sustainable manner and steadily improve the quality of life of their peoples.

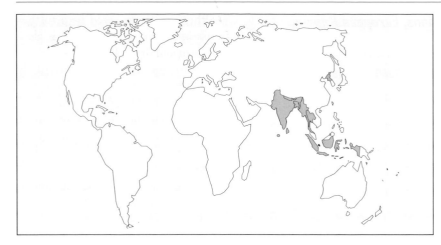

10 Member States
Population (1997): 1 457 million

GNP per capita

- Regional average (1995) $ 532
  min.: Nepal $ 200
  max.: Thailand $ 2 740

- Annual average growth rate
  (1985-1995)
  min.: Bangladesh 2.1 %
  max.: Thailand 8.4 %

Bangladesh	Indonesia
Bhutan	Maldives
Democratic	Myanmar
People's	Nepal
Republic of	Sri Lanka
Korea	Thailand
India	

South-East Asia

The health situation of the South-East Asia Region today and in the future is determined by many factors including ageing and geographical distribution of the population, poverty and economic progress, education and literacy levels, and infrastructure, functioning and interventions of the health care system.

Along with a slow decline of death rates and gradual increase in life expectancy, the process of epidemiological transition is under way in most countries. Communicable diseases are gradually being replaced by chronic and degenerative conditions (e.g. cardiovascular diseases and cancer) which in some countries are becoming the main causes of death and morbidity. Countries of the Region are thus bearing the double burden of both communicable and noncommunicable diseases.

The infant mortality rate has declined during the last decade in virtually all countries of the Region but still remains high (60-100 per 1000 live births) in some. Under-5 mortality rates show a similar pattern. The maternal mortality ratio has slowly declined overall during the last decade but remains high in most countries, and 235 000 maternal deaths (40% of

the global total) occur in the Region. Only Sri Lanka and Thailand have attained relatively low maternal mortality ratios. Maternal health data show that countries with low maternal mortality have a high proportion of deliveries by trained personnel, a well-established primary health care infrastructure and good referral systems. Management and training programmes in safe motherhood need to focus on midwives and to assign them to the community level.

Health successes

The main change in the morbidity and mortality patterns in the Region during the last 10 years results from a decline of polio, measles, neonatal tetanus and other target diseases of the Expanded Programme on Immunization.

Polio eradication activities have accelerated dramatically, particularly with the implementation of national immunization days in nine countries. Health experts are confident that they will be able to eradicate poliomyelitis through effective universal immunization and adequate epidemiological surveillance. A 70% reduction in the number of reported cases of diphtheria and whooping cough has been achieved as a result of the 90% immunization coverage. The total number of measles deaths in the Region has decreased by about 87% and

Tables concerning demography, health indicators and GNP are based on United Nations and World Bank estimates. All other information is from regional sources.

Selected health-for-all (HFA) indicators	1975			1997			2025			HFA targets	No. of Member States which have *not* met the HFA targets in 1997
	Average	Max.	Min.	Average	Max.	Min.	Average	Max.	Min.		
Life expectancy at birth (years)	52	66	42	63	73	53	72	78	67	> 60	3
Infant mortality rate (per 1000 live births)	124	171	44	68	104	15	32	41	6	< 50	5
Under-5 mortality rate (per 1000 live births)	177	240	50	85	142	18	38	50	8	< 70	5

the number of reported cases has fallen by about 67% as a result of about 80% immunization coverage. Bhutan, the Democratic People's Republic of Korea, Maldives, Sri Lanka and Thailand have achieved the target of no more than one neonatal tetanus case per 1000 live births.

Another positive epidemiological trend is the fall in the incidence and prevalence of leprosy. Multidrug therapy has proved so successful that it is expected to eliminate leprosy as a public health problem by 2000. There has also been a clear decline in the number of registered cases of guinea-worm disease in India since 1984. If the prevention and control programmes of such diseases are intensified, there is a real chance that they may be eradicated, eliminated or brought to very low levels of incidence and/or prevalence during the next few years.

Unfinished agenda

Despite overall improvements in socioeconomic status and increased life expectancy, **communicable diseases** are still deep-rooted in the Region. Old diseases like cholera and tuberculosis still dominate the disease pattern, while malaria, plague and kala-azar, which were on the verge of eradication, have reappeared. An added cause for concern is the appearance of drug-resistant strains of tuberculosis, gonococcal infections and malaria. New diseases such as cholera caused by strain O139 and HIV infections have appeared, with HIV/AIDS assuming epidemic proportions and becoming one of the most menacing health problems in some South-East Asian countries. Diseases which were not previously public health concerns are now assuming importance in association with HIV in some countries. In light of these trends, WHO has formulated a strategy to strengthen national and international capacity in the surveillance and control of communicable diseases representing new, emerging and re-emerging public health problems. The underlying factors contributing to the high prevalence of communicable diseases include poverty, malnutrition, ignorance, an insanitary environment and lack of safe drinking-water. Population growth and rapid urbanization with attendant overcrowding, poor housing and environmental deterioration have worsened the situation, and have contributed to the emergence and re-emergence of infectious diseases in the Region.

It is estimated that acute respiratory infections cause about 1.4 million deaths in children aged under 5 annually in the Region. Diarrhoeal diseases continue to be one of the leading causes of childhood death in most South-East Asian countries, accounting for about 25% of under-5 and the United States, as well as NGOs. An estimated $1 billion of external funding is needed until final eradication. The very success of the venture, which has resulted in diminishing threats from vaccine-preventable diseases, is in danger of being its downfall, as the public and donors tend to lose interest when the diseases come under control. But experience shows that the diseases return as soon as vaccine coverage drops.

Partners in response to emergencies

The traditional forms of action in response to emergency situations, due to natural or other disasters, originally consisted mainly of immediate aid in the form of urgently needed drugs, vaccines, medical equipment and other medical supplies. In the 1970s, however, WHO and the international community emphasized and developed primary health care approaches and, more recently, relief programmes focusing on preventive programmes. Technical cooperation with disaster-prone countries increasingly aimed at improving national capacity to take preventive measures and to remain more effectively in control of emergency situations. This involved Member States in activities relating to the public health management of emergencies, research on the epidemiology of disasters, studies of populations at risk, assessment of needs, priorities in the event of mass casualties, and disease control following disasters. Under WHO's impetus, several universities have established undergraduate and postgraduate programmes on health management of disasters. In collaboration with **UNHCR** and other international agencies, WHO has increasingly become involved in the health problems of refugees and has participated fully

in the provision of emergency assistance by the United Nations system.

Emergency relief, disaster preparedness and management of disasters are the three main lines of action for WHO's involvement. Emergency humanitarian action is made possible through funding from donors as extrabudgetary contributions ($25 million in 1996). The Panafrican Emergency Training Centre and the Emergency Health Management Training project based in Addis Ababa provide support to countries of the African continent. In the Americas, the Regional Emergency Programme has strengthened the capacity of emergency managers to coordinate with the national health sector, and to this end developed a computerized relief supply management system. In South-East Asia, the national capacities of Member States and their coordinating mechanisms were reinforced, especially in Bangladesh, India and Myanmar. At the global level, several sets of guidelines were issued and training programmes were implemented.

The new WHO policy for emergency and humanitarian activities is based on three concepts:
- the Organization's position as a "health facilitator";
- its complementary role, in view of its specialized health knowledge, within the UN framework of emergency management coordination (such as monitoring the distribution of drugs in certain situations, e.g. Iraq); and
- its insistence on linking emergency management policy to development in order to help affected countries to achieve long-term improvements in public health status – a prerequisite for sustainable development.

Under WHO's impetus, several universities have established undergraduate and postgraduate programmes on health management of disasters.

Box 30. Health Futures at EXPO 2000

WHO is planning to take millions of people on a fascinating journey to discover Health Futures, an exhibition presenting its vision for healthy living in the 21st century. The exhibition is being developed in cooperation with the organizers of EXPO 2000, the World Exhibition set to celebrate the third millennium in Hanover, Germany, from 1 June to 31 October 2000.

In 2000, the theme will be the future itself under the banner "Humankind – Nature – Technology". EXPO 2000 aims to stimulate people's imagination, and encourage them into actively meeting the challenges facing humankind on the eve of the 21st century. The United Nations programme of action for sustainable development which resulted from the 1992 Earth Summit in Rio de Janeiro, Brazil, will provide the framework for the many events at EXPO 2000. In the Thematic Area, Agenda 21 will be brought to life in several subexhibitions: health, humankind, environment; landscape and climate, nutrition, knowledge; information and communication, the future of work, energy, mobility, basic needs, the future of the past and the 21st century.

WHO will develop Health Futures as part of the Thematic Area, highlighting the health chapter of Agenda 21, which underlines that health and sustainable development are inextricably linked. Health Futures will make clear that the promotion and protection of health are crucial to sustainable development. Reaching millions of Expo visitors, the health exhibition is a unique opportunity to promote public awareness of the factors that influence health, positively or adversely, and to encourage people to protect and promote their health more actively in various ways.

Visitors will learn that health and well-being are the product of many factors, and that good health needs supportive environments; that given supportive environments, people have the power to improve their health; and that new knowledge and technologies are revolutionizing approaches to health, health care and health systems. Areas to be highlighted are youth and active ageing, infectious and chronic diseases, healthy cities and technology for health. The exhibition will illustrate realistic, practical, cost-effective and sustainable approaches that are available now or will be in the near future.

Based on WHO's new policy for health for all in the 21st century, the exhibition will underline the major determinants of health ranging from nutrition to the empowerment of women and will remind visitors of the equity gap in health care, and of the gap in life expectancy at birth between developing and developed countries, stressing the need for international cooperation to eliminate or eradicate infectious diseases.

Health Futures will explore the effectiveness of modern media to communicate complex health messages to a mass lay audience, combining theatre stage productions, science centre approaches and multimedia messages to form an innovative learning experience. Educational media envisaged include CD-ROMs, electronic games, health on-line systems, and an Internet site including "a virtual walk through Health Futures".

Partners for research

The *International Agency for Research on Cancer* was established in 1965. Subject to the general authority of WHO, it concentrates on environmental biology and cancer epidemiology.

In 1972, WHO launched a special programme of research, development and research training in *human reproduction* with particular reference to the needs of developing countries. In 1988 UNDP, UNFPA, and the World Bank joined as cosponsors. In the 25 years of its existence, the programme has made major contributions to the improvement of reproductive health in the world. Key achievements in the area of development and improvement of methods of fertility regulation include the development of two once-a-month injectable contraceptives, extension of the duration of effectiveness of the copper IUD to 11 years and establishment of its safety in women at low risk of sexually transmitted diseases; demonstration of the feasibility of developing steroid-based contraceptives for men; clinical studies on the various uses of antiprogestogens in

WHO is participating

in the multilateral

development of

knowledge in the

global health domain.

erning bodies in 1997. The consultation has extended beyond government and health ministries to consider the views of nongovernmental organizations, United Nations partners (including the World Bank and the World Trade Organization), the private sector, and academic and research institutions. Hundreds of individuals and organizations have been mobilized in the process. Their views have been systematically analysed and are reflected in the new health policy, *Health for all in the 21st century*, to be submitted to the 51st World Health Assembly in May 1998.

The Global Knowledge Partnership, which includes all the major United Nations agencies, is currently preparing an inventory of current "knowledge for development" activities conducted by their respective organizations. WHO is participating in the multilateral development of knowledge in the global health domain. Global knowledge builds on what began at the 1995 G7 meeting on the global information society, and continued at the more broadly-based 1996 conference on the information society and development. The Global Knowledge '97 Conference, of which WHO was a partner, was part of a much broader process of preparing

societies and individuals for the information age. Coming to terms with the knowledge revolution is a central part of rethinking development for the 21st century.

The global knowledge revolution has only just begun and we are still at the dawn of the information age, but we are already faced with a series of urgent riddles and challenges.

Many individuals and probably the world as a whole will benefit from new technology. However, if left on its present track, the revolution will probably bypass billions of people. No one actor alone has the combination of power, resources and vision necessary to guide the revolution so that it advances the general good, neither the governments, the private sector, civil society nor the voluntary community. The knowledge revolution comes at a time when traditional concepts of international development are being questioned. The developing world has fragmented into a kaleidoscope of countries and blocs, and old donor-recipient relationships have become archaic. Global problems, too big for national governments and international agencies, call for new partnerships, coalitions and networks capable of responding at an appropriate scale, speed and level.

Chapter 8
Health agenda for the 21st century

Future health challenges

During 1995, 15 000 babies were born every hour. More than 90% of them will survive their first five years to see the dawn of the new century. Half of them will live to celebrate their 75th birthday in 2070. Many will become centenarians who will live throughout the entire 21st century and into the early 22nd.

By 2025, the 1995 baby will be an adult whose own child will have a 90% chance of surviving not merely the first five years, but the first 50 years of life. Two out of every three babies born in 2025 will live to be at least 75.

The enhanced life expectancy of tomorrow's children is the harvest of health improvements witnessed in the 20th century. Another consequence is that even before 2025, for the first time, small children will be outnumbered by people over 65. While children under 5 years will represent about 8% of a global population that will have risen to 8 billion, the over-65s will represent about 10%. For every 100 adults aged 20-64 in 2025 there should be 17 older people aged 65 and above, 14 children under 5 and more than 40 older children and adolescents aged 5-19 years.

For young and old alike, the world of 2025 will be very different from that of today. This report has explained trends in health across the human life span during the past 50 years. While the conclusion overall is that health has steadily improved, the main issues now are how to sustain those improvements and how to meet the health challenges of the future.

In the early 21st century the world, already free of smallpox, should also be free of poliomyelitis, measles, and neonatal tetanus. Some other infectious and parasitic diseases will be eliminated, and the burden of many more which currently afflict tropical regions should be further reduced.

Most children should be protected from vaccine-preventable diseases through well-established and sustainable immunization programmes; deaths among small children should be further cut through a package of interventions known as the Integrated Management of Childhood Illnesses.

Most of the global population should have regular access to essential drugs. However, as shown in *Table 11*, it is disconcerting to note that in the early 21st century, it is expected that there will be 21% more deaths among adults aged 20-64 years than during the late 20th century. Given that these adults form the main foundation for any social and economic support to the young and old, it is imperative that they are protected from premature mortality and disability.

Table 11. Deaths by age group, world, 1975-2000 and 2000-2025

Age group	1975-2000		2000-2025	
	Number (000)	Percentage of total	Number (000)	Percentage of total
0-4	304 970	25	181 024	12
5-19	96 127	8	63 400	4
20-64	349 719	28	422 028	29
65+	482 479	39	787 202	54
All ages	1 233 295	100	1 453 654	100

The epidemiological assessment in this report suggests that the major health problems by the year 2025 will be diseases of the circulatory system, cancers, infectious and parasitic diseases and external causes *(Table 12)*.

Chapter 3 of this report and *The World Health Report 1997* on chronic diseases have discussed the dominant role of these diseases, musculoskeletal conditions, and mental and behavioural disorders, in defining ill-health among adults. Available data indicate that in some countries, deaths from circulatory diseases are falling while cancer deaths are increasing *(Fig. 21)*.

WHO estimates that about two-thirds of global cancer deaths, cancer incidence during 1997 and cancer prevalence in 1997 can be clustered according to just four risk factors, i.e.: diet-related (stomach, colon-rectum, liver, mouth-pharynx and prostate); tobacco-related (lung); infection-related (lymphoma and cervix); and hormone-related (breast). WHO foresees that the overeall global situation in respect of cancers of the stomach, liver, mouth and pharynx, and of the cervix and breast, will improve in the early 21st century while those related to the lung, trachea, bronchus, colon and rectum, and prostate as well as lymphoma, will worsen.

The changing world is experiencing changing patterns of health. Influences include: rapid modernization; an everyday life dependent on technological advances; changing behaviour – sedentary living, excessive or ill-balanced diets and smoking; and a deteriorating environment – air pollution, exposure to chemicals, contamination of soil and water, and hazards to food safety. Together, these are resulting in an increase in crippling chronic diseases such as diabetes, rheumatoid arthritis and low back pain. In addition, many hundreds of millions of people worldwide are affected by some form of mental disorder, from the relatively minor to the incurable and life-threatening; many individuals suffer from several simultaneously. An increase has also been observed in the incidence of suicide, associated with economic downturns.

Fig. 21. Death rates by cause, adults aged 20-64, selected countries, 1985 and 1995[a]

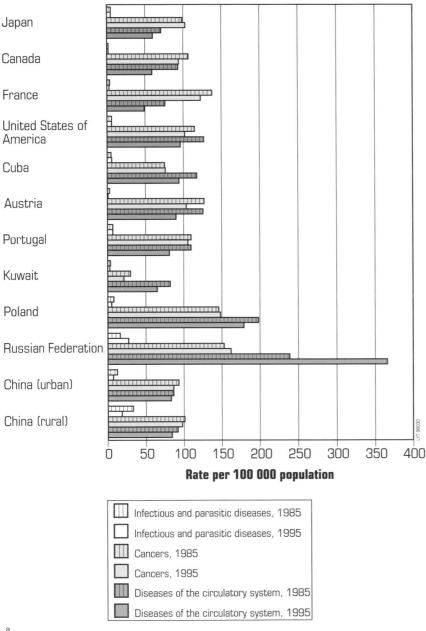

Rate per 100 000 population

Infectious and parasitic diseases, 1985
Infectious and parasitic diseases, 1995
Cancers, 1985
Cancers, 1995
Diseases of the circulatory system, 1985
Diseases of the circulatory system, 1995

[a] Ranked by decreasing order of 1985 life expectancy values.

Table 12. Leading clusters of diseases/conditions, WHO regions, selected years[a]

Disease category	1960						1980					
	Africa	The Americas	Eastern Mediterranean	Europe	South-East Asia	Western Pacific[b]	Africa	The Americas	Eastern Mediterranean	Europe	South-East Asia	Western Pacific[b]
Infectious and parasitic	1	1	1	5	1		1	1	2	5	1	
Perinatal and maternal	2	2	3		3		2	3	5		3	
Malignant neoplasms		5		2		3		5		2		2
Endocrine and nutritional	4				2		4				2	
Mental and behavioural												
Circulatory system	5	4	5	1		2	5	4	1	1		1
Respiratory system	3		2	3		1	3		3	4		3
All external causes		3	4	4		4		2	4	3		4

Disease category	1997						2025					
	Africa	The Americas	Eastern Mediterranean	Europe	South-East Asia	Western Pacific[b]	Africa	The Americas	Eastern Mediterranean	Europe	South-East Asia	Western Pacific[b]
Infectious and parasitic	1	2	2		1		1	4	4	5	3	
Perinatal and maternal	2	5	5		3		2	5				
Malignant neoplasms		4		2		2		3	5	2	2	2
Endocrine and nutritional	5						5				5	
Mental and behavioural				5						4	4	
Circulatory system	4	3	1	1	2	1	3	1	1	1	1	1
Respiratory system	3		3	4		3	4		2			4
All external causes		1	4	3		4		2	3	3		3

a Indicative list, as ranked by the respective regional offices.
b For all years, the Western Pacific Region ranked *Digestive system* in fifth position. This category was not used for the other regions.

With a better understanding of ageing and diseases processes, distinctions have become artificial between infectious and non-infectious diseases, as well as between physical and mental ill-health. Recent studies indicate for example that interruption of the blood supply to the brain has important mental and physical health consequences, producing stroke, vascular dementia and transient ischaemic attacks (mini-strokes). Every year, millions of people survive a stroke and suffer brain damage with varying degrees of continuing mental and physical disability.

Vascular dementia has a more gradual onset than stroke and is less likely to be reported as a cause of death, but it is another important cause of disability. Transient ischaemic attacks affecting the brain are important warning signs of future stroke or dementia and call for prompt preventive measures. Although most strokes and dementia occur in the elderly, they are nevertheless a significant cause of morbidity in younger populations (one-third of strokes occur in people aged under 65). Both stroke and dementia contribute significantly to the global burden of disease, and are expensive to treat. To the cost to health services should be added the financial and emotional cost to the families who provide most of the caring for those affected.

In addition to the prevention methods common to cardiovascular disease and stroke, such as smoking cessation or avoidance, hypertension treatment and diet modification, there are also now promising treatments for stroke which, if started within hours of onset, may reduce the extent of

Box 31. The brain, neurology and psychiatry

Because of the importance of the brain in controlling human activity, injury and diseases affecting the brain result in a significant proportion of all human disability. Until relatively recently, knowledge about the brain depended on crude observation and studying the effects of head injury. Study of the brain's electrical activity gave some insight into the pathology of epilepsy, but only in recent decades have scientific studies thrown light on the relationships between brain function and mental functions such as thought and emotions. The coming decades should bring better understanding of the biological or physical processes in the brain that accompany thinking and feeling.

Until recently, the physical processes of the brain were studied by neurologists and neuroscientists, whereas the mental processes (thinking and feeling) were studied by psychologists and psychiatrists, with little interaction between the two groups. In some countries, the clinical discipline of neuropsychiatry has flourished, bringing the two together, while in others they have stayed separate. Several factors are now bringing the two together. One is the advance in "noninvasive" methods of investigation. Apart form crude electroencephalographs, the only way of investigating brain function used to be to open the skull and physically probe into the brain. The technology is now available, however, to localize extremely accurately virtually every part of the brain without opening the skull. By following the changes in blood flow and chemical activity that accompany neural activity, it is possible to map the areas involved when, for instance, the subject looks at something, hears a word or experiences pain or pleasure.

Within the next 10-15 years, such methods are likely to generate new knowledge of the functional anatomy of the human brain, making possible a better understanding of how normal brain function is disturbed in conditions such as dyslexia, epilepsy and motor dysfunctions. These tools should also throw light on how the brain is altered during the disturbed thought patterns and emotions that are such a troublesome feature of schizophrenia and the affective disorders.

Another factor influencing our understanding of the relationship between brain function and mental function is the discovery in recent decades of the psychotropic drugs used to treat mental disorders. These drugs have shown that it is possible to change mental function by chemically modifying brain function. Study of their action has led to an understanding of the chemicals that carry messages from one nerve cell to another (neurotransmitters) and the chemical environment in which the brain functions. Originally, most of the drugs used to treat mental disorders were discovered almost by chance. Now, with more precise knowledge of neurotransmission, it is possible to design drugs that will block or accelerate the nervous activity causing mental disorders. It is now unscientific to argue over whether epilepsy, stroke, dementia, multiple sclerosis, schizophrenia, bipolar disorders or indeed the addictions are "neurological" or "psychiatric". All are diseases or conditions of the brain which demand investigation, treatment and care for those affected and, taken together, which contribute to an enormous amount of disability in the world.

With increasing knowledge, much of the gulf between the mind and brain, between neurology and psychiatry, between neuroscience and psychology, is fast being bridged, enabling rational research and interventions to be carried out to prevent or treat brain damage and disorders of brain function. These advances have the potential to bring about a significant reduction in the level of disability worldwide.

brain damage or even allow the brain to recover completely. For many patients, however, the brain will be irreversibly damaged unless an effective rehabilitation strategy is in place to make a timely response *(Box 31)*.

Globally there are still 21 million deaths among those aged under 50; most of them are due to infectious diseases, many of them being preventable through cost-effective interventions such as immunization and essential clinical care management, personal hygiene, public health and sanitation practices, and the safe processing, preparation and handling of foods. With increasing international travel and mass population movements due to war and internal conflicts, foodborne diseases are emerging as a major threat in the 21st century *(Box 32)*.

Globalization of trade and services also poses global threats to health. The health of the world's citizens is inextricably linked, and is less determined by events within geographical boundaries. The threat posed by emerging and re-emerging infectious diseases is accentuated by changes in human behaviour, changes in ecology and climate, in land use patterns and economic development, as well as by tourism and migration.

Despite the progress that can be achieved in a world without frontiers, there is a danger that insistence on cross-border uniformity, or even on unwarranted minimum levels, could reduce the scope of mutually beneficial trade. Countries may have failed to enforce adequate environmental standards, or (more commonly) been deterred from introducing justified improvements, by pressures arising from business concerns about international competitiveness. Attention should be paid to identifying those areas of policy where common or agreed cross-border minimum standards are justified, and those where the choice should be left to individual States and governments.

Patterns of health and disease have changed more rapidly worldwide in the last half-century than during any comparable period in history. Although survival strategies underlying health systems development during the past decades have been extremely successful in increasing the length of human life, they have not led to a corresponding reduction in morbidity and disability, or improvement in the quality of life. Available data indicate that disability-free life expectancy at birth has not significantly increased. While mortality reduction targets are achieved through disease-specific interventions, the attainment by people of their full potential for health – the main thrust of

Box 32. Foodborne diseases – A global threat

Public health officials attribute the rise in incidence of foodborne illnesses and the emergence of new foodborne diseases to a combination of different factors related to changes in demographics and consumer lifestyles, in food production, international trade and travel, and microbial adaptation. Globalization of the food supply means that people are exposed, through foods purchased locally, to pathogens native to remote parts of the world. As a result of international travel, people are exposed to foodborne hazards in foreign countries and import the disease into their home country upon their return. As a result, a person may acquire an illness in one country and expose others in a location thousands of kilometres from the original source of the infection. Changes in microbial populations can lead to the evolution of new pathogens, the development of new virulence factors for old pathogens, the development of antibiotic resistance making a disease more difficult to treat, or to changes in the ability to survive in adverse environmental conditions. People are becoming increasingly vulnerable, particularly since the number of susceptible individuals such as the elderly and people with HIV infection or other underlying medical conditions is increasing. As lifestyles change, more people eat meals prepared outside the home. Insufficient training in food handling constitutes one of the major factors responsible for the rise in foodborne disease incidence.

To deal with these problems, a comprehensive strategy is needed at national and international levels. This must be based on effective food control, improving agricultural and animal husbandry practices, applying food technologies with the potential to reduce or eliminate foodborne pathogens, and educating persons who handle food. Improved surveillance programmes are essential for early detection of foodborne disease outbreaks and for limiting their spread before they take on epidemic or pandemic proportions. Early identification of the source of the outbreak is becoming increasingly important as countries move towards industrialization. Protecting the public from emerging foodborne diseases also means keeping track of new events in agricultural and processing practices and of the origin of food, while climatic and environmental changes need to be monitored for potential negative effects on the food chain.

the health-for-all movement – is far from complete.

Outlining desirable aspirations for better health and constructing a reasonable vision for the future has become crucial for setting health objectives for the early 21st century. It is therefore time for a breakthrough in thinking and a clearly defined vision for guiding strategies to defeat the powerful enemies of positive health, and thus ensure quality of life.

Present knowledge and scientific evidence show that diseases and disabilities, which prevent many people from reaching old age in good health, can be delayed or avoided. Such prevention of major infectious and chronic diseases is however possible only if there is a shift in emphasis from the disease itself to risk factors or determinants related to the development of the disease.

A single risk factor may contribute to many diseases and different risk factors often act in combination to produce a single disease. Many of these risk factors associated with a broad spectrum of diseases – physical or mental, infectious or non-infectious – widespread in both developing and developed countries have been created by, and can be controlled by people themselves. Tackling a limited number of risk factors, over which the individual has control, and environmental hazards over which national and international communities have a say, could reduce substantially sickness and suffering caused by them.

In visualizing the future, the following fundamental points have been considered:

- The *primary focus* of health development is positive health, an enhancement of the health potential of individuals and a contributor to better quality of life in the context of human development. Health will then not be an end in itself but a resource for everyday life that enables individuals to realize aspirations and strategic needs and to change or cope with their environment. Policies and strategies for health development provide people with a positive sense of health and enable them to make full use of their physical, mental and social capacities. Positive health implies adding life to years i.e. increasing years lived free from ill-health,

reducing or minimizing adverse effects of illness and disability, and improving quality of life through a healthy lifestyle in a healthy physical, social and ecological environment.

- The *primary concern* will be to improve health potential and quality of life at all phases of the life cycle. Preventive, protective, promotive, curative and rehabilitative measures to improve health will also ensure that such improvements can be sustained, and if possible further enhanced. It will make individuals economically and socially active given their biological and chronological maturity.

- The *primary objective* of health development activities will be outcome-oriented. Various disease-specific interventions will be assessed not so much in terms of outputs, for example, improved access to health care or services, reduction in mortality, morbidity or disability from any single disease or condition. Instead they will be assessed in terms of outcomes, ensuring value for money by improving the overall health of the individual and enhancing his or her health potential. Health care should not only meet professional standards but also benefit the person who receives it. Quality assessment may become heavily biased towards reflecting consumers' needs and interests as well as their expectations and values. A major consequence of such an "outcome" perspective is the advantage of health and social interventions being integrated and inclusive. It requires and reflects the contributions of all those who provide care including self-care. However, it cannot identify which specific initiative or action was responsible for the outcome.

Many risk factors

associated with

a broad spectrum

of diseases have been

created by, and can

be controlled by

people themselves.

With these fundamentals underpinning health improvements for people-centred development, a future health picture can be envisioned and elaborated for the first quarter of the 21st century. This foresees that, worldwide, *every individual should enjoy his or her full health potential throughout the life span and be socially, economically and mentally productive and able to have a better quality of life.* Concerted efforts should be made to sustain and build on health gains in terms of increased life expectancy and reduced risk of ill-health, and to reduce and where possible eliminate premature mortality and disability.

An effective response to all these challenges requires a radically different approach and should be based on knowledge, experience and insights gained over the past 50 years.

Some of the developments in technology, and the information and knowledge that stem from them, are listed in the following section. So too are examples of advances in communication technology which allow this information and knowledge to be accessible to those who need it (*Box 33*).

Health and technology

The most significant feature of technology development in the early part of the 21st century will be the rapidly increasing knowledge-intensity of products and processes used globally. Lifelong learning will be essential for ensuring that workers remain productive, especially as populations and labour forces age over the coming decades. The emphasis will need to be on active ageing, encouraging individuals to participate fully in society regardless of their age.

The delivery of health care is dependent on past, recent and future research in biomedical science. Examples of the highly successful use of

---

Box 33. Sharing knowledge for health

A knowledge-based organization in an environment where knowledge has become a raw material must give serious consideration to how such knowledge is managed, disseminated and used. The interaction between partners in international health is influenced by the following five key factors:

1. **Globalization.** Globalization is principally about increasing interdependence – economic, political and social. It has both positive and negative influences on health. Integration at one level can be matched by marginalization and increasing inequities at others.
2. **The information revolution.** The rapid development of information and communications technology opens up new ways to produce, analyse and disseminate data and health knowledge. The challenge is to build a managed network that allows accessing and dissemination of knowledge; makes it useful and practical; and allows for debates and feedback mechanisms. Information technology also makes available new means of assistance between centres (telemedicine, Internet-based training, etc.).
3. **The health research/technology revolution.** Health information itself is subject to ever more rapid changes and updates, and WHO information (for example on drug development, safety, treatment schedules etc.) needs to be totally reliable and up to date. The average shelf-life of a health fact is currently five years.
4. **The increased privatization of health, health research and intellectual property.** Increasingly health and medical research are private, and a determining factor in one of the largest and most rapidly growing world markets. Research at university institutes is frequently dependent on significant contributions from the private sector.
5. **A broader understanding of and accountability for health.** The increased knowledge available on determinants of health and on the impact of sectors other than health calls for a broader range of information input in areas such as economics, law, human rights and ethics.

Reliable health information and knowledge are becoming a sought-after commodity not only in terms of patents and intellectual property, but also in terms of systems knowledge and comparative data. Given the increasingly fluid borders between health/biomedical research, pharmaceutical and nutrition research and agricultural research, the issues and partners WHO deals with could change significantly.

The challenge before the international community is how to best manage the intellectual capital inherent in these many partners and networks. The result of good management of intellectual capital equals health leadership. The leadership issue in this case is: who sets the "gold standard" for global health issues and the global health debate; and whose approach/paradigm on how to define health is accepted. From this follow proposals on how to manage health, pay for health, and measure the health of populations.

discoveries in basic science, or technological developments, are: molecular and cell biology; immunology and genetics; and those relevant for diagnostic and therapeutic procedures, such as magnetic resonance in ageing and the surgical applications of laser techniques. In neurobiology, understanding of the ever-increasing panoply of neurotransmitters has led to new insights into the action of psychotropic drugs and neurotoxins of dietary origin.

Applications of technology can be divided according to functional categories: for prevention, diagnosis, therapy or rehabilitation. The technologies themselves may be classified as biologicals, pharmaceuticals, medical devices and replacement and assistive devices.

Biological medicine is the basis for the fundamental understanding of disease processes. It has made possible the development of novel compounds, and has provided new methods for the large-scale production of existing biologicals. It is the basis for highly sensitive specific diagnostic tests and for the development of new vaccines. Recombinant DNA techniques are available for prenatal screening and postnatal examination, to detect errors in the formation or biological activity of peptides which could result in schizophrenia. They will also prove important in the development of new vaccines.

As a result of the molecular and cell biology revolutions, screening procedures in medical and public health diagnoses are being speeded up. A new generation of drugs is coming into use which can exercise more precise control over human body functions. Current ground-breaking genome research will shift the balance from diagnosis and treatment of disease to prediction or early detection, so that disease can be managed prior to the onset of symptoms. Al-

though it raises ethical problems, it also has the potential to offer significant benefits.

A wealth of diagnostic devices has emerged, covering virtually all branches of medicine and health care. Advances in imaging technology have brought a new dimension to diagnostic procedures. Ultrasonic techniques are cheaper (though less precise) than computer-aided tomography and magnetic resonance imaging, and are suitable for screening and fore a wide range of diagnostic work. They also have therapeutic applications. Endoscopic techniques are relatively inexpensive, and automated procedures such as cytological screening are becoming more reliable.

Lasers are being used in surgical treatment, and microsurgery has become much more sophisticated. Artificial joints and prostheses, using new materials and substitutes as well as improvements in traditional materials, have become valuable weapons against disability. The quality of these and other devices such as cardiac pacemakers is continually improving. Transplant surgery has a major future with a rapidly ageing population. Increasing efforts are also being made in the clinical application of the xenotransplantation of cells, tissues and organs from animal donors to human recipients, and in the production of biologicals for human use from transgenic and cloned animals.

Some promising possibilities in the fields of biologicals and pharmaceuticals are new vaccines against infectious diseases, including combination vaccines such as for DPT as well as oral vaccine.

Key areas for general research include sequencing genomes of major pathogens and studying the spread of antimicrobial resistance. There will be an upsurge in the development of low-cost, simple diagnostic and therapeutic devices for use in early detec-

Current ground-

breaking genome

research will shift

the balance from

diagnosis and

treatment of disease

to prediction or

early detection.

tion of disease or relief from pain. As well as continuing developments in biomaterials for prostheses, advances in robotics are expected to have a considerable impact.

In short, scientific and technological developments in the broadest sense are contributing significantly to the provision of health care. Continued investment in basic and applied science will certainly pay off. Properly planned schemes for technology transfer should make it possible for developing countries to capitalize, for health, on advances in other countries, and there is great scope for regional cooperation.

Technological advances may however raise serious ethical issues which require the urgent attention of the international community. The most recent example is the successful cloning in 1997 of a sheep by somatic cell nuclear transfer. Governments, regional groupings and international bodies worldwide have reacted by firmly opposing human reproductive cloning. WHO's governing bodies have stated categorically that the replication of human individuals is ethically unacceptable.

The information society

Individuals are being expected to assume increasing responsibility for their own health, within the supportive framework of the State. The availability of meaningful information becomes central to their ability to make choices. Each person creates health within the settings of everyday life (at school, at work, at home). Society's role is to create the conditions that allow the attainment of health by all its members.

The information society provides the tools. Sharing the world's store of global health knowledge through information and communication technology is a keystone to international health development. Rapidly developing information technologies are changing the way the world communicates, with far-reaching consequences, including in the area of public health.

Information societies have three main characteristics. They use information as an economic resource, stimulating business towards greater efficiency (e.g. through the electronic transfer of money). Individual citizens use information more intensively as consumers, to inform their choices, make their purchases and take greater control over their lives.

The capacity of information technology has been increasing at an exponential rate for nearly 20 years and shows no sign of slowing down. These new information systems – satellite broadcasting, telecommunications networks using fiberoptics and the Internet – are global.

Information technology can raise education levels, strengthen community links and stimulate public participation in decision-making. In health, it enables doctors to keep closer track of their patients' progress through sophisticated records management systems. Globally, it enables the surveillance and monitoring of disease, and facilitates the rapid international responses of organizations such as WHO to epidemics. The introduction of information technology in health care delivery and health systems management will enhance quality of care, efficiency and cost-effectiveness in the management of individual and community health.

There is concern that the shift towards information societies will widen the gap between developed and developing countries. International agencies, including WHO, have for several decades been facilitating the information flow towards developing countries, with the expansion of information systems, libraries and archives, so that poorer nations can

Properly planned schemes for technology transfer should make it possible for developing countries to capitalize, for health, on advances in other countries.

obtain information at affordable cost and build their own information infrastructures.

Advances in communications

Communication technology should be placed at the service of all, to facilitate their access to the information they need. The new networks of information that are now developing could lay the foundations of a new social structure. No previous telecommunications advance, even the telephone and television, has penetrated public consciousness as quickly as the Internet. Its integration into conventional social and economic processes is taking place at an unprecedented speed, yet it may be only the very beginning of the Internet explosion. Already, communities and nations around the globe are starting to sketch out the "cyberplaces" of the 21st century.

This technology should not only contribute to promoting economic development and improving quality of life – it could remodel society. The time and space devoted to health issues in the media are expanding. Increasingly, media institutions are playing an active role in the social affairs of the societies they serve. The media have a powerful role to play in partnership with the health sector, in the service of health goals.

Political trends affecting health

Politics involve conflicts of power and influence, and competition between interest groups. Through politics things can be done or prevented from being done, and decisions are taken about who gets what and when in society. Since the attainment of health evokes moral and emotional responses, *health policy cannot be developed in a moral vacuum.*

The commitments and interests of international agencies, foreign aid, nongovernmental organizations and community organizations shape the politics of health and health care. The business interests of pharmaceutical and medical devices companies, as well as the motivations and ideologies of health care providers, also influence health and health care.

Workers' health, for example, is subject to trade and commerce policies as well as to the process of industrialization and the power of unions. Satisfying the health demands of women, the aged, ethnic minorities, children, the disabled and those with certain diseases such as AIDS involves politics related to ideology, ethics and the lack of political influence of these groups.

The evaluation of the health-for-all strategy carried out in 1997 illustrates that in many countries progress in traditional health indicators has been insufficient to ensure the achievement of the goal. Even in countries where the targets have been reached, equity has not been achieved, irrespective of political regime or economic development level, in spite of legislation to protect political and civil rights.

The search for equity is at the heart of the political struggle. Governments, regardless of their political style, should seek to meet health needs through rearrangement of health care systems. Recently in some countries, the core public function of ensuring equity has weakened as individual States reduce emphasis on social areas and transfer some responsibilities to the private sector and to local levels where mechanisms to safeguard equity may be lacking or weak.

Reforms have affected the content and formulation of social policies as the State modifies its role as designer, financier, implementer and regulator of

Since the attainment of health evokes moral and emotional responses, health policy cannot be developed in a moral vacuum.

policies. These modifications relate to shifts in the final purpose of social policies, from universal access associated with high cost and low impact for most to a new paradigm focused on the poor. This framework includes specific targeting strategies and equity with the premise of *treating unequally those who are socially and economically unequal.*

As a result, communities have started to mobilize for their own future through grassroots movements, nongovernmental organizations, and other means. Although community-based health care has become the new rhetoric in many contexts, its effectiveness is hampered by fragmentation, lack of societal commitment and social cohesion, and the value of illness and health services as private goods.

There is a risk that the accelerating global evolution, with the riches it promises, will leave more than half a billion people in poverty in the year 2020. In spite of increasing globalization, national policies remain of paramount importance in determining levels of employment and labour standards, for example. While the current trend is towards international responsibility for standard-setting in many key areas, and towards their implementation at the local level, national governments have a role to play in policy setting and legislation, especially in the social sector. This is particularly so in cases where resources have to be diverted from the social sector because of globalization of trade and services, which may result in a decline in the provision of essential medical and health services.

While forecasters may not be expected to reach beyond the extrapolation of known factors, leaders and policy-makers are mandated to do so. They must determine the global scenario of the early 21st century and put in place the building blocks that will permit a quantum leap forward.

If the global community does not take action soon, hunger, malnutrition and resulting illnesses will persist, natural resources will continue to be degraded, and conflicts over scarce resources such as water will become even more common. For most of humanity, the world will not be a pleasant place to live. It does not have to be this way. With foresight and decisive action, we can create a better world for all people. We have the knowledge and the skills and we still have the necessary resources, including natural resources.

Health imperatives for the 21st century

On the **unfinished agenda** for health, poverty remains the main item. The priority must be to reduce it in the poorest countries of the world, and to eliminate the pockets of poverty that exist within countries, including among refugees. Policies directed at improving health and ensuring equity are the keys to economic growth and poverty reduction.

Safeguarding the gains already achieved in health depends largely on sharing health and medical knowledge, expertise and experience on a global scale. Apart from establishing and expanding national health services based on primary health care, industrialized countries can play a vital part in helping solve global health problems. It is in their own interests as well as those of developing countries to do so.

Increased international cooperation in health can be facilitated by a managed global network making use of the latest communication technologies. Global surveillance for the detection of and response to emerging infectious diseases is essential. As a result of increased global trade and travel, the prevention of foodborne

If the global community does not take action soon, hunger, malnutrition and resulting illnesses will persist, natural resources will continue to be degraded, and conflicts over scarce resources will become even more common.

infections in particular is of increasing importance. Wars, conflicts, refugee movements and environmental degradation also facilitate the spread of infections as well as being health hazards in themselves.

Enhancing health potential in the future depends on preventing and reducing premature mortality, morbidity and disability. It involves enabling people of all ages to achieve over time their maximum potential, intellectually and physically through education, the development of life skills and healthy lifestyles.

The health implications of ***healthy ageing*** – the physical and mental characteristics of old age and their associated problems – need to be better understood. Much more research is required in order to reduce disability among older age groups.

Concern for the older members of today's society is part of the intergenerational relationships that need to be developed in the 21st century. These relationships, vital for social cohesion, should be based on equity, solidarity and social justice.

The young and old must learn to understand each other's differing aspirations and requirements. The young have the skills and energies to enhance the life quality of their elders. The old have the wisdom of experience to pass on to the children of today and of coming generations.

Concern for the older members of today's society is part of the intergenerational relationships that need to be developed in the 21st century.

Annex 1

Members and Associate Members of WHO

As of 1 January 1998, WHO had 191 Members and two Associate Members. They are listed below with the date on which they became a party to the Constitution or were admitted to associate membership.

Afghanistan 19 April 1948
Albania 26 May 1947
Algeria* 8 November 1962
Andorra 15 January 1997
Angola 15 May 1976
Antigua and Barbuda* 12 March 1984
Argentina* 22 October 1948
Armenia 4 May 1992
Australia* 2 February 1948
Austria* 30 June 1947
Azerbaijan 2 October 1992
Bahamas* 1 April 1974
Bahrain* 2 November 1971
Bangladesh 19 May 1972
Barbados* 25 April 1967
Belarus* 7 April 1948
Belgium* 25 June 1948
Belize 23 August 1990
Benin 20 September 1960
Bhutan 8 March 1982
Bolivia 23 December 1949
Bosnia and Herzegovina*
    10 September 1992
Botswana* 26 February 1975
Brazil* 2 June 1948
Brunei Darussalam 25 March 1985
Bulgaria* 9 June 1948
Burkina Faso* 4 October 1960
Burundi 22 October 1962
Cambodia* 17 May 1950
Cameroon* 6 May 1960
Canada 29 August 1946
Cape Verde 5 January 1976
Central African Republic*
    20 September 1960
Chad 1 January 1961
Chile* 15 October 1948
China* 22 July 1946
Colombia 14 May 1959
Comoros 9 December 1975
Congo 26 October 1960
Cook Islands 9 May 1984
Costa Rica 17 March 1949
Côte d'Ivoire* 28 October 1960
Croatia* 11 June 1992
Cuba* 9 May 1950
Cyprus* 16 January 1961
Czech Republic* 22 January 1993

Democratic People's Republic of Korea
    19 May 1973
Democratic Republic of the Congo*
    24 February 1961
Denmark* 19 April 1948
Djibouti 10 March 1978
Dominica* 13 August 1981
Dominican Republic 21 June 1948
Ecuador* 1 March 1949
Egypt* 16 December 1947
El Salvador 22 June 1948
Equatorial Guinea 5 May 1980
Eritrea 24 September 1993
Estonia 31 March 1993
Ethiopia 11 April 1947
Fiji* 1 January 1972
Finland* 7 October 1947
France 16 June 1948
Gabon* 21 November 1960
Gambia* 26 April 1971
Georgia 26 May 1992
Germany* 29 May 1951
Ghana* 8 April 1957
Greece* 12 March 1948
Grenada 4 December 1974
Guatemala* 26 August 1949
Guinea* 19 May 1959
Guinea-Bissau 29 July 1974
Guyana* 27 September 1966
Haiti* 12 August 1947
Honduras 8 April 1949
Hungary* 17 June 1948
Iceland 17 June 1948
India* 12 January 1948
Indonesia* 23 May 1950
Iran (Islamic Republic of)*
    23 November 1946
Iraq* 23 September 1947
Ireland* 20 October 1947
Israel 21 June 1949
Italy* 11 April 1947
Jamaica* 21 March 1963
Japan* 16 May 1951
Jordan* 7 April 1947
Kazakstan 19 August 1992
Kenya* 27 January 1964
Kiribati 26 July 1984
Kuwait* 9 May 1960

---

* Member States that have acceded to the Convention on the Privileges and Immunities of the Specialized Agencies and its Annex VII.

Kyrgyzstan 29 April 1992
Lao People's Democratic Republic*
    17 May 1950
Latvia 4 December 1991
Lebanon 19 January 1949
Lesotho* 7 July 1967
Liberia 14 March 1947
Libyan Arab Jamahiriya*
    16 May 1952
Lithuania 25 November 1991
Luxembourg* 3 June 1949
Madagascar* 16 January 1961
Malawi* 9 April 1965
Malaysia* 24 April 1958
Maldives* 5 November 1965
Mali* 17 October 1960
Malta* 1 February 1965
Marshall Islands 5 June 1991
Mauritania 7 March 1961
Mauritius* 9 December 1968
Mexico 7 April 1948
Micronesia (Federated States of)
    14 August 1991
Monaco 8 July 1948
Mongolia* 18 April 1962
Morocco* 14 May 1956
Mozambique 11 September 1975
Myanmar 1 July 1948
Namibia 23 April 1990
Nauru 9 May 1994
Nepal* 2 September 1953
Netherlands* 25 April 1947
New Zealand* 10 December 1946
Nicaragua* 24 April 1950
Niger* 5 October 1960
Nigeria* 25 November 1960
Niue 4 May 1994
Norway* 18 August 1947
Oman 28 May 1971
Pakistan* 23 June 1948
Palau 9 March 1995
Panama 20 February 1951
Papua New Guinea 29 April 1976
Paraguay 4 January 1949
Peru 11 November 1949
Philippines* 9 July 1948
Poland* 6 May 1948
Portugal 13 February 1948
Qatar 11 May 1972
Republic of Korea* 17 August 1949
Republic of Moldova 4 May 1992
Romania* 8 June 1948
Russian Federation* 24 March 1948
Rwanda* 7 November 1962
Saint Kitts and Nevis
    3 December 1984
Saint Lucia* 11 November 1980
Saint Vincent and the
    Grenadines 2 September 1983

Samoa 16 May 1962
San Marino 12 May 1980
Sao Tome and Principe
    23 March 1976
Saudi Arabia 26 May 1947
Senegal* 31 October 1960
Seychelles* 11 September 1979
Sierra Leone* 20 October 1961
Singapore* 25 February 1966
Slovakia* 4 February 1993
Slovenia* 7 May 1992
Solomon Islands 4 April 1983
Somalia 26 January 1961
South Africa 7 August 1947
Spain* 28 May 1951
Sri Lanka 7 July 1948
Sudan 14 May 1956
Suriname 25 March 1976
Swaziland 16 April 1973
Sweden* 28 August 1947
Switzerland 26 March 1947
Syrian Arab Republic
    18 December 1946
Tajikistan 4 May 1992
Thailand* 26 September 1947
The Former Yugoslav Republic
    of Macedonia* 22 April 1993
Togo* 13 May 1960
Tonga* 14 August 1975
Trinidad and Tobago* 3 January 1963
Tunisia* 14 May 1956
Turkey 2 January 1948
Turkmenistan 2 July 1992
Tuvalu 7 May 1993
Uganda* 7 March 1963
Ukraine* 3 April 1948
United Arab Emirates 30 March 1972
United Kingdom of Great Britain and
    Northern Ireland* 22 July 1946
United Republic of Tanzania*
    15 March 1962
United States of America
    21 June 1948
Uruguay* 22 April 1949
Uzbekistan 22 May 1992
Vanuatu 7 March 1983
Venezuela 7 July 1948
Viet Nam 17 May 1950
Yemen 20 November 1953
Yugoslavia* 19 November 1947
Zambia* 2 February 1965
Zimbabwe* 16 May 1980

Associate Members

Puerto Rico 7 May 1992
Tokelau 8 May 1991

* Member States that have acceded to the Convention on the Privileges and Immunities of the Specialized Agencies and its Annex VII.

Annex 2
Statistics

Explanatory notes

The *World Health Report 1998 – Life in the 21st century, a vision for all* presents an overview of the global health situation and trends from the 1950s to 2025. Results are based on an assessment carried out in 1997 using 1997 or latest available data. The content of the report was determined essentially by its theme as well as by the availability of information concerning key health and health-related indicators. The majority of Member States still experience great difficulty in obtaining valid and timely data on many indicators such as disease morbidity and health-care coverage.

Since 1979, the Member States of WHO have carried out monitoring and evaluation of the Global Strategy for Health for All by the Year 2000 three times. However, data coverage varies for the different indicators in the short list which is used for this purpose.

In general, official statistics reported to WHO are incomplete, and are often not comparable among countries, nor up to date. Therefore this report is also based on the best available and reasonably reliable data from all sources, which have been duly validated. Sources include national reports, reports of all WHO offices and information from WHO collaborating centres, as well as personal communications.

Reference has also been made to publications and documents of other international bodies such as the United Nations, World Bank, FAO,

ILO, UNESCO, UNCTAD and intergovernmental organizations such as OECD. The main source of estimates relating to demographic indicators, including life expectancy at birth, fertility and infant mortality as well as the number of deaths and population by age, was the Population Division, Department for Economic and Social Information and Policy Analysis, United Nations, hereinafter referred to as United Nations Population Division (UNPD). A number of statistical values such as the under-5 mortality rate were derived from those estimates, but otherwise no attempt was made, for the present report, to refine figures taken from recognized international sources and research publications.

Surveillance data for a number of diseases (communicable and non-communicable) of major public health concern are lacking. Global and regional estimates of prevalence, incidence and even mortality are not available for many of the diseases including some of those targeted for eradication, elimination or control. Using whatever reliable estimates were available, diseases/conditions were assessed according to their effect on people's health at different stages of life (i.e. infants and small children, older children and adolescents, adults and older people) in order to provide an overview of the situation and trends.

Because many of WHO's activities in different fields are interdependent, programmes have been clustered and their activities, products and other outputs synthesized according to their

---

Notes

... Data not available or not applicable.

"Billion" means a thousand million.

$ denotes United States dollars.

Unless specified otherwise, data refer to 1997.

target age groups. The aim is to provide a global overview of WHO's work during the year 1997, irrespective of the organizational level at which activities were carried out, i.e. country, regional or interregional.

As of 1 January 1998 WHO had 191 Member States and two Associate Members (see *Annex 1*). The global health assessment relates only to Member States. For analytical purposes they have been grouped according to the United Nations classification and are described below.

Least developed countries (LDCs) are defined as "Those low-income countries that are suffering from long-term handicaps to growth, in particular, low levels of human resources development and/or structural weakness". To reflect the three-pronged approach that would cover more aspects of the development process, the Committee for Development Planning of the United Nations has used the following criteria for an initial selection:

(i) *GDP per capita;*
(ii) *augmented physical quality of life index (APQL)* consisting of life expectancy at birth, per capita calorie supply, combined primary and secondary school enrolment ratios and adult literacy; and
(iii)*economic diversification index (EDI)* consisting of the share of manufacturing in GDP, share of employment in industry, per capita electricity consumption and the export concentration ratio.

The Committee then took into consideration other special circumstances such as trade and exchange rate fluctuations and made a subjective assessment and judgement when arriving at a final list. The list of 48 LDCs approved by the United Nations General Assembly in 1994 is given below.

Least developed countries:
Afghanistan, Angola, Bangladesh, Benin, Bhutan, Burkina Faso, Burundi, Cambodia, Cape Verde, Central African Republic, Chad, Comoros, Democratic Republic of the Congo, Djibouti, Equatorial Guinea, Eritrea, Ethiopia, Gambia, Guinea, Guinea-Bissau, Haiti, Kiribati, Lao People's Democratic Republic, Lesotho, Liberia, Madagascar, Malawi, Maldives, Mali, Mauritania, Mozambique, Myanmar, Nepal, Niger, Rwanda, Samoa, Sao Tome and Principe, Sierra Leone, Solomon Islands, Somalia, Sudan, Togo, Tuvalu, Uganda, United Republic of Tanzania, Vanuatu, Yemen, Zambia.

Developing countries – excluding least developed countries:
Algeria, Antigua and Barbuda, Argentina, Bahamas, Bahrain, Barbados, Belize, Bolivia, Bosnia and Herzegovina, Botswana, Brazil, Brunei Darussalam, Cameroon, Chile, China, Colombia, Congo, Cook Islands, Costa Rica, Côte d'Ivoire, Croatia, Cuba, Cyprus, Democratic People's Republic of Korea, Dominica, Dominican Republic, Ecuador, Egypt, El Salvador, Fiji, Gabon, Ghana, Grenada, Guatemala, Guyana, Honduras, India, Indonesia, Iran (Islamic Republic of), Iraq, Israel, Jamaica, Jordan, Kenya, Kuwait, Lebanon, Libyan Arab Jamahiriya, Malaysia, Malta, Marshall Islands, Mauritius, Mexico, Micronesia (Federated States of), Mongolia, Morocco, Namibia, Nauru, Nicaragua, Nigeria, Niue, Oman, Pakistan, Palau, Panama, Papua New Guinea, Paraguay, Peru, Philippines, Qatar, Republic of Korea, Saint Kitts and Nevis, Saint Lucia, Saint Vincent and the Grenadines, Saudi Arabia, Senegal, Seychelles, Singapore, Slovenia, South Africa, Sri Lanka, Suriname, Swaziland, Syrian Arab Republic, Thailand, The Former Yugoslav Republic of Macedonia, Tonga, Trinidad and Tobago, Tunisia, Turkey, United Arab Emirates, Uruguay, Venezuela, Viet Nam, Yugoslavia, Zimbabwe.

Economies in transition:
Albania, Armenia, Azerbaijan, Belarus, Bulgaria, Czech Republic, Estonia, Georgia, Hungary, Kazakstan, Kyrgyzstan, Latvia, Lithuania, Poland, Republic of Moldova, Romania, Russian Federation, Slovakia, Tajikistan, Turkmenistan, Ukraine, Uzbekistan.

Developed market economies:
Andorra, Australia, Austria, Belgium, Canada, Denmark, Finland, France, Germany, Greece, Iceland, Ireland, Italy, Japan, Luxembourg, Monaco, Netherlands, New Zealand, Norway, Portugal, San Marino, Spain, Sweden, Switzerland, United Kingdom, United States of America.

Throughout the report "developed world" refers to countries classified as developed market economies and economies in transition; and "developing world" to LDCs and other developing countries. In some cases the developed world has also been referred to as the "industrialized countries" or "developed countries" in the text.

The designations used for groupings of countries in the text and tables are intended solely for statistical and analytical purposes and do not necessarily express a judgement about the stage reached by a particular country in the development process.

As countries are added to or removed from a particular group, revised estimates are computed for the groups and subgroups of countries retroactively to ensure their comparability over time. Accordingly, data by WHO region or by the United Nations classification in this report may differ from comparable figures presented in earlier World Health Reports (1995, 1996 and 1997) and in other WHO and UN publications, because of variations in base values, country groupings and reference years.

A major constraint in the assessment of the global health situation relates to data on **health status**. There are no clear positive measures of health. Even in respect of negative ill-health measures, little information is at present available on disability, and the data on incidence and prevalence of diseases, particularly in the developing world, are notoriously unreliable and enormously variable. Although mortality data are imperfect, they are nevertheless used to illustrate general patterns and orders of magnitude of major health problems. This report, based primarily on four distinct measures of ill-health – mortality, incidence, prevalence and severe activity limitation (permanent and long-term) – uses reasonably reliable data and estimates from a variety of statistical sources. For example, the United Nations Population Division biennially assesses the global demographic situation and makes estimates of numbers of deaths by age and sex for many countries. This report uses the 1996 assessment. While major differences may be considered indicative of actual disparities and trends, caution is necessary in interpreting small differences in values of different groups.

Country data on **causes of death**, in respect of communicable and noncommunicable diseases and conditions, pose a problem. Underreporting, imprecise listing of causes and inaccurate diagnosis complicate both national and international studies of mortality. Furthermore, attributing death to specific causes often results in epidemiological and clinical judgement in identifying underlying causes. Following the rules and procedures of the *International statistical classification of diseases and related health problems, tenth revision* (ICD-10), unique causes were assigned to deaths and thereby double counting was avoided. Efforts

were made to reduce the paucity of data by preparing "guesstimates" in accordance with epidemiological and statistical principles and procedures while ensuring a reasonable degree of reliability, and of international comparability. Similarly in respect of incidence and prevalence some of the estimates reflect comorbidity of diseases and conditions.

Global values for mortality, morbidity and disability from a large number of diseases and conditions were determined following extensive consultation on the quality and consistency of the estimates with experts within the Organization and at WHO collaborating centres. Judicious use was made of available data from a variety of sources and the most recent data were reviewed, interpreted and extrapolated in a global context. Coverage of diseases and conditions is restricted to those of major public health concern and falls far short of the total spectrum of such diseases covered by the ICD-10. The resulting figures relating to 1997 indicate orders of magnitude of health problems associated with these selected diseases, but they lack the degree of precision necessary for any more in-depth disease-specific analysis. In spite of all these efforts, it is to be recognized that the uncertainties associated with the statistical information and the epidemiological assumptions add to the margin of error that would in any event be involved in estimation procedures.

To carry out its *directing* and *co-ordinating* functions at international and regional levels, WHO has since 1990 been incrementally developing its database on global and regional estimates of mortality and morbidity by diseases/conditions, based on official country data supplemented by reliable national and international estimates. The extensive use, in this report, of data based on estimates and

other indirect approaches should not, however, give the mistaken impression that the necessary data are already being collected by all developing and developed countries; rather, it is a matter of concern that use of such estimates may detract from the current efforts being made to compile accurate and timely data on health indicators in the developing world. Empirical data continue to be essential for assessing health situations, identifying problems and working out solutions in the area of health development. It would thus be appreciated if readers would send their comments and suggestions for improving the quality of the estimates used in this report and assist WHO by suggesting more reliable data sources for use in the future.

The World Health Report makes prudent use of the limited number of pages available for producing a comprehensive summary related to a specific theme. We present information only once in the report in the form of a table, graph or map, whichever is most appropriate to convey the finding, unless the finding is of such importance and complexity as to warrant presentation in more than one form.

Primary sources of data

Table A – Basic indicators gives data on key health and health-related indicators relating to the world health situation. It contains data for 1997 or for the latest available year in respect of WHO's 191 Member States. As far as possible data are given for the early 1950s, late 1990s and for 2025 to reflect the global assessment of the past, present and future situation.

The following indicators which were used in the 1997 report have been updated: life expectancy at birth; under-5 mortality rate; infant mortality rate; age- and sex- standardized death rate; GNP per capita;

population (total and growth rate per annum); adult literacy; reported cases of leprosy, AIDS, tuberculosis, malaria, measles and neonatal tetanus; immunization coverage (BCG, DPT3, OPV3, measles and tetanus toxoid 2).

New indicators added this year are: ratio of female to male life expectancy at birth; ratio of female to male under-5 mortality rate; deaths under age 50 (as a percentage of the total); population: age 15-49 (females), ratio of age 65+ to age <5 (both sexes), in urban areas and in urban agglomerations >1 million; total fertility rate (per woman); antenatal care and deliveries in health facilities.

Data for most of the indicators were assembled by WHO from national reports on monitoring and evaluation of the Strategy and from various sources listed; data concerning health status and health care were taken from WHO publications or are estimates made by WHO programmes on the basis of information supplied by Member States. Although every effort was made to standardize the data for international comparison, care must be taken in using them for comparative analysis and in interpreting the results. ***Table B – Analytical tabulations*** are primarily based on the values given in *Table A*. In addition, the following health-related indicators appear only in *Table B*: death rates for the age group 20-64 (ratio female to male). Figures refer to all 191 Member States, which in 1997 had an estimated population of 5833 million, or 99.7% of the world population. The population data and other demographic data are estimates of the UNPD following the 1996 population assessment. These figures serve as denominators for various rates and weights used for computing the aggregate values in *Table B*. Further details are given in the reference publications and documents listed in each case under *Source*.

All tables, figures and maps are compiled especially for the *World Health Report 1998* on the basis of data provided by WHO regional offices and technical programmes, IARC and UNPD, except for *Fig. 7* (source: REVES), *Fig. 12* (source: National Long Term Care Surveys, United States), *Fig. 19* (source: UNESCO), and *Table 7* (source: United Nations Department of Economic and Social Affairs – DESA).

1. Population and demography

1.1 ***Population size, growth rate, age and sex distribution, urbanization***.
Sources:
(a) *World population prospects 1950-2050 (with supplementary tabulations), 1996 revision.* New York, United Nations, forthcoming.
(b) *Demographic indicators 1950-2050, 1996 revision; Sex and age annual 1950-2050, 1996 revision; Annual populations, 1950-2050, 1996 revision; Urban and rural areas, 1950-2030, 1996 revision; Urban agglomerations, 1950-2015, 1996 revision;* and *Age patterns of fertility, 1990-1995, 1996 revision.* New York, United Nations, 1996 (databases) .

2. Health status

2.1 ***Global health situation: mortality, morbidity and disability, selected diseases, all ages, 1997 estimates***.
Source: WHO.

2.2 ***Number of deaths and age and sex distribution, infant mortality rate and life expectancy at birth***.
Sources: see section 1 – Population and demography, above.

2.3 ***Under-5 mortality rate*** refers to the probability of dying between birth and exactly 5 years of age ex-

pressed per 1000 live births.
Source: Office of World Health Reporting, using data given in the *World population prospects, 1996 revision* and the formula provided by the United Nations Population Division.

2.4 ***Age- and sex-standardized death rate*** is obtained by applying the age- and sex-specific death rates of a given population for a country or group of countries to a standard population, the standard population being the 1990 world population, estimated at 5.3 billion (*sources 1a and 1b*).
Source: WHO.

2.5 ***Age-specific death rates*** refer to the number of deaths in the age groups 0-4, 5-19, 20-64 and 65+, per 100 000 population in the same age groups (*sources 1a and 1b*).
Source: WHO.

2.6 ***Annual number of reported cases*** refers to the number of cases of selected diseases reported by Member States to WHO as of 31 December 1997 for the year concerned: leprosy, AIDS, tuberculosis, malaria, measles, neonatal tetanus and poliomyelitis. In view of possible delay in the reporting of these data to WHO, numbers given in this report may differ from national values.
Source: WHO.

2.7 ***Yellow fever, measles, neonatal tetanus elimination status, hepatitis B, hepatitis C.***
Source: WHO.

2.8 ***Life expectancy without severe disability.***
Source: Réseau Espérance de Vie en Santé (REVES). Contribution of the international network on health expectancy and the disability process. Montpellier, 1997 (personal communication).

2.9 ***Underweight prevalence among preschool children*** refers to the percentage of children under 5 years who have a weight that is below

minus two standard deviations from the median weight-for-age of the reference population.
Source: WHO.

2.10 *Cancer*.
Sources: International Agency for Research on Cancer (IARC), WHO.

2.11 *Diabetes mellitus* refers to the number of persons with diabetes in 1997 and 2025.
Source: WHO.

2.12 *Acquired immune deficiency syndrome (AIDS)/ human immunodeficiency virus (HIV)*.
Source: WHO.

2.13 *Regular access to essential drugs* refers to the percentage of the population with regular financial and geographical access to the most needed essential drugs (20-30), whether generic or non-generic, in the public or private sector.
Source: WHO.

2.14 *Micronutrient malnutrition*.
Source: WHO.

2.15 *Percentage of population underweight and overweight.*
Source: WHO.

2.16 *Neonatal, perinatal and maternal mortality.*
Source: WHO.

3. Health care and environment

3.1 *Immunization coverage for BCG, DPT3, OPV3 and measles* refers respectively to the percentages of infants surviving to age 1 who have been fully immunized with BCG, a third dose of diphtheria-pertussis-tetanus vaccine, a third dose of oral polio vaccine and measles vaccine. *Immunization coverage for TT2* refers to the percentage of pregnant women immunized with two or more doses of tetanus toxoid given during pregnancy.
Source: WHO.

3.2 *Antenatal care (% of live births)* refers to the percentage of women attended at least once during pregnancy by skilled health personnel for reasons related to pregnancy (doctors and/or persons with midwifery skills who can diagnose and manage obstetrical complications as well as normal deliveries). Live births is used as a proxy for the total number of pregnancies.
Source: WHO.

3.3 *Deliveries in health facilities (% of live births)* refers to the percentage of deliveries in public and private hospitals, clinics and health centres, irrespective of who attended the delivery at these facilities. Live births is used as a proxy for the total number of pregnancies.
Source: WHO.

3.4 *Water supply and sanitation coverage*. *Access to safe water* refers to the percentage of the population with safe drinking-water available in the home or with reasonable access to treated surface waters and untreated but uncontaminated water such as that from protected boreholes, springs and sanitary wells. *Access to adequate sanitation* refers to the percentage of the population with at least adequate excreta-disposal facilities which can effectively prevent human, animal and insect contact with excreta.
Source: WHO/UNICEF joint monitoring programme. *Water supply and sanitation sector monitoring report 1996*. Geneva, WHO, 1996.

4. Education

4.1 *Adult literacy rate*.
Source: UNESCO. *World education report 1998*. Paris, UNESCO, 1998.

5. Economy

5.1 *Gross national product (GNP) per capita*.
Source: World Bank. *World development report 1997*. New York, Oxford University Press, 1997.

5.2 *Growth of gross domestic product (GDP) and GDP per capita*.
Sources:
(a) United Nations. *World economic and social survey 1997*. New York, United Nations, 1997.
(b) United Nations Department of Economic and Social Affairs (DESA) – *personal communication*.

Table A1. Basic indicators
Estimates are obtained or derived from relevant WHO programmes or from responsible international agencies for the areas of their concern

Member States[a]	Life expectancy at birth (years)			Under-5 mortality rate			Infant mortality rate		Age and sex standardized death rate (per 100 000 population)		Deaths under age 50 as % of total		GNP per capita
	Both sexes		Ratio female/male	Both sexes		Ratio female/male							US$
	1997	2025	1997	1997	2025	1997	1997	2025	1997	2025	1997	2025	1995
WHO Member States with values above all three health-for-all targets in 1997[b]													
Africa													
Algeria	69	75	1.04	52	18	0.83	45	16	794	528	46	16	1 600
Cape Verde	67	73	1.03	57	26	0.97	42	22	893	611	51	33	960
Mauritius	72	77	1.10	16	7	0.83	16	7	684	469	21	6	3 380
South Africa	65	74	1.10	68	23	0.81	48	20	926	582	47	21	3 160
Americas													
Argentina	73	78	1.10	25	14	0.79	22	12	597	436	18	11	8 030
Bahamas	74	79	1.09	17	9	0.63	14	6	586	419	31	11	11 940
Barbados	76	80	1.07	12	7	0.68	9	6	493	377	9	5	6 560
Belize	75	79	1.04	36	21	1.00	30	18	531	406	40	21	2 630
Brazil	67	74	1.12	45	23	0.76	43	21	834	569	40	20	3 640
Canada	79	81	1.08	7	7	0.90	6	5	401	334	9	4	19 380
Chile	75	79	1.08	15	9	0.82	13	8	522	408	21	10	4 160
Colombia	71	76	1.08	30	20	0.75	23	17	680	482	40	19	1 910
Costa Rica	77	80	1.06	14	8	0.78	12	8	460	372	25	10	2 610
Cuba	76	79	1.05	11	7	0.71	9	5	492	394	16	7	...
Dominican Republic	71	77	1.06	43	20	0.79	34	15	673	462	44	18	1 460
Ecuador	70	75	1.08	56	30	0.81	46	23	706	532	48	25	1 390
El Salvador	70	75	1.09	48	25	0.88	39	20	723	517	50	29	1 610
Guatemala	67	73	1.08	63	35	0.89	41	23	820	609	61	39	1 340
Honduras	70	75	1.07	47	24	0.80	35	18	706	513	59	35	600
Jamaica	75	79	1.06	20	9	0.63	12	6	547	413	21	10	1 510
Mexico	72	77	1.09	36	22	0.85	31	18	617	465	42	20	3 320
Nicaragua	68	75	1.07	57	30	0.83	45	23	778	533	62	36	380
Panama	74	78	1.06	26	13	0.89	22	10	557	435	31	13	2 750
Paraguay	70	75	1.07	47	27	0.80	39	23	738	514	47	27	1 690
Peru	68	75	1.07	60	29	0.81	46	21	770	517	47	23	2 310
Suriname	72	77	1.07	25	10	0.71	24	9	672	470	27	11	880
Trinidad and Tobago	74	78	1.07	15	7	0.58	14	6	578	416	18	7	3 770
United States of America	77	80	1.09	9	7	0.71	7	5	475	376	11	6	26 980
Uruguay	73	75	1.09	19	15	0.84	17	13	616	541	12	10	5 170
Venezuela	73	77	1.08	24	14	0.79	21	12	604	444	37	17	3 020
Eastern Mediterranean													
Bahrain	73	77	1.06	20	8	0.65	18	7	618	422	38	6	7 840
Cyprus	78	80	1.06	8	7	0.70	7	5	444	354	8	5	...
Iran, Islamic Republic of	69	76	1.02	57	20	1.05	39	15	742	507	52	27	...
Jordan	70	76	1.06	36	13	0.73	30	11	753	510	49	21	1 510
Kuwait	76	79	1.06	15	7	0.67	15	6	490	371	34	8	17 390
Lebanon	70	75	1.05	33	15	0.78	29	13	737	535	30	13	2 660
Oman	71	76	1.06	31	11	0.69	25	10	696	476	51	22	4 820
Qatar	72	77	1.08	23	8	0.67	17	7	1 075	444	41	4	11 600
Saudi Arabia	71	77	1.05	28	8	0.77	24	7	675	428	44	12	7 040
Syrian Arab Republic	69	75	1.07	39	14	0.71	33	13	787	530	48	21	1 120
Tunisia	70	76	1.03	46	16	0.88	38	13	754	508	36	12	1 820
United Arab Emirates	75	79	1.04	18	7	0.71	15	6	547	365	32	4	17 400
Europe													
Albania	71	75	1.09	49	25	0.93	32	17	675	543	32	13	670
Armenia	71	75	1.10	27	19	0.82	25	17	706	521	22	10	730
Austria	77	80	1.09	7	6	0.69	6	5	466	363	7	3	26 890

Member States[a]	Life expectancy at birth (years)			Under-5 mortality rate			Infant mortality rate		Age and sex standardized death rate (per 100 000 population)		Deaths under age 50 as % of total		GNP per capita
	Both sexes		Ratio female/ male	Both sexes		Ratio female/ male							US$
	1997	2025	1997	1997	2025	1997	1997	2025	1997	2025	1997	2025	1995
Azerbaijan	71	76	1.12	39	25	0.85	34	22	701	520	31	15	480
Belarus	70	75	1.16	19	10	0.69	15	8	762	562	16	8	2 070
Belgium	77	80	1.09	7	6	0.76	7	5	457	364	6	3	24 710
Bosnia and Herzegovina	73	77	1.08	20	9	0.70	14	8	629	477	14	4	...
Bulgaria	71	76	1.10	18	8	0.73	16	8	688	510	10	4	1 330
Croatia	72	76	1.12	16	7	0.58	10	6	664	497	10	4	3 250
Czech Republic	73	77	1.09	9	6	0.41	9	6	656	489	7	3	3 870
Denmark	76	78	1.07	8	6	0.71	7	5	517	417	7	3	29 890
Estonia	69	75	1.17	18	8	0.64	12	6	782	543	14	6	2 860
Finland	77	80	1.10	6	5	0.92	5	5	484	369	8	3	20 580
France	79	81	1.11	8	7	0.73	7	5	414	342	10	5	24 990
Georgia	73	77	1.12	23	16	0.75	23	16	624	482	15	8	440
Germany	77	80	1.09	7	5	0.76	6	5	481	378	6	3	27 510
Greece	78	81	1.07	10	7	0.99	8	6	428	353	6	3	8 210
Hungary	69	74	1.14	16	8	0.75	14	8	796	579	13	6	4 120
Iceland	79	82	1.05	6	5	1.07	5	5	385	319	8	4	24 950
Ireland	77	80	1.07	6	5	0.70	6	5	482	368	6	3	14 710
Israel	78	80	1.05	9	7	0.73	7	5	·442	353	10	7	15 920
Italy	78	82	1.08	8	6	0.88	7	5	420	329	6	3	19 020
Kazakstan	68	74	1.15	39	23	0.78	35	21	844	575	29	14	1 330
Kyrgyzstan	68	74	1.14	46	27	0.80	40	24	824	567	38	21	700
Latvia	68	74	1.19	21	10	0.62	16	9	825	600	15	7	2 270
Lithuania	70	75	1.17	16	9	0.74	13	6	722	550	17	8	1 900
Luxembourg	76	80	1.09	7	5	0.77	6	5	489	378	7	3	41 210
Malta	77	80	1.06	10	6	0.50	8	5	464	365	7	3	...
Netherlands	78	81	1.08	8	7	0.82	6	5	437	351	7	3	24 000
Norway	78	79	1.08	6	6	0.83	5	5	443	383	6	4	31 250
Poland	71	76	1.14	18	8	0.70	13	7	702	514	14	6	2 790
Portugal	75	79	1.10	10	6	0.63	8	5	523	394	8	3	9 740
Republic of Moldova	68	73	1.13	27	17	0.71	27	17	852	599	20 ·	11	920
Romania	70	75	1.11	32	15	0.76	24	11	750	549	15	7	1 480
Russian Federation	64	72	1.23	36	16	0.67	19	9	1 009	672	22	9	2 240
Slovakia	71	76	1.13	13	7	0.77	13	7	696	506	14	6	2 950
Slovenia	74	77	1.12	11	6	0.61	7	5	606	459	10	3	8 200
Spain	78	81	1.09	9	7	0.86	7	6	429	354	8	4	13 580
Sweden	79	82	1.06	6	6	0.89	5	5	414	321	5	3	23 750
Switzerland	79	81	1.09	7	6	0.83	5	5	413	342	8	4	40 630
The Former Yugoslav Republic of Macedonia	72	77	1.06	35	15	0.82	24	10	621	461	17	6	860
Turkey	69	75	1.08	58	22	0.79	45	16	754	514	38	15	2 780
Ukraine	69	75	1.16	21	10	0.69	18	9	805	563	15	7	1 630
United Kingdom	77	80	1.07	7	6	0.78	6	5	464	367	5	3	18 700
Uzbekistan	67	74	1.10	57	34	0.81	43	26	824	583	46	25	970
South-East Asia													
Democratic People's Republic of Korea	72	77	1.09	25	13	0.91	22	11	659	456	27	8	...
Indonesia	65	73	1.06	59	20	0.81	49	18	949	597	43	15	980
Maldives	65	74	0.96	65	16	1.45	50	15	1 070	593	58	26	990
Sri Lanka	73	78	1.06	18	8	0.93	15	6	600	428	24	8	700
Thailand	69	76	1.09	36	14	0.92	30	10	733	499	39	16	2 740
Western Pacific													
Australia	78	81	1.08	8	6	0.82	6	5	420	343	9	5	18 720
Brunei Darussalam	76	79	1.06	12	6	0.53	9	6	457	381	28	6	...
China	70	75	1.05	40	17	1.24	38	16	737	537	24	8	620
Fiji	73	77	1.06	23	8	0.65	20	8	618	444	29	8	2 440
Japan	80	82	1.08	6	6	0.83	4	4	370	318	6	3	39 640
Malaysia	72	77	1.06	21	8	0.85	11	7	648	449	30	10	3 890
New Zealand	77	80	1.07	8	6	0.77	7	5	458	366	9	5	14 340

Member States[a]	Life expectancy at birth (years)			Under-5 mortality rate			Infant mortality rate		Age and sex standardized death rate (per 100 000 population)		Deaths under age 50 as % of total		GNP per capita
	Both sexes		Ratio female/male	Both sexes		Ratio female/male							US$
	1997	2025	1997	1997	2025	1997	1997	2025	1997	2025	1997	2025	1995
Philippines	68	75	1.05	42	16	0.80	36	14	804	536	44	16	1 050
Republic of Korea	72	77	1.10	12	5	1.04	10	5	652	456	20	5	9 700
Singapore	77	81	1.06	6	6	0.88	5	5	458	335	14	4	26 730
Solomon Islands	72	77	1.06	27	10	0.69	23	9	628	467	43	17	910
Vanuatu	67	75	1.06	46	16	0.79	39	14	1 148	562	47	21	1 200
Viet Nam	67	75	1.07	51	21	1.04	38	18	828	543	43	20	240

WHO Member States with values below all three health-for-all targets in 1997[b]

Africa

Member States[a]	1997	2025	Ratio	1997	2025	Ratio	1997	2025	1997	2025	1997	2025	1995
Angola	46	60	1.07	191	91	0.89	126	64	1 954	1 144	80	67	410
Benin	55	68	1.09	120	46	0.82	86	37	1 427	787	75	54	370
Botswana	50	66	1.06	94	46	0.89	57	29	1 795	856	72	55	3 020
Burkina Faso	46	60	1.04	161	79	0.94	98	51	1 999	1 175	79	68	230
Burundi	47	60	1.07	167	88	0.89	116	65	1 900	1 152	79	64	160
Cameroon	56	70	1.05	104	34	0.91	59	27	1 367	699	69	45	650
Central African Republic	49	62	1.10	148	69	0.82	96	47	1 799	1 033	71	56	340
Chad	48	60	1.07	167	88	0.89	116	67	1 850	1 153	74	61	180
Comoros	58	68	1.02	109	40	1.01	83	34	1 305	800	72	43	470
Congo	51	65	1.10	129	56	0.80	91	42	1 665	922	73	59	680
Côte d'Ivoire	51	64	1.04	128	58	0.89	87	44	1 658	939	74	53	660
Democratic Republic of the Congo	53	66	1.06	125	56	0.88	90	42	1 534	895	76	61	120
Equatorial Guinea	50	61	1.07	162	85	0.90	108	60	1 688	1 099	72	58	380
Eritrea	51	65	1.06	143	58	0.90	99	44	1 674	916	75	53	...
Ethiopia	50	64	1.06	166	71	0.89	109	51	1 737	983	79	63	100
Gabon	55	67	1.06	126	55	0.88	86	38	1 410	854	58	43	3 490
Gambia	47	58	1.07	185	102	0.89	123	72	1 907	1 235	77	57	320
Ghana	58	69	1.07	107	43	0.87	74	34	1 263	755	71	45	390
Guinea	46	58	1.02	190	106	0.98	125	74	1 939	1 268	82	69	550
Guinea-Bissau	44	56	1.07	195	111	0.89	133	80	2 115	1 367	73	64	250
Kenya	54	69	1.07	101	43	0.95	66	32	1 444	743	73	51	280
Lesotho	59	70	1.05	94	34	0.92	73	28	1 226	701	63	40	770
Liberia	51	68	1.06	200	65	0.98	160	52	1 564	784	80	59	...
Madagascar	59	69	1.05	103	38	0.88	78	33	1 277	784	70	44	230
Malawi	41	57	1.02	221	114	0.98	143	77	2 384	1 257	82	73	170
Mali	48	59	1.07	178	97	0.89	150	93	1 852	1 192	82	68	250
Mauritania	53	64	1.06	137	66	0.89	93	49	1 509	940	73	52	460
Mozambique	47	60	1.06	163	85	0.89	112	61	1 908	1 146	76	64	80
Namibia	56	68	1.03	98	41	0.94	61	31	1 379	791	66	46	2 000
Niger	49	60	1.07	176	94	0.89	115	66	1 828	1 168	82	70	220
Nigeria	52	64	1.06	141	70	0.91	78	42	1 563	978	77	58	260
Rwanda	42	57	1.06	197	96	0.90	126	72	2 391	1 267	82	67	180
Senegal	51	62	1.04	153	77	0.95	63	32	1 641	1 031	76	58	600
Sierra Leone	38	51	1.08	251	139	0.89	172	99	2 686	1 601	81	71	180
Togo	50	65	1.06	130	57	0.89	87	42	1 722	934	73	59	310
Uganda	41	59	1.05	180	84	0.91	114	59	2 442	1 207	82	73	240
United Republic of Tanzania	51	65	1.05	123	54	0.89	81	41	1 638	897	76	57	120
Zambia	43	61	1.04	149	66	0.96	105	46	2 357	1 100	78	68	400
Zimbabwe	49	64	1.04	108	55	0.90	69	36	1 889	947	73	57	540

Americas

Member States[a]	1997	2025	Ratio	1997	2025	Ratio	1997	2025	1997	2025	1997	2025	1995
Haiti	54	64	1.06	109	54	0.79	84	44	1 512	981	61	46	250

Eastern Mediterranean

Member States[a]	1997	2025	Ratio	1997	2025	Ratio	1997	2025	1997	2025	1997	2025	1995
Afghanistan	45	57	1.02	246	142	0.98	156	105	2 131	1 328	82	63	...
Djibouti	50	62	1.07	162	82	0.88	107	59	1 685	1 072	75	53	...
Somalia	49	60	1.07	174	91	0.89	113	64	1 810	1 144	81	68	...
Sudan	55	66	1.05	108	48	0.89	72	36	1 435	876	69	43	...
Yemen	58	70	1.02	109	34	1.00	81	29	1 317	746	74	47	260

Member States[a]	Life expectancy at birth (years)			Under-5 mortality rate			Infant mortality rate		Age and sex standardized death rate (per 100 000 population)		Deaths under age 50 as % of total		GNP per capita
	Both sexes		Ratio female/ male	Both sexes		Ratio female/ male							US$
	1997	2025	1997	1997	2025	1997	1997	2025	1997	2025	1997	2025	1995
South-East Asia													
Bangladesh	58	70	1.00	104	34	1.07	80	29	1 300	738	60	28	240
Bhutan	53	67	1.06	142	50	0.87	105	41	1 587	877	70	43	420
Nepal	57	70	0.99	108	33	1.11	83	30	1 331	744	63	33	200
Western Pacific													
Cambodia	54	67	1.05	131	44	0.90	104	40	1 508	839	69	33	270
Lao People's Democratic Republic	53	67	1.06	140	46	0.89	87	39	1 560	862	72	43	350
Papua New Guinea	58	68	1.03	80	34	1.10	62	30	1 370	799	57	30	1 160
Other WHO Member States													
Africa													
Sao Tome and Principe	...	...	...	...	...	...	...	...	...	...	...	...	*350*
Seychelles	...	...	...	...	...	...	...	...	...	...	...	...	*6 620*
Swaziland	60	71	1.08	95	33	0.81	66	28	1 161	679	70	38	1 170
Americas													
Antigua and Barbuda	...	...	...	...	...	...	...	...	...	...	...	...	...
Bolivia	61	72	1.06	84	34	0.90	67	25	1 097	624	60	36	800
Dominica	...	...	...	...	...	...	...	...	...	...	...	...	*2 990*
Grenada	...	...	...	...	...	...	...	...	...	...	...	...	*2 980*
Guyana	64	72	1.11	71	38	0.72	59	32	959	632	48	19	590
Saint Kitts and Nevis	...	...	...	...	...	...	...	...	...	...	...	...	*5 170*
Saint Lucia	...	...	...	...	...	...	...	...	...	...	...	...	*3 370*
Saint Vincent and the Grenadines	...	...	...	...	...	...	...	...	...	...	...	...	*2 280*
Eastern Mediterranean													
Egypt	66	74	1.04	66	22	0.90	56	19	898	565	47	17	790
Iraq	62	75	1.05	113	20	0.96	103	17	1 047	538	67	27	...
Libyan Arab Jamahiriya	65	74	1.06	75	24	0.87	57	19	918	572	64	31	...
Morocco	67	74	1.06	64	22	0.86	52	18	865	558	47	18	1 110
Pakistan	64	73	1.03	99	45	0.97	75	39	978	586	64	31	460
Europe													
Andorra	...	...	...	...	...	...	...	...	...	...	...	...	...
Monaco	...	...	...	...	...	...	...	...	...	...	...	...	...
San Marino	...	...	...	...	...	...	...	...	...	...	...	...	...
Tajikistan	67	74	1.09	75	42	0.81	57	33	822	574	53	30	340
Turkmenistan	65	72	1.11	74	42	0.81	58	33	959	642	50	26	920
Yugoslavia	...	...	...	...	...	...	...	...	...	...	...	...	...
South-East Asia													
India	62	71	1.01	90	45	1.17	73	38	1 045	657	48	22	340
Myanmar	60	71	1.06	90	29	0.86	79	25	1 183	696	53	22	...
Western Pacific													
Cook Islands	...	...	...	...	...	...	...	...	...	...	...	...	...
Kiribati	...	...	...	...	...	...	...	...	...	...	...	...	*920*
Marshall Islands	...	...	...	...	...	...	...	...	...	...	...	...	...
Micronesia, Federated States of	...	...	...	...	...	...	...	...	...	...	...	...	...
Mongolia	66	74	1.05	69	33	1.04	53	28	915	584	46	21	310
Nauru	...	...	...	...	...	...	...	...	...	...	...	...	...
Niue	...	...	...	...	...	...	...	...	...	...	...	...	...
Palau	...	...	...	...	...	...	...	...	...	...	...	...	...
Samoa	69	76	1.05	68	38	0.93	58	35	736	503	45	23	1 120
Tonga	...	...	...	...	...	...	...	...	...	...	...	...	*1 630*
Tuvalu	...	...	...	...	...	...	...	...	...	...	...	...	...

[a] Italics indicate less populous Member States (under 150 000 population in 1997).

[b] The three targets in WHO's strategy for health for all by the year 2000 relating to health status are: life expectancy at birth above 60 years; under-5 mortality rate below 70 per 1 000 live births; infant mortality rate below 50 per 1 000 live births.

...Data not available or not applicable.

Table A2. Basic indicators

Estimates are obtained or derived from relevant WHO programmes or from responsible international agencies for the areas of their concern

Member States[a]	Female Age 15-49 (000) 1997	Both sexes All ages (000) 1997	Population								Adult literacy rate	Total fertility rate	
			Average annual growth rate (%) Both sexes			Age 65 + to age < 5 (ratio)		In urban areas (%)		In urban agglom- erations > 1 million (%)			
			1955-1975	1975-1995	1995-2025	1997	2025	1997	2025	1995	1995	1997	2025
WHO Member States with values above all three health-for-all targets in 1997[b]													
Africa													
Algeria	7 463	29 473	2.5	2.9	1.8	0.3	0.8	57	72	13	61.6	3.8	2.1
Cape Verde	109	406	2.5	1.7	1.9	0.3	0.5	58	77	0	71.6	3.6	2.1
Mauritius	320	1 141	2.3	1.1	0.9	0.6	1.6	41	55	0	82.9	2.3	2.1
South Africa	10 842	43 336	2.6	2.4	1.8	0.3	0.7	50	62	30	81.8	3.8	2.2
Americas													
Argentina	8 862	35 671	1.6	1.5	1.0	1.0	1.6	89	93	41	96.2	2.6	2.1
Bahamas	85	288	3.8	2.0	1.1	0.6	1.7	88	92	0	98.2	2.0	2.1
Barbados	72	262	0.4	0.3	0.4	1.6	2.6	49	64	0	97.4	1.7	2.1
Belize	54	224	2.6	2.3	1.9	0.3	0.7	47	57	0	...	3.7	2.1
Brazil	45 582	163 132	2.7	1.9	1.0	0.5	1.4	80	88	33	83.3	2.2	2.1
Canada	7 878	29 943	2.0	1.2	0.7	1.9	3.5	77	82	36	...	1.6	2.0
Chile	3 865	14 625	2.1	1.6	1.1	0.7	1.7	84	89	34	95.2	2.4	2.1
Colombia	10 074	37 068	2.8	2.1	1.3	0.4	1.2	74	83	35	91.3	2.7	2.1
Costa Rica	922	3 575	3.3	2.8	1.7	0.4	1.1	51	65	0	94.8	2.9	2.3
Cuba	3 033	11 068	1.9	0.8	0.2	1.3	3.2	77	85	20	95.7	1.6	1.9
Dominican Republic	2 114	8 097	3.1	2.2	1.2	0.4	1.2	64	76	57	82.1	2.8	2.1
Ecuador	3 090	11 937	2.9	2.6	1.5	0.4	1.1	61	74	27	90.1	3.1	2.1
El Salvador	1 570	5 928	3.1	1.6	1.6	0.3	0.8	46	59	21	71.5	3.1	2.1
Guatemala	2 569	11 241	2.9	2.9	2.4	0.2	0.4	40	54	21	55.6	4.9	2.7
Honduras	1 408	5 981	3.2	3.2	2.1	0.2	0.6	45	62	0	72.7	4.3	2.3
Jamaica	677	2 515	1.3	1.0	1.0	0.6	1.3	55	68	0	85.0	2.4	2.1
Mexico	25 391	94 281	3.2	2.2	1.2	0.4	1.2	74	81	27	89.6	2.8	2.1
Nicaragua	1 067	4 351	3.2	2.7	2.1	0.2	0.6	63	75	27	65.7	3.9	2.2
Panama	714	2 722	2.9	2.1	1.2	0.5	1.4	57	69	0	90.8	2.6	2.1
Paraguay	1 226	5 088	2.4	3.0	2.2	0.2	0.6	54	69	22	92.1	4.2	2.7
Peru	6 413	24 367	2.8	2.2	1.4	0.4	1.1	72	81	28	88.7	3.0	2.1
Suriname	115	437	1.9	0.8	1.2	0.4	1.0	51	66	0	93.0	2.4	2.1
Trinidad and Tobago	334	1 307	1.7	1.2	0.9	0.8	1.7	73	82	0	97.9	2.1	2.1
United States of America	69 405	271 648	1.3	1.0	0.7	1.7	2.8	77	83	38	...	2.0	2.1
Uruguay	794	3 221	0.9	0.6	0.5	1.5	1.9	91	94	42	97.3	2.3	2.1
Venezuela	5 881	22 777	3.6	2.7	1.6	0.3	1.1	87	92	28	91.1	3.0	2.1
Eastern Mediterranean													
Bahrain	138	582	3.6	3.6	1.5	0.3	1.8	91	96	0	85.2	3.0	2.1
Cyprus	187	766	0.7	1.0	0.8	1.3	2.5	55	69	0	...	2.3	2.1
Iran, Islamic Republic of	16 159	71 518	2.8	3.7	2.1	0.2	0.6	60	73	19	...	4.8	2.1
Jordan	1 323	5 774	3.0	3.7	2.7	0.2	0.3	73	82	22	86.6	5.1	2.8
Kuwait	456	1 731	8.4	2.6	1.8	0.2	1.4	97	98	64	78.6	2.8	2.1
Lebanon	853	3 144	2.7	0.4	1.3	0.5	1.0	89	93	61	92.4	2.7	2.1
Oman	469	2 401	2.8	4.7	3.7	0.1	0.2	80	94	0	...	7.2	4.1
Qatar	101	569	8.3	6.0	1.2	0.2	2.6	92	95	0	79.4	3.8	2.1
Saudi Arabia	3 907	19 494	3.6	4.7	2.8	0.2	0.5	84	91	23	62.8	5.9	3.3
Syrian Arab Republic	3 538	14 951	3.2	3.3	2.1	0.2	0.5	53	67	27	70.8	4.0	2.1
Tunisia	2 462	9 326	1.9	2.3	1.4	0.4	1.1	64	77	19	66.7	2.9	2.1
United Arab Emirates	431	2 308	9.7	7.7	1.3	0.2	2.5	85	90	0	79.2	3.5	2.1
Europe													
Albania	879	3 422	2.8	1.7	0.8	0.5	1.4	38	54	0	...	2.6	2.1
Armenia	991	3 642	3.0	1.3	0.5	1.1	2.3	69	78	35	...	1.7	2.0
Austria	2 020	8 161	0.4	0.3	0.1	2.6	4.5	64	73	26	...	1.4	1.7

Member States[a]	Female Age 15-49 (000) 1997	Both sexes All ages (000) 1997	Population Average annual growth rate (%) Both sexes 1955-1975	1975-1995	1995-2025	Age 65 + to age < 5 (ratio) 1997	2025	In urban areas (%) 1997	2025	In urban agglom-erations > 1 million % 1995	Adult literacy rate 1995	Total fertility rate 1997	2025
Azerbaijan	2 051	7 655	2.7	1.4	0.9	0.6	1.4	56	69	25	...	2.3	2.1
Belarus	2 653	10 339	0.9	0.5	-0.2	2.4	3.7	73	83	17	99.5	1.4	1.7
Belgium	2 497	10 188	0.5	0.2	0.0	2.8	4.0	97	98	11	...	1.6	2.0
Bosnia and Herzegovina	1 045	3 784	1.2	-0.2	0.6	1.6	4.0	42	57	0	...	1.4	1.7
Bulgaria	2 070	8 427	0.8	-0.1	-0.4	3.0	4.0	69	79	14	98.3	1.5	1.8
Croatia	1 117	4 498	0.4	0.3	-0.2	2.5	3.6	57	69	0	97.6	1.6	1.9
Czech Republic	2 647	10 237	0.4	0.1	-0.2	2.2	3.9	66	74	12	...	1.4	1.7
Denmark	1 271	5 248	0.7	0.2	0.1	2.3	3.2	85	89	25	...	1.8	2.1
Estonia	366	1 455	1.1	0.2	-0.6	2.8	4.5	74	81	0	99.8	1.3	1.6
Finland	1 257	5 142	0.5	0.4	0.1	2.3	3.7	64	75	21	...	1.8	2.1
France	14 585	58 542	1.0	0.5	0.1	2.6	4.1	75	82	21	...	1.6	1.9
Georgia	1 380	5 434	1.2	0.5	0.2	1.7	2.4	60	72	25	...	1.9	2.1
Germany	19 802	82 190	0.6	0.2	0.0	3.2	5.0	87	91	41	...	1.3	1.6
Greece	2 590	10 522	0.6	0.7	-0.1	3.4	5.2	60	70	30	96.7	1.4	1.8
Hungary	2 537	9 990	0.3	-0.2	-0.5	2.6	3.9	66	77	20	99.2	1.4	1.7
Iceland	70	274	1.6	1.1	0.7	1.3	2.6	92	95	0	...	2.2	2.1
Ireland	911	3 559	0.4	0.6	0.2	1.7	3.0	58	69	0	...	1.8	2.1
Israel	1 455	5 781	3.5	2.4	1.2	1.0	1.8	91	93	36	...	2.8	2.1
Italy	14 317	57 241	0.7	0.2	-0.3	3.6	7.0	67	74	20	98.1	1.2	1.5
Kazakstan	4 462	16 832	2.9	0.9	0.6	0.8	1.6	61	72	7	...	2.3	2.1
Kyrgyzstan	1 124	4 481	2.8	1.5	1.0	0.5	1.0	39	54	0	...	3.2	2.1
Latvia	618	2 474	1.0	0.1	-0.6	2.7	3.7	74	82	0	99.7	1.4	1.7
Lithuania	933	3 719	1.2	0.6	-0.2	2.2	3.3	73	83	0	99.5	1.5	1.8
Luxembourg	103	417	0.9	0.6	0.5	2.3	3.3	90	95	0	...	1.8	2.1
Malta	94	371	-0.2	0.9	0.5	1.6	3.0	90	94	0	...	2.1	2.1
Netherlands	4 008	15 661	1.2	0.6	0.1	2.2	4.2	89	92	14	...	1.6	1.9
Norway	1 057	4 364	0.8	0.4	0.2	2.3	3.1	74	81	0	...	1.9	2.1
Poland	10 143	38 635	1.1	0.6	0.1	1.9	3.0	65	75	17	...	1.7	2.0
Portugal	2 510	9 802	0.3	0.4	-0.1	2.7	4.2	37	53	19	89.6	1.5	1.8
Republic of Moldova	1 180	4 448	1.9	0.7	0.3	1.3	2.1	53	69	0	98.9	1.8	2.1
Romania	5 807	22 606	1.0	0.3	-0.2	2.4	3.7	57	70	9	97.9	1.4	1.7
Russian Federation	38 914	147 708	0.9	0.5	-0.4	2.6	3.9	77	84	19	99.5	1.4	1.7
Slovakia	1 424	5 355	1.1	0.6	0.1	1.7	3.1	60	72	0	...	1.5	1.8
Slovenia	494	1 922	0.6	0.5	-0.3	2.8	5.1	52	64	0	...	1.3	1.6
Spain	10 310	39 717	1.0	0.5	-0.2	3.2	5.9	77	84	17	97.1	1.2	1.5
Sweden	2 017	8 844	0.6	0.4	0.3	2.6	3.5	83	87	18	...	1.8	2.1
Switzerland	1 800	7 276	1.2	0.6	0.2	2.5	4.6	62	72	0	...	1.5	1.8
The Former Yugoslav Republic of Macedonia	571	2 190	1.1	1.3	0.5	1.2	2.5	61	73	0	...	1.9	2.1
Turkey	16 951	62 774	2.6	2.1	1.2	0.5	1.3	72	86	25	82.3	2.5	2.1
Ukraine	12 883	51 424	1.1	0.3	-0.4	2.7	4.0	71	81	15	...	1.4	1.7
United Kingdom	14 023	58 200	0.5	0.2	0.1	2.5	3.4	89	92	23	...	1.7	2.1
Uzbekistan	5 898	23 656	3.3	2.5	1.6	0.3	0.8	42	56	10	...	3.5	2.1
South-East Asia													
Democratic People's Republic of Korea	6 497	22 837	3.1	1.5	1.0	0.5	1.5	62	73	11	...	2.1	2.1
Indonesia	54 967	203 480	2.3	1.9	1.1	0.4	1.1	38	58	8	83.8	2.6	2.1
Maldives	59	273	2.1	3.1	2.8	0.2	0.4	28	43	0	93.2	6.8	2.5
Sri Lanka	5 093	18 273	2.2	1.4	1.0	0.7	1.7	23	39	0	90.2	2.1	2.1
Thailand	17 071	59 159	3.0	1.7	0.6	0.7	1.9	21	36	11	93.8	1.7	2.1
Western Pacific													
Australia	4 723	18 250	2.1	1.3	1.0	1.6	2.7	85	88	58	...	1.9	2.1
Brunei Darussalam	81	307	4.8	3.0	1.4	0.3	1.6	71	81	0	88.2	2.7	2.1
China	341 244	1 243 738	2.1	1.4	0.6	0.8	1.9	32	52	11	81.5	1.8	2.1
Fiji	211	809	2.7	1.6	1.3	0.4	1.2	41	56	0	91.6	2.8	2.1
Japan	30 439	125 638	1.1	0.6	-0.1	3.1	5.8	78	84	38	...	1.5	1.8
Malaysia	5 277	21 018	2.8	2.5	1.5	0.3	1.0	55	71	6	83.5	3.2	2.1
New Zealand	943	3 641	1.9	0.7	1.1	1.4	2.3	86	91	0	...	2.0	2.1

Member States[a]	Female Age 15-49 (000) 1997	Both sexes All ages (000) 1997	Population								Adult literacy rate	Total fertility rate	
			Average annual growth rate (%) Both sexes			Age 65 + to age < 5 (ratio)		In urban areas (%)		In urban agglom- erations > 1 million %			
			1955- 1975	1975- 1995	1995- 2025	1997	2025	1997	2025	1995	1995	1997	2025
Philippines	17 867	70 724	3.0	2.3	1.5	0.3	0.9	56	72	15	94.6	3.6	2.1
Republic of Korea	13 161	45 717	2.5	1.2	0.5	0.8	2.6	84	93	52	98.0	1.7	2.0
Singapore	1 005	3 439	2.8	1.9	0.8	0.8	3.1	100	100	100	91.1	1.8	2.1
Solomon Islands	92	404	3.2	3.5	2.7	0.2	0.4	18	35	0	...	5.0	2.7
Vanuatu	42	178	3.1	2.6	2.3	0.2	0.5	19	33	0	...	4.4	2.6
Viet Nam	20 087	76 548	2.0	2.2	1.3	0.4	0.9	20	30	6	93.7	3.0	2.1
WHO Member States with values below all three health-for-all targets in 1997[b]													
Africa													
Angola	2 513	11 569	1.6	2.9	2.9	0.1	0.2	33	51	19	...	6.7	3.9
Benin	1 294	5 720	1.9	2.9	2.8	0.2	0.3	40	59	0	37.0	5.8	3.3
Botswana	375	1 518	2.8	3.3	1.9	0.2	0.4	67	90	0	69.8	4.5	2.3
Burkina Faso	2 426	11 087	2.1	2.7	2.7	0.1	0.2	17	34	0	19.2	6.6	3.7
Burundi	1 488	6 398	1.6	2.5	2.4	0.2	0.3	8	19	0	35.3	6.3	3.4
Cameroon	3 176	13 937	2.2	2.8	2.6	0.2	0.3	47	64	18	63.4	5.3	3.1
Central African Republic	818	3 416	1.9	2.3	2.0	0.2	0.4	40	56	0	60.0	5.0	3.0
Chad	1 541	6 702	1.8	2.3	2.3	0.2	0.3	23	37	0	48.1	5.5	3.4
Comoros	144	651	2.5	3.4	2.7	0.1	0.3	32	49	0	57.3	5.5	2.8
Congo	625	2 745	2.5	3.0	2.7	0.2	0.2	60	74	39	74.9	5.9	3.6
Côte d'Ivoire	3 219	14 300	3.8	3.6	1.9	0.2	0.4	45	61	20	40.1	5.1	2.2
Democratic Republic of the Congo	10 486	48 040	2.7	3.4	2.9	0.1	0.2	30	46	9	77.3	6.2	3.7
Equatorial Guinea	96	420	-0.3	2.9	2.3	0.2	0.3	45	66	0	78.5	5.5	3.4
Eritrea	786	3 409	2.6	2.1	2.4	0.2	0.4	18	32	0	...	5.3	2.8
Ethiopia	12 972	60 148	2.3	2.8	3.0	0.1	0.2	17	32	4	35.5	7.0	4.0
Gabon	258	1 138	1.1	3.0	2.3	0.4	0.4	53	71	0	63.2	5.4	3.1
Gambia	284	1 169	2.8	3.6	2.0	0.2	0.4	31	49	0	38.6	5.2	3.1
Ghana	4 240	18 338	2.7	2.9	2.5	0.2	0.4	37	54	10	64.5	5.3	2.9
Guinea	1 664	7 614	1.9	2.9	2.5	0.1	0.2	31	49	21	35.9	6.6	3.8
Guinea-Bissau	255	1 112	0.9	2.7	2.0	0.3	0.3	23	38	0	54.9	5.4	3.4
Kenya	6 665	28 414	3.3	3.5	2.1	0.2	0.4	31	51	7	78.1	4.9	2.1
Lesotho	500	2 131	2.0	2.7	2.3	0.3	0.4	26	46	0	71.3	4.9	3.0
Liberia	571	2 467	2.9	1.4	3.8	0.2	0.3	46	62	0	38.3	6.3	3.7
Madagascar	3 566	15 845	2.5	3.3	2.8	0.1	0.3	28	46	0	...	5.7	3.2
Malawi	2 275	10 086	2.6	3.1	2.5	0.1	0.2	14	29	0	56.4	6.7	3.9
Mali	2 571	11 480	2.3	2.8	2.8	0.1	0.2	28	47	0	31.0	6.6	3.9
Mauritania	571	2 392	2.1	2.6	2.3	0.2	0.4	54	73	0	37.7	5.0	3.0
Mozambique	4 137	18 265	2.2	2.5	2.4	0.2	0.2	37	57	13	40.1	6.1	3.6
Namibia	377	1 613	2.4	2.7	2.3	0.2	0.4	38	59	0	...	4.9	3.0
Niger	2 137	9 788	2.9	3.3	3.0	0.1	0.2	19	36	0	13.6	7.1	4.0
Nigeria	26 873	118 369	2.7	2.9	2.6	0.2	0.3	42	61	11	57.1	6.0	3.3
Rwanda	1 371	5 883	3.1	0.8	3.1	0.1	0.2	6	12	0	60.5	6.0	2.9
Senegal	2 019	8 762	2.7	2.8	2.4	0.2	0.3	45	62	21	33.1	5.6	3.2
Sierra Leone	1 032	4 428	1.7	1.8	2.3	0.2	0.2	35	53	0	31.4	6.1	3.6
Togo	966	4 317	2.4	2.9	2.6	0.2	0.2	32	49	0	51.7	6.1	3.3
Uganda	4 578	20 791	3.6	2.9	2.8	0.1	0.1	13	26	0	61.8	7.1	3.7
United Republic of Tanzania	7 273	31 507	2.9	3.2	2.5	0.1	0.3	26	45	6	67.8	5.5	3.2
Zambia	1 970	8 478	2.9	2.6	2.3	0.1	0.2	44	57	16	78.2	5.5	2.8
Zimbabwe	2 805	11 682	3.2	3.0	1.8	0.2	0.4	34	52	13	85.1	4.7	2.1
Americas													
Haiti	1 826	7 395	1.7	1.9	1.9	0.3	0.3	33	51	21	45.0	4.6	3.5
Eastern Mediterranean													
Afghanistan	5 247	22 132	2.3	1.2	2.8	0.2	0.3	21	37	10	31.5	6.9	3.6
Djibouti	156	634	5.6	5.5	2.1	0.2	0.4	83	88	0	46.2	5.4	3.1
Somalia	2 253	10 217	2.4	2.8	3.1	0.1	0.2	27	43	0	...	7.0	4.0
Sudan	6 853	27 899	2.3	2.6	1.9	0.2	0.5	34	55	8	46.1	4.6	2.5
Yemen	3 542	16 294	2.0	3.9	3.3	0.1	0.2	36	55	0	...	7.6	4.2

Member States[a]	Female Age 15-49 (000) 1997	Both sexes All ages (000) 1997	Population								Adult literacy rate	Total fertility rate	
			Average annual growth rate (%) Both sexes			Age 65 + to age < 5 (ratio)		In urban areas (%)		In urban agglomerations > 1 million %			
			1955-1975	1975-1995	1995-2025	1997	2025	1997	2025	1995	1995	1997	2025
South-East Asia													
Bangladesh	30 099	122 013	2.6	2.2	1.4	0.3	0.7	20	37	10	38.1	3.1	2.1
Bhutan	425	1 862	1.9	2.1	2.4	0.2	0.3	7	16	0	42.2	5.9	3.3
Nepal	5 252	22 591	2.1	2.6	2.1	0.2	0.5	11	23	0	27.5	5.0	2.3
Western Pacific													
Cambodia	2 582	10 516	1.9	1.7	1.8	0.2	0.6	22	40	0	...	4.5	2.3
Lao People's Democratic Republic	1 179	5 194	2.2	2.4	2.5	0.2	0.3	22	39	0	56.6	6.7	2.5
Papua New Guinea	1 079	4 500	2.3	2.3	1.9	0.2	0.5	17	30	0	72.2	4.7	2.3
Other WHO Member States													
Africa													
Sao Tome and Principe	...	*138*	*1.3*	*2.5*	*1.6*	...	...	*45*	*62*	*0*	...	...	...
Seychelles	...	*75*	*2.2*	*1.1*	*0.9*	...	...	*56*	*71*	*0*	...	...	...
Swaziland	235	906	2.6	2.9	2.3	0.2	0.4	33	53	0	76.7	4.5	2.3
Americas													
Antigua and Barbuda	...	*67*	*0.6*	*0.6*	*0.8*	...	...	*36*	*50*	*0*	...	...	...
Bolivia	1 886	7 774	2.3	2.2	1.9	0.3	0.6	63	77	17	83.1	4.4	2.4
Dominica	...	*71*	*1.2*	*-0.1*	*0.5*	...	...	*70*	*79*	*0*	...	...	...
Grenada	...	*93*	*0.4*	*0.0*	*0.7*	...	...	*37*	*53*	*0*	...	...	...
Guyana	245	847	2.1	0.6	1.0	0.4	1.2	37	54	0	98.1	2.3	2.1
Saint Kitts and Nevis	...	*41*	*-0.5*	*-0.5*	*0.5*	...	...	*34*	*46*	*0*	...	...	...
Saint Lucia	...	*146*	*1.3*	*1.4*	*1.1*	...	...	*37*	*50*	*0*	...	...	...
Saint Vincent and the Grenadines	...	*114*	*1.2*	*0.9*	*0.9*	...	...	*51*	*72*	*0*	...	...	...
Eastern Mediterranean													
Egypt	15 890	64 465	2.3	2.4	1.5	0.4	1.0	45	59	23	51.4	3.4	2.1
Iraq	4 966	21 177	3.2	3.0	2.5	0.2	0.5	76	84	30	58.0	5.3	2.8
Libyan Arab Jamahiriya	1 251	5 784	4.0	4.0	2.9	0.2	0.3	86	91	31	76.2	5.9	3.3
Morocco	7 237	27 518	2.7	2.2	1.4	0.3	1.0	54	69	17	43.7	3.1	2.1
Pakistan	32 761	143 831	2.7	3.0	2.3	0.2	0.5	36	53	17	37.8	5.0	2.3
Europe													
Andorra	...	*74*	*7.4*	*5.1*	*2.7*	...	...	*95*	*96*	*0*	...	...	...
Monaco	...	*32*	*1.1*	*1.2*	*1.0*	...	...	*100*	*100*	*0*	...	...	...
San Marino	...	*26*	*0.9*	*1.4*	*1.0*	...	...	*95*	*98*	*0*	...	...	...
Tajikistan	1 454	6 046	3.3	2.7	1.7	0.3	0.7	33	47	0	...	3.9	2.1
Turkmenistan	1 073	4 235	3.1	2.4	1.6	0.3	0.8	45	58	0	...	3.6	2.1
Yugoslavia	...	...	...	...	...	...	...	...	...	...	...	...	...
South-East Asia													
India	236 115	960 178	2.3	2.0	1.2	0.4	1.1	28	43	10	52.0	3.1	2.1
Myanmar	12 213	46 765	2.2	2.0	1.4	0.4	0.8	27	43	9	83.1	3.3	2.1
Western Pacific													
Cook Islands	...	*20*	*0.9*	*0.0*	*0.9*	...	...	*62*	*74*	*0*	...	...	...
Kiribati	...	*81*	*2.1*	*1.8*	*1.8*	...	...	*37*	*51*	*0*	...	...	...
Marshall Islands	...	*59*	*3.5*	*3.1*	*3.0*	...	...	*70*	*81*	*0*	...	...	...
Micronesia, Federated States of	...	*130*	*3.2*	*2.8*	*2.4*	...	...	*29*	*46*	*0*	...	...	...
Mongolia	660	2 568	2.7	2.7	1.7	0.3	0.7	62	74	0	82.9	3.3	2.1
Nauru	...	*11*	*2.0*	*3.1*	*1.8*	...	...	*100*	*100*	*0*	...	...	...
Niue	...	*2*	*-2.0*	*-3.4*	*-2.3*	...	...	*29*	*40*	*0*	...	...	...
Palau	...	*17*	*3.1*	*2.2*	*1.7*	...	...	*72*	*81*	*0*	...	...	...
Samoa	39	168	2.3	0.4	1.5	0.4	0.9	21	33	0	...	3.8	2.1
Tonga	...	*99*	*2.6*	*0.5*	*0.4*	...	...	*44*	*63*	*0*	...	...	...
Tuvalu	...	*10*	*0.9*	*2.6*	*0.9*	...	...	*49*	*69*	*0*	...	...	...

[a] Italics indicate less populous Member States (under 150 000 population in 1997).

[b] The three targets in WHO's strategy for health for all by the year 2000 relating to health status are: life expectancy at birth above 60 years; under-5 mortality rate below 70 per 1 000 live births; infant mortality rate below 50 per 1 000 live births.

... Data not available or not applicable.

Table A3. Basic indicators
Estimates are obtained or derived from relevant WHO programmes or from responsible international agencies for the areas of their concern

Member States[a]	Reported cases of selected diseases during the specified year						Immunization coverage (%) 1996					% of live births	
							Children immunized by age 12 months				Pregnant women	Antenatal care	Deliveries in health facilities
	Leprosy 1996	AIDS 1996	Tuberculosis 1996	Malaria 1995	Measles 1996	Neonatal tetanus 1996	BCG	DPT3	OPV3	Measles	Tetanus toxoid 2	1996	1996
WHO Member States with values above all three health-for-all targets in 1997[b]													
Africa													
Algeria	...	44	...	18	21 003	16	94	77	77	75	36	58	76
Cape Verde	...	36	...	305	0	0	80	73	73	66	4	99	...
Mauritius	...	5	...	...	0	0	86	89	89	85	78	99	95
South Africa	280	729	91 578	9 287	6 501	9	95	73	73	76	26	89	79
Americas													
Argentina	565	2 067	13 397	1 065	59	3	100	83	90	100	...	...	90
Bahamas	...	374	59	...	0	0	...	85	85	92	...	100	99
Barbados	...	130	3	...	0	0	...	85	85	100	...	98	98
Belize	...	38	53	9 413	0	1	90	85	85	80	...	96	76
Brazil	39 792	16 469	87 254	565 727	580	51	99	74	97	77	...	74	81
Canada	...	797	...	...	327	...	...	...	...	...	...	100	99
Chile	...	323	4 038	...	0	0	91	91	91	93	...	91	98
Colombia	709	1 042	9 702	49 669	160	27	99	99	97	97	...	83	77
Costa Rica	15	192	162	...	24	...	91	84	84	86	...	95	98
Cuba	262	94	1 579	20	0	...	99	97	95	98	...	100	99
Dominican Republic	229	367	6 006	1 808	0	0	72	85	84	81	...	97	92
Ecuador	115	67	6 327	18 128	42	34	100	88	89	79	...	75	64
El Salvador	...	417	1 686	3 362	1	5	100	98	96	96	...	69	51
Guatemala	...	831	3 496	24 178	1	12	77	73	73	70	...	53	23
Honduras	...	797	4 176	59 446	4	4	98	95	95	91	...	73	45
Jamaica	...	527	121	10	4	0	98	92	92	96	...	98	79
Mexico	523	4 216	10 852	7 316	180	60	99	100	95	93	...	71	63
Nicaragua	...	25	3 003	69 444	0	1	100	91	99	90	...	71	59
Panama	...	243	1 099	730	0	0	100	92	92	90	...	72	84
Paraguay	401	50	2 148	898	13	8	89	80	81	81	...	83	55
Peru	90	998	41 739	192 629	105	45	100	100	100	87	...	64	46
Suriname	64	2	53	6 606	0	1	...	80	79	78	...	100	...
Trinidad and Tobago	...	412	205	35	0	0	...	89	90	88	...	98	96
United States of America	157	36 693	21 337	700	489	...	...	...	...	...	...	94	99
Uruguay	...	156	701	...	2	0	100	86	86	84	...	80	96
Venezuela	534	634	5 576	16 371	89	12	89	57	73	64	...	74	97
Eastern Mediterranean													
Bahrain	...	5	156	192	74	0	...	98	98	95	54	96	97
Cyprus	...	4	24	1	55	0	...	98	98	90	...	100	98
Iran, Islamic Republic of	54	35	14 189	67 532	2 329	21	90	96	97	95	50	62	65
Jordan	...	4	474	197	448	2	...	100	100	98	41	80	78
Kuwait	...	5	400	654	14	1	...	100	100	99	21	99	97
Lebanon	...	6	836	27	2	4	...	94	94	85	...	85	...
Oman	...	12	222	1 801	24	0	96	100	100	98	51	98	82
Qatar	...	2	257	475	38	0	98	92	92	86	...	100	87
Saudi Arabia	112	100	...	18 751	2 407	28	91	93	93	92	60	87	86
Syrian Arab Republic	...	9	5 200	626	2 060	61	100	96	96	95	78	33	37
Tunisia	...	55	2 387	49	533	2	87	91	91	86	48	71	86
United Arab Emirates	...	0	507	2 914	425	0	98	90	90	90	...	95	95
Europe													
Albania	...	1	738	...	1 203	0	94	98	100	92	...	...	95
Armenia	...	6	928	...	2 061	0	82	85	97	89	...	95	95
Austria	...	130	1 375	...	0	...	...	...	...	...	...	100	99

Member States[a]	Reported cases of selected diseases during the specified year						Immunization coverage (%) 1996					% of live births	
							Children immunized by age 12 months				Pregnant women	Antenatal care	Deliveries in health facilities
	Leprosy 1996	AIDS 1996	Tuberculosis 1996	Malaria 1995	Measles 1996	Neonatal tetanus 1996	BCG	DPT3	OPV3	Measles	Tetanus toxoid 2	1996	1996
Azerbaijan	...	2	2 480	2 844	151	2	90	95	97	99	...	95	95
Belarus	...	0	5 598	...	395	0	...	95	94	74	...	100	100
Belgium	...	147	1 348	304	3	0	...	...	...	...	...	90	99
Bosnia and Herzegovina	...	3	2 220	...	...	...	...	...	...	...	...	...	...
Bulgaria	...	10	3 109	...	749	0	...	...	...	...	...	100	100
Croatia	...	16	2 174	...	123	1	90	91	91	91	...	...	...
Czech Republic	...	18	1 969	...	10	0	96	97	98	97	...	99	99
Denmark	...	155	484	...	118	0	...	...	...	...	...	100	99
Estonia	...	7	521	...	34	0	99	90	93	86	...	95	95
Finland	...	22	645	...	0	...	100	100	100	98	...	100	99
France	...	3 684	7 656	977	66 000	0	83	96	97	82	...	99	99
Georgia	...	3	3 522	...	67	...	...	...	...	...	...	95	95
Germany	...	1 169	11 814	...	812	0	...	45	80	75	...	98	99
Greece	...	208	...	...	6 239	0	70	78	95	90	...	95	99
Hungary	...	46	4 403	...	26	0	100	100	100	100	...	...	...
Iceland	...	3	11	...	...	...	...	...	...	...	...	100	99
Ireland	...	49	434	...	53	0	...	...	...	...	...	95	95
Israel	...	39	369	...	25	0	...	...	...	...	...	90	99
Italy	...	4 891	4 155	...	29 099	0	...	50	98	50	...	100	99
Kazakstan	1	2	13 944	...	146	0	93	94	98	97	...	92	95
Kyrgyzstan	...	0	4 093	...	73	...	...	...	...	...	...	90	95
Latvia	...	5	1 761	...	3	0	100	64	77	82	...	95	95
Lithuania	...	2	2 608	...	36	0	98	91	93	96	...	95	95
Luxembourg	...	12	41	...	25		...	...	...	...	...	98	99
Malta	...	4	28	...	16	0	96	84	92	51	...	99	98
Netherlands	...	377	1 678	312	57	0	...	97	97	94	...	95	69
Norway	...	50	217	...	10	...	...	...	...	...	...	99	99
Poland	...	96	15 358	...	669	...	...	...	95	...	...	99	99
Portugal	1	720	5 248	...	111	2	91	95	...	99	...	95	94
Republic of Moldova	...	1	2 922	...	344	0	98	97	99	98	...	90	95
Romania	...	554	24 189	...	940	0	100	98	...	94	...	94	99
Russian Federation	...	46	111 075	...	8 184	0	97	87	97	95	...	95	95
Slovakia	...	0	1 503	...	0	0	...	98	98	99	...	95	95
Slovenia	...	8	563	...	8	0	...	...	...	...	...	98	100
Spain	12	5 678	8 331	...	4 457	...	...	...	...	...	...	96	96
Sweden	...	133	497	...	...	...	...	...	...	...	...	100	99
Switzerland	...	322	764	...	1	0	...	...	...	...	...	99	99
The Former Yugoslav Republic of Macedonia	...	2	724	...	846	...	...	...	...	...	...	90	91
Turkey	...	37	20 212	82 096	27 171	61	69	84	83	84	...	62	60
Ukraine	...	146	23 414	...	8 607	0	...	...	...	...	...	100	95
United Kingdom	...	1 214	6 238	...	2 569	0	...	94	96	92	...	99	99
Uzbekistan	...	1	11 919	...	893	0	...	...	...	...	...	90	90
South-East Asia													
Democratic People's Republic of Korea	...	0	...	...	0	2	99	99	99	99	...	100	100
Indonesia	15 071	32	24 647	1 460 569	15 339	814	100	93	90	93	...	82	18
Maldives	...	2	212	17	0	0	98	95	95	94	...	95	...
Sri Lanka	1 528	11	5 439	142 294	158	7	88	92	90	86	81	100	94
Thailand	1 197	17 942	39 871	82 743	5 677	32	98	96	96	...	88	77	...
Western Pacific													
Australia	...	573	...	623	...	...	...	...	...	...	...	100	99
Brunei Darussalam	...	2	...	46	...	...	...	...	...	...	...	100	98
China	1 845	38	469 358	...	68 404	2 543	97	95	96	97	13	79	51
Fiji	...	0	200	...	39	0	100	97	99	94	82	100	95
Japan	...	294	42 122	...	...	...	...	...	...	...	...	99	99
Malaysia	293	300	12 902	59 208	...	...	...	...	...	...	...	90	90
New Zealand	...	56	323	...	...	...	...	...	...	...	...	95	95

The World Health Report 1998

Member States[a]	Leprosy 1996	AIDS 1996	Tuberculosis 1996	Malaria 1995	Measles 1996	Neonatal tetanus 1996	BCG	DPT3	OPV3	Measles	Tetanus toxoid 2	Antenatal care 1996	Deliveries in health facilities 1996
Philippines	4 051	51	276 295	366 844	...	...	...	...	...	...	43	83	28
Republic of Korea	39	22	31 134	131	71	0	...	...	...	...	...	96	99
Singapore	...	92	737	316	...	...	...	...	...	...	...	100	99
Solomon Islands	...	0	289	118 521	0	1	96	97	98	90	...	71	80
Vanuatu	...	0	126	8 318	4	2	72	67	68	61	15	90	65
Viet Nam	2 883	375	74 711	666 153	5 156	257	95	94	94	96	96	78	70

WHO Member States with values below all three health-for-all targets in 1997[b]

Africa

Member States[a]	Leprosy 1996	AIDS 1996	Tuberculosis 1996	Malaria 1995	Measles 1996	Neonatal tetanus 1996	BCG	DPT3	OPV3	Measles	Tetanus toxoid 2	Antenatal care 1996	Deliveries in health facilities 1996
Angola	157	115	15 424	156 603	251	116	74	42	42	65	28	25	16
Benin	592	503	2 372	579 300	1 365	16	90	80	80	74	75	60	20
Botswana	...	1 511	6 636	17 599	1 096	0	67	83	81	82	61	92	66
Burkina Faso	668	972	1 814	501 020	18 534	15	61	48	48	54	27	59	43
Burundi	...	576	3 796	932 794	16 099	21	77	63	63	50	33	88	20
Cameroon	707	1 485	3 049	221 017	7 108	126	54	46	46	46	12	73	62
Central African Republic	468	2 077	...	127	248	17	94	53	53	46	15	67	50
Chad	982	1 242	1 936	...	9 223	219	41	20	20	31	19	30	15
Comoros	...	0	140	187 082	0	1	55	60	60	43	25	69	20
Congo	317	0	...	...	3 897	7	58	50	50	39	16	55	...
Côte d'Ivoire	1 734	6 000	13 104	4 515	20 858	351	68	55	55	65	22	83	45
Democratic Republic of the Congo	5 526	0	45 999	...	9 546	194	51	36	36	41	20	66	...
Equatorial Guinea	...	74	...	12 530	1	2	99	64	64	61	63	37	5
Eritrea	8	896	5 220	...	1 783	2	52	46	46	38	23	19	5
Ethiopia	4 747	832	171 033	...	1 586	5	87	67	67	54	36	20	10
Gabon	26	318	891	...	70	0	54	41	41	38	4	86	79
Gambia	...	78	1 242	...	15	1	99	97	97	89	92	91	...
Ghana	1 451	1 166	10 449	1 175 000	34 273	108	65	51	52	53	14	86	42
Guinea	3 326	922	4 286	512 814	9 334	289	59	48	48	49	43	59	25
Guinea-Bissau	67	37	1 728	...	73	8	68	53	54	49	20	50	...
Kenya	234	6 520	34 980	4 343 190	3 572	23	52	46	43	38	21	95	44
Lesotho	...	352	4 361	...	...	...	55	58	58	82	10	91	50
Liberia	1 003	18	840	...	1 570	74	84	45	45	44	35	83	...
Madagascar	3 921	5	12 718	...	5 961	61	87	73	73	68	17	78	45
Malawi	509	4 158	20 630	...	9 120	1	95	90	82	89	56	90	55
Mali	1 581	594	3 655	...	10 846	37	76	52	52	55	19	25	24
Mauritania	36	14	...	...	...	...	93	50	50	53	28	49	40
Mozambique	4 225	2 086	18 443	...	9 251	37	83	60	60	67	...	54	27
Namibia	...	2 615	6 773	105 593	4 901	20	79	70	71	61	75	88	67
Niger	1 219	652	...	822 305	64 723	40	50	23	23	43	36	30	16
Nigeria	6 871	308	24 063	...	88 675	1 117	43	24	26	38	34	60	31
Rwanda	...	0	3 535	...	3 988	1	93	95	99	36	43	94	25
Senegal	427	141	8 516	...	2 243	22	90	80	80	80	39	74	47
Sierra Leone	571	43	3 241	...	...	...	77	65	65	79	70	30	20
Togo	327	1 527	1 654	...	...	...	63	82	82	39	43	43	8
Uganda	886	3 021	27 356	...	26 198	167	100	79	79	79	77	87	30
United Republic of Tanzania	2 747	0	44 416	2 438 040	5 049	19	90	82	82	78	31	92	53
Zambia	511	4 552	40 417	2 742 118	9 459	15	100	83	83	93	85	92	51
Zimbabwe	54	9 129	35 735	330 002	35 328	5	79	76	76	77	65	93	69

Americas

Member States[a]	Leprosy 1996	AIDS 1996	Tuberculosis 1996	Malaria 1995	Measles 1996	Neonatal tetanus 1996	BCG	DPT3	OPV3	Measles	Tetanus toxoid 2	Antenatal care 1996	Deliveries in health facilities 1996
Haiti	72	0	6 632	23 140	1	...	...	...	...	...	...	68	20

Eastern Mediterranean

Member States[a]	Leprosy 1996	AIDS 1996	Tuberculosis 1996	Malaria 1995	Measles 1996	Neonatal tetanus 1996	BCG	DPT3	OPV3	Measles	Tetanus toxoid 2	Antenatal care 1996	Deliveries in health facilities 1996
Afghanistan	27	0	...	...	...	...	...	...	...	42	...	8	5
Djibouti	...	358	3 071	3 359	410	0	58	49	49	47	47	76	75
Somalia	38	0	3 251	...	1 830	102	...	...	...	...	...	40	2
Sudan	2 126	221	20 280	232 177	2 559	40	96	79	80	75	44	54	18
Yemen	456	60	14 364	...	...	...	50	54	54	46	19	26	12

Member States[a]	Reported cases of selected diseases during the specified year						Immunization coverage (%) 1996					% of live births	
							Children immunized by age 12 months				Pregnant women	Antenatal care	Deliveries in health facilities
	Leprosy 1996	AIDS 1996	Tuberculosis 1996	Malaria 1995	Measles 1996	Neonatal tetanus 1996	BCG	DPT3	OPV3	Measles	Tetanus toxoid 2	1996	1996
South-East Asia													
Bangladesh	11 225	0	63 471	152 729	4 929	759	100	97	98	96	90	23	5
Bhutan	37	0	1 271	23 195	9	0	98	87	86	85	15	51	11
Nepal	6 602	37	22 970	9 718	8 513	171	92	75	77	80	18	15	6
Western Pacific													
Cambodia	2 404	300	14 857	...	2 814	9	90	75	76	72	36	52	7
Lao People's Democratic Republic	298	16	1 440	311 593	917	17	61	58	68	73	31	25	7
Papua New Guinea	231	69	5 087	926 206	...	...	78	55	57	44	50	70	...
Other WHO Member States													
Africa													
Sao Tome and Principe	...	*6*	...	...	*0*	*0*	*85*	*68*	*68*	*57*	*49*	...	...
Seychelles	...	*2*	*15*	...	*2*	*0*	*100*	*100*	*100*	*98*	*100*	...	...
Swaziland	...	249	3 893	...	2 199	1	68	70	71	59	65	70	56
Americas													
Antigua and Barbuda	...	*13*	*5*	...	*0*	*1*	...	*100*	*100*	*100*	...	...	...
Bolivia	32	28	10 194	46 911	7	14	98	82	82	98	...	52	42
Dominica	...	*14*	*10*	...	*0*	*0*	*100*	*100*	*100*	*100*	...	...	...
Grenada	...	*18*	...	*1*	*0*	*0*	...	*80*	*80*	*85*	...	...	...
Guyana	...	144	314	59 311	0	0	88	83	83	91	...	95	90
Saint Kitts and Nevis	...	*6*	*3*	...	*0*	*0*	...	*100*	*98*	*100*	...	...	...
Saint Lucia	...	*14*	...	...	*0*	*0*	*89*	*88*	*88*	*95*	...	...	...
Saint Vincent and the Grenadines	...	*19*	...	...	*0*	*0*	*100*	*100*	*100*	*100*	...	...	...
Eastern Mediterranean													
Egypt	1 332	14	12 338	322	4 403	643	98	91	91	92	57	53	27
Iraq	...	15	29 196	89 984	256	74	99	94	95	97	65	59	49
Libyan Arab Jamahiriya	14	0	1 282	30	...	0	99	96	96	92	...	100	...
Morocco	79	66	31 771	197	1 324	14	96	95	95	93	46	45	37
Pakistan	1 405	19	4 307	111 836	1 090	2 012	93	77	77	78	54	27	13
Europe													
Andorra	...	...	*17*	...	...	...	...	...	...	...	...	...	...
Monaco	...	*1*	*0*	...	...	...	...	...	...	...	...	...	...
San Marino	...	*3*	*0*	...	...	...	...	...	...	...	...	...	...
Tajikistan	...	*0*	*1 647*	*6 144*	*21*	...	...	...	...	...	...	*90*	*92*
Turkmenistan	...	*0*	*2 072*	...	*96*	...	...	...	...	...	...	*90*	*90*
Yugoslavia	...	...	...	...	...	...	...	...	...	...	...	...	...
South-East Asia													
India	415 302	901	1 300 935	2 800 000	47 072	1 313	96	88	90	81	75	62	26
Myanmar	6 935	690	22 201	642 751	1 684	61	92	88	87	86	63	80	...
Western Pacific													
Cook Islands	...	*0*	*0*	*28 008*	*0*	*0*	*90*	*75*	*75*	*72*	*62*	...	...
Kiribati	...	*0*	*327*	...	*13*	*0*	*100*	*79*	*82*	*64*	*41*	...	...
Marshall Islands	...	*0*	*56*	...	*0*	*0*	*98*	*78*	*77*	*69*	*59*	...	...
Micronesia, Federated States of	*288*	*0*	*94*	...	...	...	...	...	...	...	...	...	...
Mongolia	...	*0*	*2 987*	...	*128*	*0*	*92*	*90*	*90*	*88*	...	*90*	*97*
Nauru	...	*0*	...	...	...	...	...	...	...	...	...	...	...
Niue	...	...	*2*	...	*0*	*0*	*100*	*100*	*100*	*100*	...	...	...
Palau	...	*0*	*5*	...	*0*	*0*	*0*	*98*	*100*	*99*	...	...	...
Samoa	...	*2*	*37*	...	*87*	*0*	*98*	*95*	*95*	*96*	*98*	*52*	...
Tonga	...	*1*	*22*	...	*0*	*0*	*100*	*99*	*99*	*95*	*95*	...	...
Tuvalu	...	*0*	...	...	*51*	*0*	*88*	*87*	*85*	*94*	...	...	...

[a] Italics indicate less populous Member States (under 150 000 population in 1997).

[b] The three targets in WHO's strategy for health for all by the year 2000 relating to health status are: life expectancy at birth above 60 years; under-5 mortality rate below 70 per 1 000 live births; infant mortality rate below 50 per 1 000 live births.

... Data not available or not applicable.

Table B. Analytical tabulations

Indicator	Year	Unit	WHO Member States	Developed world			Developing world		
				Total	Developed market economies	Economies in transition	Total	Developing countries other than LDCs	Least developed countries (LDCs)
Life expectancy at birth									
Both sexes	1997	years	66	74	78	68	65	67	53
	2025	years	73	78	81	74	72	73	65
Ratio female/male	1997		1.06	1.11	1.09	1.17	1.05	1.05	1.04
Under-5 mortality rate									
Both sexes	1997	per 1000 live births	75	17	8	35	83	68	144
	2025	per 1000 live births	37	10	7	19	40	31	67
Ratio female/male	1997	years	0.99	0.75	0.76	0.75	1.00	1.03	0.93
Infant mortality rate	1997	per 1000 live births	57	13	6	26	62	53	100
	2025	per 1000 live births	29	8	5	15	32	25	50
Age and sex standardized death rate	1997	per 100 000 population	888	568	442	871	987	887	1 616
	2025	per 100 000 population	608	423	357	604	655	596	952
Death rate 20-64: ratio female/male	1997		0.68	0.45	0.51	0.40	0.75	0.72	0.90
Deaths under age 50 as % of total	1997	% total deaths	40	13	8	20	49	42	73
	2025	% total deaths	20	6	4	9	25	18	53
GNP per capita	1995	US dollars	4 880	18 295	26 042	1 972	1 125	1 240	215
Population									
Total	1997	millions	5 833	1 227	835	392	4 606	3 996	610
Average annual growth rate	1955-1975	percentage	2.0	1.1	1.0	1.2	2.4	2.4	2.4
	1975-1995	percentage	1.7	0.6	0.6	0.6	2.0	1.9	2.6
	1995-2025	percentage	1.2	0.2	0.3	0.01	1.4	1.2	2.3
Ratio age 65+/age <5	1997		0.6	2.2	2.4	1.8	0.4	0.5	0.2
	2025		1.2	3.5	3.8	2.8	0.9	1.1	0.3
In urban areas	1997	% total population	47	74	78	67	39	41	25
	2025	% total population	59	81	84	75	55	57	41
In urban agglomerations>1 million	1995	% total population	16	26	32	15	14	15	6
Females aged 15-49	1997	millions	1 487	310	209	101	1 177	1 034	142
Adult literacy rate	1995	percentage	77	99	...	...	70	73	49
Total fertility rate	1997	per woman	2.8	1.7	1.6	1.7	3.1	2.8	5.3
	2025	per woman	2.3	1.9	1.9	1.8	2.4	2.2	3.2
Reported cases of selected diseases during the specified year									
Leprosy	1996	thousands	566	0.2	0.2	0.001	565	501	64
AIDS	1996	thousands	167	58	57	1	108	81	27
Tuberculosis	1996	thousands	3 798	355	115	240	3 443	2 832	611
Malaria	1995	thousands	24 672	12	3	9	24 660	14 250	10 411
Measles	1996	thousands	792	135	110	25	657	419	238
Neonatal tetanus	1996	thousands	12.5	0.004	0.002	0.002	12.5	10.0	2.5
Coverage									
Children immunized by age 12 months									
BCG[a]	1996	percentage	90	93[b]	84[b]	96	90	92	82
DPT3[a]	1996	percentage	82	82[b]	75[b]	91	82	85	69
OPV3[a]	1996	percentage	84	95[b]	93[b]	97	83	86	69
Measles[a]	1996	percentage	81	86[b]	79[b]	95	80	84	67
Pregnant women									
Tetanus toxoid 2[a]	1996	% pregnant women	...	...	...	...	47	47	45
Antenatal care	1996	% live births	68	97	97	95	65	69	48
Deliveries in health facilities	1996	% live births	46	98	98	96	40	44	21

[a] Figures based on updated values and 1996 revision of population estimates.
[b] Data available for less than 50% of Member States.
... Data not available or not applicable.

Index

Page numbers in **bold type** indicate main discussions.